CAFFEINE AND HEALTH RESEARCH

CAFFEINE AND HEALTH RESEARCH

KENNETH B. CHAMBERS
EDITOR

Nova Biomedical Books
New York

For permission to use material from this book please contact us:
Telephone 631-231-7269; Fax 631-231-8175
Web Site: http://www.novapublishers.com

Library of Congress Cataloging-in-Publication Data

Caffeine and health research / Kenneth P. Chambers (editor).
p. ; cm.
Includes bibliographical references and index.
ISBN 978-1-60456-437-2 (hardcover)
1. Caffeine--Health aspects. I. Chambers, Kenneth P.
[DNLM: 1. Caffeine--pharmacokinetics. 2. Caffeine--pharmacology. QV 107 C128514 2008]
QP801.C24C333 2008
613.8'4--dc22

2008010238

Published by Nova Science Publishers, Inc. ✦ New York

Contents

Preface

Caffeine is the most widely consumed drug in the world, most commonly from the beverages coffee, tea and soda. An estimated 80% of the world's population consumes a caffeine-containing substance daily. A typical 8-ounce (240-ml) cup of instant coffee contains about 100 mg of caffeine – about twice as much as a cup of tea or a 12-ounce (360-ml) can/bottle of soda. A 30-gram chocolate bar might contain as much caffeine as half a cup of tea. More than 99% of orally ingested caffeine is absorbed – with peak plasma levels obtained in 15 to 45 minutes. Caffeine is soluble in both water and oil and can readily cross the blood-brain barrier. Caffeine potentially has pharmacological actions other than blockage of adenosine receptors, but it requires 20 times as much caffeine to inhibit phosphodiesterase, 40 times as much caffeine to block GABAA receptors and 100 times as much caffeine to mobilize intracellular calcium as is required to block adenosine receptors. Caffeine acts primarily by the direct action of blocking adenosine receptors and by the indirect action upon the receptors for neurotransmitters. This new book presents important research on this fascinating and relevant field of research.

Expert Commentary - Coffee is one of the most common beverages consumed by millions of people all over the world and results in stimulant effects on central nervous and cardiovascular systems. In people who are not habitual consumers, caffeine increases blood pressure, plasma catecholamine levels, plasma renin activity, serum free fatty acid levels, urine production, and gastric acid secretion. It also alters the electroencephalographic pattern, affect, and sleep patterns of normal volunteers. It can precipitate or increase anxiety in normal controls or patients suffering from anxiety disorders depending on the amount of intake. On the other hand, chronic caffeine consumption has no such significant effects on blood pressure, plasma catecholamine levels, plasma renin activity, or blood glucose levels. Caffeine does not seem to be associated with myocardial infarction. However, caffeine may be associated with serious ventricular arrhythmias in susceptible people. Caffeine may increase beat-to-beat heart rate variability and also QT interval variability during rapid eye movement sleep. This commentary mainly focuses on the cardiovascular effects of caffeine in normal people and also people with anxiety, especially highlighting possible detrimental effects on beat-to-beat QT interval variability as such measures are important in relation to cardiac mortality. Future studies should also focus on the effects of caffeine on linear and nonlinear measures of respiration and also blood pressure.

Short Communication - Parkinson's disease (PD) is a common neurodegenerative disorder. It has been thought that hypofunction of nigrostriatal dopaminergic systems causes these symptoms, and levodopa has been considered the gold standard drug therapy for this disease. During long-term therapy with levodopa, however, wearing-off fluctuations and dyskinesias develop in many patients. Recently the adenosine A2A receptor selective antagonist has been a novel nondopaminergic therapy for PD, because dopamine D2 receptors and adenosine A2A receptors have opposing actions in the striatum. Caffeine is the most widely consumed behaviorally active substance, and the CNS effects of caffeine are mediated primarily by its antagonistic actions at the A1 and A2A subtypes of adenosine receptors. The neuroprotection and the motor stimulation by caffeine has been reported in patients with PD. Recent large epidemiological studies have established that the incidence of PD declines steadily with increasing levels of coffee intake. Low doses of caffeine (100-200 mg/day) can improve akinesia and walking in the patients with PD, but chronic caffeine administration induces tolerance to motor stimulant effects of caffeine. Caffeine may improve excessive daily somnolence associated with dopaminergic treatment. Neuroprotection by caffeine and motor stimulant effect of low doses of caffeine suggest that caffeine can be an adjuvant nondopaminergic therapy for PD.

Chapter I - Fecal pollution can not only impair the quality of freshwater intended for drinking, recreation, aquaculture and irrigation but also pose a significant threat to public and environmental health by contributing pathogenic microorganisms. With the increase in human development, population growth and drastic changes in climate, it is expected that the source waters are more vulnerable to known as well as emerging pathogens. In order to sustain the integrity of source water and implementation of better management practices to reduce the environmental loading of pathogens associated with waterborne disease transmission, it is essential to identify the origin of fecal pollution source(s). Several microbial source tracking (MST) phenotypic and genotypic methods have been developed to discriminate the animal and human sources of fecal pollution. However, the standardization of these methods pertaining to operations, expenses, reproducibility and global use has been a problem for reliable field application. Recently, caffeine (1, 3, 7, trimethylxanthine) has been emerging as an important chemical tracer for surveillance of human fecal waste input into source water. This chapter provides an overview on the health implications of caffeine in source water by integrating the occurrence of enteric pathogens in aquatic environment associated with waterborne disease transmission, and the genotypic and phenotypic tracking of human versus animal sources of fecal bacteria with the detection and monitoring of caffeine in source water. Additionally, a description of the application of a novel analytical technique developed using gas chromatography (GC) coupled with ion-trap tandem mass spectrometry detection system (IT-MS/MS) for determination of caffeine in aquatic systems is presented.

Chapter II - There are distinct advantages for clinicians to have at their disposal products for the effective delivery of caffeine into and across skin and some 200 research articles having been published on the subject to date. For example, topical application of caffeine has been shown to confer protection from photodamage and inhibit UVB-induced skin carcinogenesis. Furthermore, delivery of therapeutic levels of caffeine into the systemic circulation via the transdermal route from a patch device has advantages including the ability to provide controlled, sustained release of drug through the skin, directly into the bloodstream and limiting the probability of caffeine intoxication occurrence. Another advantage of the transdermal route is that it bypasses first pass hepatic metabolism, whereby caffeine is caffeine is metabolized to three primary metabolites: paraxanthine (84%), theobromine (12%), and theophylline (4%). This article seeks to review the current status of topical and transdermal delivery for caffeine and other xanthine derivatives in terms of potential for the development of therapeutic systems and their scope of applicability.

Chapter III - Despite little literature on coffee lipids, it has been hypothesized that they lower coffee quality through hydrolysis of the triacylglycerols during storage releasing free fatty acids, which are in turn oxidized to produce compounds producing off-flavour. Coffee is stored for extended periods by small producers in Brazil to fetch better market prices. As a part of our coffee-breeding program aiming to improve the quality of Brazilian coffee, the authors plan to evaluate the role of lipids during storage, developing initially methods (TLC-thin layer chromatography, HLPC-LSD-high performance liquid chromatography with light sensitive detection and HPLC with refractive index detection) for their determination. In this study experiments were carried out to evaluate the variation of lipid classes (free fatty acids, fatty acids after oil hydrolysis, triacylglycerols-TAG and terpene esters-TE) during coffee storage. Three types of coffee beans (immature, random mixture and cherry) picked in Viçosa, MG, Brazil (a region traditionally considered to be a producer of low quality coffee), were dried by two widely used procedures (dryer and open air cement patio) and stored on wood shelves in a house without neither temperature nor humidity control for 19 months. The authors tried to reproduce storage conditions used by small farmers in Brazil. At 4, 7, 10, 13, 16 and 19 months of storage, a part of samples was withdrawn and lipid classes were analyzed using the methods developed in our laboratory. The experiment consisted of thirty-six treatments in a randomised block design with three repetitions. The following treatments (T) were used: immature coffee beans dried in a dryer (T_1) and on a patio (T_2); a random mixture of coffee beans dried in a dryer (T_3) and on a patio (T_4) and cherry coffee beans dried in a dryer (T_5) and on a patio (T_6). In these treatments, samples were stored for four months followed by analysis of lipid classes. The procedure was repeated for immature, random and cherry coffee beans after 7, 10, 13, 16 and 19 months of storage corresponding to treatments T_7-T_{12}, T_{13}-T_{18}, T_{19}-T_{24}, T_{25}-T_{30} and T_{31}-T_{36}, respectively. Lipid class data were statistically analyzed through variance and regression. The qualitative factors (type of coffee and type of drying) and the averages were compared by the Tukey test at 5% probability. The quantitative factor (months of storage) and the averages were chosen based on the significance of regression coefficients using the t test at 5% probability and determination coefficients (r^2). While apparently random variation was observed in a few cases, no effects of storage time, storage type and coffee type were found on the lipid classes. These results contradict literature studies where a small number of samples were studied utilizing short storage times.

Chapter IV - Caffeine's psychostimulatory effects are well known. These are mediated by the blockage of adenosine A2A receptors on the surface of nerve cells. However, caffeine can also enter the cells and affect a number of intracellular proteins. Some of these proteins are involved in the replication of the human immunodeficiency virus type 1 (HIV-1). As a consequence, caffeine may affect the HIV-1 life-cycle at at least three steps (integration, expression and Vpr-mediated growth arrest). Several caffeine-related compounds have been shown to have similar effects. Some of these compounds are used for the treatment of diseases other than HIV-1 infection. In this article, the authors summarize the current evidence for each of the described effects of caffeine and caffeine-related compounds, as published by us and others, as well as future directions of the field. In addition, they include new results addressing and explaining the underlying reasons behind some of the controversies in the field. Finally, the authors discuss the molecular mechanism underlying the described effects of caffeine and caffeine-related compounds on HIV-1 replication and potential consequences for the treatment of HIV-1 infection.

Chapter V - Although much is known about the pharmacokinetics of caffeine (i.e., what the body does to the drug), its pharmacodynamics (i.e., what the drug does to the body) are less well understood. Specifically, the psychological effects associated with caffeine intake may often run counter to what might be expected pharmacologically. Being one of the most consumed stimulants worldwide the instrumental value of caffeine covers a broad range of partially opposing ends. For example, the effect (caffeinated) coffee exerts on human functioning depends to a great deal on the expectation of the consumer. People drink coffee to get started in morning, to enhance performance, or even to unwind after straining experiences. Likewise, the instrumental value of coffee consumption may be bound to psychosocial factors, such as enhancing group coherence. Also, coffee may be consumed for diet-related health issues to prevent diseases like diabetes, cancer, heart diseases, or gastrointestinal problems.

In this chapter, an overview of placebo studies is given to demonstrate the importance of psychological factors. Specifically, results from the so called placebo caffeine paradigm will be discussed to show that the study of the placebo caffeine effect lends itself to a better understanding of the psychological factors involved with caffeine effects. Several ways to methodologically disentangle pharmacologic and psychological effects will be introduced. From this, it will be concluded that the widely employed way of testing drug effects (the Randomized Control Trial) is insufficient to fully understand the health effect of caffeine since it is aimed at minimizing psychological factors enhancing the effect (e.g., learning effects, expectation, context). It will be shown that the health effects of caffeine are brought about by synergistically intertwined specific and non-specific factors, which, in real-life situations, always work together and make up the totality of effects. Finally, a functionally oriented psychological theory will be introduced helping to explore the psychological mechanisms associated with unspecific effects.

Chapter VI - Pharmacokinetics has had a considerable effect in enhancing our understanding of what happens to drug within the body, and has opened a way to safer and more effective drug administration to the body. Caffeine produces central stimulation because of its effect on the central nervous system. Caffeine is also used for therapeutic purposes, and is included in a wide variety of fixed combination prescription drugs and over-the-counter medications. In the present review we discuss the pharmacokinetics of caffeine. Caffeine is rapidly and completely absorbed from the gastrointestinal tract; peak plasma caffeine concentration reaches in about 15 to 120 min after oral ingestion in humans without any significant first-pass effect. Caffeine is rapidly distributed, which poorly binds to plasma albumin and there is no specific binding to tissue. Caffeine is distributed into all body tissues, rapidly crosses the blood-brain barrier and the placenta, and is also found in breast milk. The human cytochrome p450 monoxygenase metabolizes caffeine yielding trimethyl uric acid, paraxanthine and theobromine. Caffeine is efficiently eliminated through liver biotransformation to several metabolites; only a small percentage of ingested doses in humans are excreted unchanged in urine. People with some liver disorders have a significant prolongation of the half-life and a reduction in plasma clearance. In a healthy subject, the mean elimination half-life of caffeine is around 5 hr. Physiological and environmental factors that alter caffeine metabolism included age, sex, pregnancy, smoking and ingestion of drug.

Chapter VII - Caffeine is a widely used psychoactive substance consumed daily by the majority of Americans. Saletu showed that 250 mg of caffeine can produce a transient reduction of EEG total absolute power in normal persons. Additional studies have confirmed this phenomenon. Overall, however, studies of EEG changes following caffeine exposure have reported variable results. Studies have been done in individuals who are not caffeine naïve and the effect of previous caffeine usage (often for years) on EEG is unknown. It is postulated that this confound may contribute to the variations in results between studies of caffeine exposure.

Several studies have shown that persons consuming even low or moderate amounts of caffeine (in some cases, as low as 100 mg per day) may develop a withdrawal syndrome with caffeine cessation with symptoms such as headaches, lethargy, muscle pain, impaired concentration, and physiological complaints such as nausea or yawning. Preliminary studies of individuals abstaining from caffeine have demonstrated significant changes relative to when they were consuming the drug in a number of EEG variables, including: 1.) increases in theta absolute power over all cortical areas, 2.) increases in delta absolute power over the frontal cortex, 3.) decreases in the mean frequency of both the alpha and beta rhythm, 4.) increase in theta relative power and decrease in beta relative power, and 5.) significant changes in interhemispheric coherence. Additionally, caffeine cessation appears to increase firing rates of diffuse paroxysmal dysrhythmias in some individuals. Preliminary data also suggests that caffeine withdrawal has some effect on cognitive P300 auditory and visual evoked potentials.

Chapter VIII - Various positive effects on the human body have been attributed through time to diverse beverages commonly consumed in the Western world. The purpose of this paper is to examine the extent to which popular beliefs regarding certain drinks have a scientific basis. A historical description of the putative therapeutic and/or preventive characteristics of four widely consumed beverages will be presented, followed by a discussion of the state-of-the-art biomedical knowledge regarding them. The importance of wine on human health has been affirmed from time immemorial, and today, in an evidence-based nutritional perspective, the beneficial properties on the vascular system of red wine consumed in moderate quantities have been confirmed both on pathophysiological and clinical grounds. The relevance of voices of the past claiming the favourable effects of coffee, tea and chocolate on human health is also examined. Current evidence documents the beneficial effects, not only on the cardiocirculatory system, but also on other human apparati, including the respiratory and the gastrointestinal ones, of the methylxanthines, polyphenols and flavonoids contained in coffee, green tea and chocolate when assumed by healthy subjects in appropriate dosages.

This historical perspective evidences the continuing pertinence of past traditions regarding major beverages, even when compared with up-dated scientific information. The adage that one never learns enough from the past therefore holds true, though the learning may be as easy as drinking a glass of wine, sipping a cup of tea or enjoying a cup of coffee or chocolate.

In: Caffeine and Health Research
Editor: Kenneth P. Chambers

ISBN 978-1-60456-437-2

Expert Commentary

Caffeine and Cardiovascular Health: What Do We Know?

***Vikram Kumar Yeragani**[*a,b], **Shravya Yeragani**,[b] **Pratap Chokka**[b], **Karl J Bar**[c], and **Manuel Tancer**[a]*

[a]Department of Psychiatry and Behavioral Neurosciences, Wayne State University School of Medicine, Detroit, Michigan, USA.

[b]University of Alberta, Edmonton, Canada

[c]Friedrich Schiller University, Germany

Abstract

Coffee is one of the most common beverages consumed by millions of people all over the world and results in stimulant effects on central nervous and cardiovascular systems. In people who are not habitual consumers, caffeine increases blood pressure, plasma catecholamine levels, plasma renin activity, serum free fatty acid levels, urine production, and gastric acid secretion. It also alters the electroencephalographic pattern, affect, and sleep patterns of normal volunteers. It can precipitate or increase anxiety in normal controls or patients suffering from anxiety disorders depending on the amount of intake. On the other hand, chronic caffeine consumption has no such significant effects on blood pressure, plasma catecholamine levels, plasma renin activity or blood glucose levels. Caffeine does not seem to be associated with myocardial infarction. However, caffeine may be associated with serious ventricular arrhythmias in susceptible people. Caffeine may increase beat-to-beat heart rate variability and also QT interval variability during rapid eye movement sleep. This commentary mainly focuses on the cardiovascular effects of caffeine in normal people and also people with anxiety, especially highlighting possible detrimental effects on beat-to-beat QT interval variability as such measures are important in relation to cardiac mortality. Future studies should also focus on the effects of caffeine on linear and nonlinear measures of respiration and also blood pressure.

* Address correspondence to Dr. V.K. Yeragani, Professor of Psychiatry, #411, 11135-83 Ave, Edmonton, Alberta, Canada; Tel # 780-434-1986; Fax: 011-91-80-23610508, E-mail: Vikramyershr@yahoo.com

Key Words: caffeine, cardiac, autonomic, mortality, ECG, QT.

Caffeine is one of the most commonly consumed substances all over the world in various drinks including coffee and various soft drinks. Caffeine has a stimulating effect in people who are not habituated to its effects and it can produce insomnia if consumed before going to sleep. When administered acutely, caffeine produces modest increases in blood pressure, plasma catecholamine levels, plasma renin activity, serum free fatty acid levels, and gastric acid secretion. Caffeine can result in palpitations and acute anxiety in people with anxiety disorders. However, chronic caffeine consumption has no noticeable effect on blood pressure, plasma catecholamine levels, serum cholesterol concentration, and blood glucose levels. Consumption of caffeine alone may not increase the risk for hypertension. Coffee is also commonly consumed along with nicotine in habitual smokers and this group of subjects should be evaluated separately when one examines the effects of caffeine on cardiovascular system as nicotine has considerable deleterious effects in this regard. The role of caffeine in the production of cardiac arrhythmias or the effects on cardiovascular mortality needs further investigation.

Caffeine use during exposure to mental stress is extremely common. One study has examined the synergistic effects of caffeine and a demanding task in young men (1). Changes in heart rate, BP and noninvasive thoracic impedance measures of left ventricular function were examined in young men at rest and during a demanding behavioral task performed after predosing with caffeine (3.3 mg/kg, equivalent to 2 to 3 cups of coffee) or placebo in a double-blind crossover design. Systolic and diastolic BP were elevated by both caffeine and the behavioral task alone; when combined, caffeine's pressor effects were additive to those of the behavioral task. However, caffeine's pressor effect was produced by different mechanisms depending on the behavioral state. Caffeine increased systemic vascular resistance under resting conditions, but it enhanced cardiac output during behavioral arousal associated with the task. The combined influence of caffeine and the task resulted in an increase in the number of men in who peak systolic BP reached hypertensive levels, and also synergistically increased cardiac minute work and the rate-pressure product estimate of myocardial oxygen demand.

In another population-based case-control study (2), the authors identified 362 primary cardiac arrest cases without a history of clinical heart disease or major comorbidity through paramedic incident reports to evaluate the association between usual caffeine intake and primary cardiac arrest. The investigators also identified 581 controls, individually matched to cases on age and gender and meeting the same general health criteria. They obtained information on usual caffeine intake from coffee, tea, and cola during the prior year. After adjusting for cigarette smoking and other risk factors, they observed little association between daily consumption of caffeine equivalent of fewer than 5 cups per day of drip coffee (< 687 mg per day) and primary cardiac arrest. However, high usual caffeine consumption (> or = 687 mg per day) was associated with a modestly elevated risk of primary cardiac arrest (odds ratio = 1.44; 95% confidence interval (CI) = 0.82-2.53). The elevated risk associated with high caffeine consumption also appeared to be restricted to never-smokers (odds ratio for > or = 687 mg per day = 3.2; 95% CI = 1.3-8.1). This is an important study that suggests that one should take a closer look at the effects of caffeine on variables such as beat-to-beat heart rate variability and QT interval variability, which are useful noninvasive markers of cardiovascular mortality and sudden death. Low-frequency power of HRV (0.04–0.15 Hz) is related to baroreceptor sensitivity mediated by vagal as well as sympathetic systems while the HF (0.15-0.5 Hz) power is influenced by respiratory sinus arrhythmia (RSA). A decrease in beat-to-beat heart rate variability (HRV) and an increase in QT interval variability (QTV) are useful noninvasive predictors of cardiac mortality and sudden death (3-6). Linear as well as nonlinear indices of HR and QT interval variability are useful measures in this regard. Several studies have shown that HRV is related to cardiac vagal function and QTV, which primarily reflects cardiac repolarization lability reflects cardiac sympathetic activity to some extent (7).

It is important to note that anxiety, depression and schizophrenia are associated with an increased risk for cardiovascular mortality (8-11). Several studies have also shown decreased HRV and increased QTV in patients with anxiety, depression and schizophrenia (10, 12, 13). A sizeable number of these patients are also habitual caffeine consumers. Hence, the effect of caffeine on cardiac autonomic function is of special importance.

Caffeine intake results in an increase in HR and HR variability, especially the LF power during rest and also during aerobic exercise. It should be noted that if the increase in HR variability is predominantly from the contribution of LF power, it may reflect in higher LF/HF ratios, and this could be detrimental to patients at risk for cardiovascular disease. There is evidence that caffeine may exaggerate sympathetic adrenal medullary responses to the stressful events of normal day life, suggesting that excessive caffeine intake may have detrimental effects in patients with cardiac illness.

We have examined the effects of caffeine on HRV during exercise and also the effects of caffeine on QTV during sleep (14, 15). We have found that caffeine increases HR variability at rest, which includes a significant increase in HF power. After progressive exercise, caffeine resulted in a higher decrease of HF power and HR approximate entropy, a measure of regularity, which suggests that there is an exaggerated vagal withdrawal. The increase in HF power at rest after caffeine should caution investigators about the absolute association of HF power with cardiac vagal function as one of our previous reports on the effects of yohimbine, an adrenergic agent, on HR variability also showed a significant increase of HF power at rest in normal controls (16).

The other finding of a higher decrease of HF power during exercise is most likely related to the higher baseline level of HR HF power leading to an exaggerated vagal withdrawal. The higher LF power after caffeine during exercise may also suggest an increased cardiac sympathetic responsiveness. Thus, the net effect of caffeine on exercise appears to be an increase in cardiac sympathovagal interaction, which is usually associated with significant cardiac events. This is especially important in view of an increase in sudden death in psychiatric patients with anxiety disorders, depression, and psychosis. This becomes even more significant as some of these groups of patients seem to consume high levels caffeinated beverages as mentioned above. Finally, these groups of patients exhibit a decrease in HR HF power, an indicator of cardiac vagal function, which may make the myocardium more vulnerable to sympathetic stimulation.

There are other reports showing an increase of HR LF and HF powers and total power in humans after caffeine consumption. Modest amounts of caffeine improved autonomic function in diabetic patients and healthy volunteers. For individuals with abnormal HRV, regular caffeine use may have the potential to reduce the risk of cardiovascular events in certain disease groups such as patients with diabetes (17). These authors concluded that the caffeinated beverages have the potential to be useful supplements to exercise. However, in vulnerable populations such as patients with the psychiatric conditions mentioned earlier and also diabetes, one should be cautious about the increase in LF power associated with caffeine and the more exaggerated decrease in HF power that we have seen especially after exercise. Thus, the findings in normal controls may have different implications for caffeine use than for vulnerable groups for cardiac events.

Our study on sleep and QTV has shown significant increases QTV after caffeine administration during REM sleep. This can be explained on the basis that the relative increase in sympathetic activity during REM sleep has made the subjects more sensitive to the sympathomimetic effects of caffeine. At the cellular level, caffeine is a competitive antagonist of adenosine receptors, causing increased lipolysis, and facilitates central nervous system transmission. However, the relationship between adenosine receptors, caffeine, and cardiac function is unclear and deserves further investigation.

Generally, sleep is considered to be a condition associated with a relatively high vagal activity. However, this increase in vagal activity may be blunted in patients with coronary artery disease. Our findings of significant increases in LF/HF ratios of HR variability, as well as QTvi, suggesting sympathetic predominance, have implications for excessive intake of caffeine and the nocturnal occurrence of sudden death.

Further studies are needed to study the effects of caffeine on QTvi during sleep in patients with coronary artery disease. We should also comment on acute versus chronic intake of caffeine, especially of more than 400 mg. If this is an acute intake, it can lead to a significant increase in cardiac sympathetic activity and can be detrimental, especially in patients with other cardiac risk factors and who are not habitual caffeine consumers. This includes situations, where the effects of caffeine are compounded by mental stress and other physiological challenges.

Future studies should systematically and carefully examine the effect of different doses of caffeine in habitual and nonhabitual consumers on QTV and HRV and respiratory variability in normal controls and vulnerable populations at rest, during sleep and also during and after exercise. Irregular respiration and increased variability of respiratory measures are also associated with a higher risk for cardiovascular mortality. It is best to avoid including the high risk patients in these studies in view of the ethical considerations.

References

[1] Pincomb, G.A., Lovallo, W.R., Passey, R.B., and Wilson, M.F. (1988). Effect of behavior state on caffeine's ability to alter blood pressure. *The American Journal of Cardiology*; 61:798-802.

[2] Weinmann, S., Siscovick, D.S., Raghunathan, T.E., Arbogast, P., Smith, H., Bovbjerg, V.E., Cobb, L.A., and Psaty, B.M. (1997). Caffeine intake in relation to the risk of primary cardiac arrest. *Epidemiology* (Cambridge, Mass. 8:505-8.

[3] Malliani, A., Pagani, M., Lombardi, F., and Cerutti, S. (1991). Cardiovascular neural regulation explored in the frequency domain. *Circulation*; 84:482-92.

[4] Lombardi, F., Sandrone, G., Mortara, A., Torzillo, D., La Rovere, M.T., Signorini, M.G., Cerutti, S., and Malliani, A. (1996). Linear and nonlinear dynamics of heart rate variability after acute myocardial infarction with normal and reduced left ventricular ejection fraction. *The American Journal of Cardiology*; 77:1283-8.

[5] Berger, R.D., Kasper, E.K., Baughman, K.L., Marban, E., Calkins, H., and Tomaselli, G.F. (1997). Beat-to-beat QT interval variability: novel evidence for repolarization lability in ischemic and nonischemic dilated cardiomyopathy. *Circulation*; 96:1557-65.

[6] Berger, R.D. (2003). QT variability. *Journal of Electrocardiology*; 36 Suppl:83-7.

[7] Yeragani, V.K., Pohl, R., Jampala, V.C., Balon, R., Kay, J., and Igel, G. (2000). Effect of posture and isoproterenol on beat-to-beat heart rate and QT variability. *Neuropsychobiology*; 41:113-23.

[8] Kawachi, I., Sparrow, D., Vokonas, P.S., and Weiss, S.T. (1994). Symptoms of anxiety and risk of coronary heart disease. The Normative Aging Study. *Circulation,* 90:2225-9.

[9] Kawachi, I., Colditz, G.A., Ascherio, A., Rimm, E.B., Giovannucci, E., Stampfer, M.J., and Willett, W.C. (1994). Prospective study of phobic anxiety and risk of coronary heart disease in men. *Circulation*; 89:1992-7.

[10] Jindal, R., MacKenzie, E.M., Baker, G.B., and Yeragani, V.K. (2005). Cardiac risk and schizophrenia. *J Psychiatry Neurosci.* 30:393-5.

[11] Carney, R.M. and Freedland, K.E. (2003). Depression, mortality, and medical morbidity in patients with coronary heart disease. *Biological Psychiatry;* 54:241-7.

[12] Rao, R.K. and Yeragani, V.K. (2001). Decreased chaos and increased nonlinearity of heart rate time series in patients with panic disorder. *Auton Neurosci.* 88:99-108.

[13] Yeragani, V.K., Rao, K.A., Smitha, M.R., Pohl, R.B., Balon, R., and Srinivasan, K. (2002). Diminished chaos of heart rate time series in patients with major depression. *Biological Psychiatry*, 51:733-44.

[14] Bonnet, M., Tancer, M., Uhde, T., and Yeragani, V.K. (2005). Effects of caffeine on heart rate and QT variability during sleep. *Depression and Anxiety,* 22:150-5.

[15] Yeragani, V.K., Krishnan, S., Engels, H.J., and Gretebeck, R. (2005). Effects of caffeine on linear and nonlinear measures of heart rate variability before and after exercise. *Depression and Anxiety*; 21:130-4.

[16] Yeragani, V.K., Berger, R., Pohl, R., Srinivasan, K., Balon, R., Ramesh, C., Weinberg, P., and Berchou, R. (1992). Effects of yohimbine on heart rate variability in panic disorder patients and normal controls: a study of power spectral analysis of heart rate. *Journal of Cardiovascular Pharmacology;* 20:609-18.

[17] Richardson, T., Rozkovec, A., Thomas, P., Ryder, J., Meckes, C., and Kerr, D. (2004). Influence of caffeine on heart rate variability in patients with long-standing type 1 diabetes. *Diabetes Care*; 27:1127-31.

In: Caffeine and Health Research
Editor: Kenneth P. Chambers

ISBN 978-1-60456-437-2

Short Communication

Caffeine and Parkinson's Disease

Mayumi Kitagawa*
Department of Neurology, Sapporo Azabu Neurosurgical Hospital, Sapporo, Japan

Abstract

Parkinson's disease (PD) is a common neurodegenerative disorder. It has been thought that hypofunction of nigrostriatal dopaminergic systems causes these symptoms, and levodopa has been considered the gold standard drug therapy for this disease. During long-term therapy with levodopa, however, wearing-off fluctuations and dyskinesias develop in many patients. Recently the adenosine A2A receptor selective antagonist has been a novel nondopaminergic therapy for PD, because dopamine D2 receptors and adenosine A2A receptors have opposing actions in the striatum. Caffeine is the most widely consumed behaviorally active substance, and the CNS effects of caffeine are mediated primarily by its antagonistic actions at the A1 and A2A subtypes of adenosine receptors. The neuroprotection and the motor stimulation by caffeine has been reported in patients with PD. Recent large epidemiological studies have established that the incidence of PD declines steadily with increasing levels of coffee intake. Low doses of caffeine (100-200 mg/day) can improve akinesia and walking in the patients with PD, but chronic caffeine administration induces tolerance to motor stimulant effects of caffeine. Caffeine may improve excessive daily somnolence associated with dopaminergic treatment. Neuroprotection by caffeine and motor stimulant effect of low doses of caffeine suggest that caffeine can be an adjuvant nondopaminergic therapy for PD. (203 words)

* Tel: +81 (Japan) 11 731 2321.

Introduction

Parkinson's disease (PD) is a common degenerative disorder characterized by muscle rigidity, tremor, difficulty initiating movements, slowing of movement and postural instability. These symptoms are related to dopaminergic hypofunction in nigrostriatal systems. Levodopa entered clinical practice in 1967, and the first study reporting improvements in patients with PD resulting from treatment with levodopa was published in 1968 [8]. However, long-term therapy with levodopa is associated with motor complications such as wearing-off fluctuations and dyskinesias [25]. Many studies suggested that pulsatile stimulation of dopamine receptors by levodopa having a short half-life might relate motor complications [20, 27]. Dopamine agonists are currently used as the first line treatment of PD, and a selective A2A receptor antagonist KW-6002 has also been focused on as a novel nondopaminergic approach to PD therapy.

Dopamine D2 receptors and adenosine A2A receptors are coexpressed on striatopallidal and mesocortical dopaminergic systems [10], and they have opposing actions on neurotransmitter release and gene expression in these dopaminergic systems [17]. Dopamine causes an increase in locomotor behavior mediated by D2 receptor, and low doses of caffeine induces the same behavioral change mediated by A2A receptor blockade [31]. Caffeine-induced stimulation of locomotion may be non-dopaminergic, because selective A2A receptor antagonists produced locomotor stimulation in mice lacking the D2 receptors [1]. In animal studies, a selective A2A receptor antagonist KW-6002 ameliorated the hypolocomotion at minimum effective dose (0.16 mg/kg) induced by nigral dopaminergic dysfunction with 1-methyl-4-phenyl-1,2,3,6-tetrahydropyridine hydrochloride (MPTP) or reserpine treatment [22]. KW6002 prolongs the efficacy halftime of levodopa in patients with advanced PD, and enhances the antiparkinsonian response of lower doses of levodopa with 45% less dyskinesias compared with that induced by optimal dose levodopa alone [4]. In an animal study, A2A angagonists inhibited the development of sensitized responses to levodopa in mouse models of levodopa-induced dyskinesias [30]. Increased synthesis of adenosine A2A receptors in striatopallidal pathway neurons by chronic levodopa treatment may be associated with the development of dyskinesias [5]. The effect of theophylline, which is a nonspecific adenosine antagonist, was not strong enough to enhance clearly the antiparkinsonian action of levodopa or to increase ON time in patients with advanced PD [16].

Caffeine is the most widely used psychoactive drug, and the effects of caffeine are mediated primarily by antagonistic actions at the A1 and A2A subtypes of adenosine receptors [11]. Caffeine activates the raphe nuclei and the locus coeruleus associated with mood and alertness, and the caudate nucleus associated with locomotion at 1 mg/kg [19]. Caffeine at 2.5 and 5 mg/kg activates other components of the nigrostriatal dopaminergic system, the thalamus, ventral tegmental area and amygdala. The shell of the nucleus accumbens (NAc) associated with addiction and reward was activated by caffeine at the higher dose (10 mg/kg). In animal studies, the effect of caffeine on spontaneous locomotion is markedly biphasic. Low doses of caffeine (6.25-25 mg/kg) induce spontaneous locomotion and rotation in animals with unilateral nigrostriatal lesions as dopamine receptor agonists [12], but the high doses of caffeine (100 mg/kg) lead to a behavioral depression. Chronic exposure to caffeine resulted in tolerance to the motor effects of an acute administration of caffeine. The involvement of adenosine A1 and A2A receptors in these effects of caffeine is still a matter of debate. Previous studies reported as follows:

1. Systemic administration of high doses of caffeine increased extracellular levels of dopamine and glutamate in the shell of the NAc, which may be mediated by A1 receptor blockade [28]. In contrast, acute systemic administration of motor-activating doses of the A2A receptor antagonist significantly decreased extracellular levels of dopamine and glutamate in the shell of the NAc [23].
2. The stimulant effect of low doses of caffeine may be mediated by A2A receptor blockade while the depressant effect seen at higher doses under some conditions is explained by A1 receptor blockade [31].
3. Development of the tolerance to the motor-activating effects of caffeine may be mostly because of A1 receptor blockade [13].

In rats, the reserpine-induced hypokinesia was reversed by the combination of subthreshold doses of caffeine plus trihexyphenidyl [18]. Is caffeine useful in treatment of PD? In the present article, I summarize the previously reported studies about the efficacy of caffeine in patients with PD.

Beneficial Effects of Caffeine on Parkinson's Disease

1. Neuroprotection

In animal models of focal and global ischemia, pharmacological blockade or gene disruption of A2A receptor markedly reduced cerebral ischemic damage [29]. In the 1-methyl-4-phenyl-1,2,3,6-tetrahydropyridine (MPTP) neurotoxin model of PD, caffeine attenuated MPTP toxicity by A2A receptor blockade [7]. Recent large epidemiological studies have established that the incidence of PD declines steadily with increasing levels of coffee intake, with the relative risk reduced as much as fivefold over a typical range of caffeine consumption [3].

2. Effects of Caffeine on Parkinsonian Motor Symptoms

Early studies of chronically administration of the high doses of caffeine (800- 1,400 mg) failed to enhance the antiparkinsonian action of dopamine receptor agonists (bromocriptine and piribedil) and developed severe psychiatric and cardiovascular adverse effects in patients with PD [14, 26]. However, recent studies evaluated that the low doses of caffeine (100-200 mg) can improve akinesia and walking in patients with PD [9, 15]. Inappropriate dosage of caffeine may account for its clinical ineffectiveness in early studies. In addition, it is not easy to evaluate the effect of drugs on akinesia and freezing phenomenon. For example, freezing of gait (FOG) that is a common and disabling symptom of PD can be distinguished by three subtypes in relation to leg motion; (i) shuffling with small steps, (ii) trembling in place and (iii) total akinesia. Different subtypes of FOG may have different therapeutic response and pathopysiologic origins, but have been lumped together into one group or one symptom. Previously we have studied the effect of low doses of caffeine on FOG, taking into account the differences among patients and the tolerance to the locomotor stimulant effect of caffeine [15]. We instructed the patients to stop intake of caffeine-containing beverages and foods from one month before, as well as during the study. 100 mg of caffeine per day could improve the inability of heel-off of the first swing leg at gait initiation, which resulted in the improvement of "total akinesia" type of FOG, but had no effect on "trembling in place" type of FOG. The tolerance to the effects on "total akinesia" type of FOG developed within a few months, and a two-week caffeine withdrawal period could restore the effect of caffeine without any withdrawal syndrome. 150 ml of coffee contains 100 mg of caffeine, and caffeine consumption from all sources may be more than 200 mg/day in the US and Europe. The chronic caffeine exposure may induce tolerance to the effect of caffeine and a selective A2A receptor antagonist KW6002 on FOG.

3. Effects of Caffeine on Somnolence

Excessive daytime somnolence (EDS) is common in patients with PD [21], and relates to levodopa dose and the use of a dopamine agonist. The pharmacological mechanism by which dopamine generate EDS is unknown, because mesolimbic dopamine transmission has been implicated in behavioral and cortical arousal. There are a large number of studies showing that caffeine increases alertness. Some studies suggested that adenosine promotes sleepiness by targeting arousal networks in the brain such as cholinergic system [2, 24]. The oral administration of caffeine dose-dependently (3-30 mg/kg) increased the extracellular levels of acetylcholine in the hippocampus of rats via A1 receptor [6]. Because the extensive loss of cortical acetylcholine may associate with cognitive dysfunction and hallucinations in the patients with PD with dementia (PDD) and those with diffuse Lewy body disease (DLBD), caffeine may improve not only excessive daily sleepiness but also cognitive dysfunction in patients with PD.

Conclusion

In conclusion, the common consumption of coffee may reduce risk of developing PD, and low doses of caffeine can be a nondopaminergic drug for some PD symptoms. However, it should be noted that the dosage of caffeine accounts for its clinical effectiveness and that chronic administration of caffeine induces tolerance to its motor stimulant effects. (1326 words)

References

[1] Aoyama S, Kase H, Borrelli E. (2000). Rescue of locomotor impairment in dopamine D2 receptor-deficient mice by an adenosine A2A receptor antagonist. *J Neurosci.* 1, 20, 5848-5852.

[2] Arrigoni E, Chamberlin NL, Saper CB, McCarley RW. (2006). Adenosine inhibits basal forebrain cholinergic and noncholinergic neurons in vitro. *Neuroscience.*140, 403-413.

[3] Ascherio A, Weisskopf MG, O'Reilly EJ, McCullough ML, Calle EE, Rodriguez C, Thun MJ. (2004). Coffee consumption, gender, and Parkinson's disease mortality in the cancer prevention study II cohort: the modifying effects of estrogen. *Am. J. Epidemiol.* 160, 977-984.

[4] Bara-Jimenez W, Sherzai A, Dimitrova T, Favit A, Bibbiani F, Gillespie M, Morris MJ, Mouradian MM, Chase TN. (2003). Adenosine A(2A) receptor antagonist treatment of Parkinson's disease. *Neurology.* 61, 293-296.

[5] Calon F, Dridi M, Hornykiewicz O, B_dard PJ, Rajput AH, Di Paolo T. (2004). Increased adenosine A2A receptors in the brain of Parkinson's disease patients with dyskinesias. *Brain.* 127, 1075-1084.

[6] Carter AJ, O'Connor WT, Carter MJ and Ungerstedt U. (1995). Caffeine enhances acetylcholine release in the hippocampus in vivo by a selective interaction with adenosine A1 receptors. *J. Pharmacol. Exp. Ther.* 273, 637-642.

[7] Chen JF, Xu K, Petzer JP, Staal R, Xu YH, Beilstein M, Sonsalla PK, Castagnoli K, Castagnoli N Jr, Schwarzschild MA. (2001). Neuroprotection by caffeine and A (2A) adenosine receptor inactivation in a model of Parkinson's disease. *J. Neurosci.* 21, RC143.

[8] Cotzias, G. (1968). N Engl J Med, 278, 630.

[9] Deleu D, Jacob P, Chand P, Sarre S, Colwell. Effects of caffeine on levodopa pharmacokinetics and pharmacodynamics in Parkinson disease. *A. Neurology.* 2006; 67:897-9.

[10] Fink JS, Weaver DR, Rivkees SA, Peterfreund RA, Pollack AE, Adler EM, Reppert SM. (1992). Molecular cloning of the rat A2 adenosine receptor: selective co-expression with D2 dopamine receptors in rat striatum. *Brain Res. Mol. Brain Res.*14, 186-195.

[11] Fredholm BB, Battig K, Holmen J, Nehlig A, Zvartau EE. (1995). Actions of caffeine in the brain with special reference to factors that contribute to its widespread use. *Pharmacol. Rev.* 51, 83-133.

[12] Garrett BE, Holtzman SG. (1995). The effects of dopamine agonists on rotational behavior in non-tolerant and caffeine-tolerant rats. *Behav. Pharmacol.* 6, 843-851.

[13] Karcz-Kubicha M, Antoniou K, Terasmaa A, Quarta D, Solinas M, Justinova Z, Pezzola A, Reggio R, Muller CE, Fuxe K, Goldberg SR, Popoli P, Ferre S. (2003). Involvement of adenosine A1 and A2A receptors in the motor effects of caffeine after its acute and chronic administration. *Neuropsychopharmacology.* 28,1281-1291.

[14] Kartzinel R, Shoulson I, Calne DB. (1976). Studies with bromocriptine: III. Concomitant administration of caffeine to patients with idiopathic parkinsonism. *Neurology*. 26, 741-743.

[15] Kitagawa M, Houzen H, Tashiro K. (2007). Effects of caffeine on the freezing of gait in Parkinson's disease. *Mov. Disord.* 22, 710-712.

[16] Kulisevsky J, Barbanoj M, Gironell A, Antonijoan R, Casas M, Pascual-Sedano B. (2002). A double-blind crossover, placebo-controlled study of the adenosine A2A antagonist theophylline in Parkinson's disease. *Clin. Neuropharmacol.* 25, 25-31.

[17] Le Moine C, Svenningsson P, Fredholm BB, Bloch B. (1997). Dopamine-adenosine interactions in the striatum and the globus pallidus: inhibition of striatopallidal neurons through either D2 or A2A receptors enhances D1 receptor-mediated effects on c-fos expression. *J. Neurosci.* 17, 8038-8048.

[18] Moo-Puc RE, Villanueva-Toledo J, Arankowsky-Sandoval G, Alvarez-Cervera F, Gongora-Alfaro JL. (2004). Treatment with subthreshold doses of caffeine plus trihexyphenidyl fully restores locomotion and exploratory activity in reserpinized rats. *Neurosci. Lett.* 367, 327-331.

[19] Nehlig A, Boyet S. (2000). Dose-response study of caffeine effects on cerebral functional activity with a specific focus on dependence. *Brain Res.* 858, 71-77.

[20] Olanow W, Schapira AH, Rascol O. (2000). Continuous dopamine-receptor stimulation in early Parkinson's disease. *Trends Neurosci.* 23, S117-126.

[21] O'Suilleabhain PE, Dewey RB Jr. (2002). Contributions of dopaminergic drugs and disease severity to daytime sleepiness in Parkinson disease. Arch Neurol. 59, 986-989.

[22] Pinna A, Pontis S, Borsini F, Morelli M. (2007). Adenosine A2A receptor antagonists improve deficits in initiation of movement and sensory motor integration in the unilateral 6-hydroxydopamine rat model of Parkinson's disease. *Synapse.* 61, 606-614.

[23] Quarta D, Ferre S, Solinas M, You ZB, Hockemeyer J, Popoli P, Goldberg SR. (2004). Opposite modulatory roles for adenosine A1 and A2A receptors on glutamate and dopamine release in the shell of the nucleus accumbens. Effects of chronic caffeine exposure. *J. Neurochem.* 88, 1151-1158.

[24] Rainnie DG, Grunze HC, McCarley RW, Greene RW. (1994). Adenosine inhibition of mesopontine cholinergic neurons: implications for EEG arousal. Science. 263, 689-692.

[25] Schrag A, Quinn N. Dyskinesias and motor fluctuations in Parkinson's disease. (2000). A community-based study. *Brain.* 123, 2297-2305.

[26] Shoulson I, Chase T. (1975). Caffeine and the antiparkinsonian response to levodopa or piribedil. *Neurology.* 25, 722-724.

[27] Smith LA, Jackson MJ, Hansard MJ, Maratos E, Jenner P. (2003). Effect of pulsatile administration of levodopa on dyskinesia induction in drug-na_ve MPTP-treated common marmosets: effect of dose, frequency of administration, and brain exposure. *Mov. Disord.* 18, 487-495.

[28] Solinas M, Ferre S, You ZB, Karcz-Kubicha M, Popoli P. (2002). Caffeine induces dopamine and glutamate release in the shell of the nucleus accumbens. *J. Neurosci.* 22, 6321-6324.

[29] Wardas J. (2002). Neuroprotective role of adenosine in the CNS. *Pol. J. Pharmacol.* 54, 313-326.

[30] Xiao D, Bastia E, Xu YH, Benn CL, Cha JH, Peterson TS, Chen JF, Schwarzschild MA. (2006). Forebrain adenosine A2A receptors contribute to L-3,4-dihydroxyphenylalanine-induced dyskinesia in hemiparkinsonian mice. *J. Neurosci.* 26,13548-13555.

[31] Yacoubi M, Ledent C, Menard JF, Parmentier M, Costentin J, Vaugeois JM. (2000). The stimulant effects of caffeine on locomotor behaviour in mice are mediated through its blockade of adenosine A(2A) receptors. *Br. J. Pharmacol.* 129,1465-1473.

In: Caffeine and Health Research
Editor: Kenneth P. Chambers

ISBN 978-1-60456-437-2

Chapter I

Caffeine as an Indicator of Fecal Contamination in Source Water: Health Implications, Detection and Monitoring

Sergei S. Verenitch*[*]*, Bidyut R. Mohapatra and Asit Mazumder
Water and Aquatic Sciences Research Program, University of Victoria,
PO Box 3020 STN CSC, Victoria, British Columbia V8W 3N5, Canada

Abstract

Fecal pollution can not only impair the quality of freshwater intended for drinking, recreation, aquaculture and irrigation but also pose a significant threat to public and environmental health by contributing pathogenic microorganisms. With the increase in human development, population growth and drastic changes in climate, it is expected that the source waters are more vulnerable to known as well as emerging pathogens. In order to sustain the integrity of source water and implementation of better management practices to reduce the environmental loading of pathogens associated with waterborne disease transmission, it is essential to identify the origin of fecal pollution source(s). Several microbial source tracking (MST) phenotypic and genotypic methods have been developed to discriminate the animal and human sources of fecal pollution. However, the standardization of these methods pertaining to operations, expenses, reproducibility and global use has been a problem for reliable field application. Recently, caffeine (1, 3, 7, trimethylxanthine) has been emerging as an important chemical tracer for surveillance of human fecal waste input into source water. This chapter provides an overview on the health implications of caffeine in source water by integrating the occurrence of enteric pathogens in aquatic environment associated with waterborne disease transmission, and the genotypic and phenotypic tracking of human versus animal sources of fecal bacteria with the detection and monitoring of caffeine in source water. Additionally, a description of the application of a novel analytical technique developed using gas chromatography

[*] Fax: 250-721-7120, E-mail: ssv@uvic.ca

(GC) coupled with ion-trap tandem mass spectrometry detection system (IT-MS/MS) for determination of caffeine in aquatic systems is presented.

1. Introduction

The increase in urbanization, agricultural and industrial activities possesses an unprecedented threat to the sustainability of freshwater used for drinking, recreation, aquaculture and crop irrigation (Davies and Mazumder 2003; Vitousek et al., 1997). The freshwater quality is deteriorated by contamination of pathogens through point and non-point sources of fecal pollution including direct discharge of municipal waste effluents, leaching from poorly maintained septic tanks, sewer line leakage, inefficient sewage treatment, agricultural and urban runoff, storm water drainage, combined sewer and sanitary sewer overflows, and defecation of domestic- and wild-animals (WHO, 2003).

Generally, contamination of source water by human fecal input has been considered to be a threat to public and environmental health because it is a vector for propagation and/or transmission of an array of human-specific bacterial, viral and protozoan pathogens associated with waterborne diseases (WHO, 1993). A number of studies reported that animal fecal wastes are also the carriers of enteric pathogens responsible for gastrointestinal illness (Craun et al., 2004). However, some quantitative risk assessment studies have indicated that the public health risk from animal-derived fecal contamination is lesser than that from human feces because the disease-causing viruses are mostly human-specific (Levy et al., 1998; Upton 1999). Therefore, to maximize the integrity of source water and to minimize the public and environmental health risk associated with fecal pollution; significant efforts have been made worldwide to develop efficient techniques to distinguish the animal versus human sources of fecal pollution (USEPA, 2002a).

Fecal indicator bacteria have been used by the regulatory agencies for assessing fecal pollution in waterways (Clesceri et al., 1998). Elevated levels of fecal indicator bacteria in water bodies primarily provide evidence of fecal pollution and secondarily indicate the vulnerability of water bodies to enteric pathogens. In recent years several cultivation methods have been developed to enumerate fecal indicator bacteria from water samples. However, these methods do not provide information about the source(s) of fecal pollution. Tracking the origins of fecal contamination, commonly known as microbial source tracking (MST), is paramount for assessing the health risk posed to public and environment and for implementing better management practices to reduce, and/or abate the environmental loading of pathogens responsible for waterborne disease transmission (USEPA, 2005).

Several MST methods have been developed in recent years to identify the potential fecal source(s) in waterways either by using host-specific molecular markers or by comparing the phenotypic and genotypic fingerprints with a reference library composing of the fingerprints of fecal indicator bacteria derived from the known sources of fecal contamination (Meays et al., 2004; Mohapatra et al., 2007a, b; Scott et al., 2002; Simpson et al., 2002). The standardization of these methods pertaining to operations, expenses, reproducibility and global use has been currently under development (USEPA, 2005). A series of human-specific chemical markers, such as metabolites, pharmaceuticals, personal care products and foods have also been used in MST studies to trace the human input (Eaganhouse, 1997; Scott et al., 2002). As these chemical markers are present in trace quantities in the waterways, analytical quantification of these markers are a great challenge for reliable identification of the fecal sources (Scott et al., 2002; Simpson et al., 2002).

Recently, caffeine (1, 3, 7, trimethylxanthine) was used as a potential chemical marker for surveillance of human fecal input into source water (Buerge et al., 2003; Peeler et al., 2006; Piocos et al., 2000; Seiler et al., 1999; Siegener et al., 2002; Standley et al., 2000). Having been an active ingredient in many beverages, pharmaceuticals and numerous food products, and being partially metabolized in human body, caffeine has been found in different aquatic ecosystems: wastewater at the level of $\mu g\ l^{-1}$ (Metcalfe et al., 2003; Ternes et al., 2001), surface water at the concentrations between 10 to 100 $ng\ l^{-1}$ (Buerge et al., 2003, Kolpin et al., 2004, Togola et al., 2007), groundwater from 40 to 230 $ng\ l^{-1}$ (Seiler et al., 1999) and seawater at the levels from 5 to 71 $ng\ l^{-1}$ (Siegener et al., 2002, Weigel et al., 2002). Furthermore, the stability of caffeine under variable environmental stressors, its source-specificity and its long term persistence in water environment insist to consider caffeine as an ideal surrogate of human-derived fecal pollution of source water. In view of the potential of caffeine as a chemical tracer of fecal contamination, it is essential to develop robust analytical method for its monitoring in aquatic environment.

This chapter provides an overview on the health implications of caffeine in source water by integrating the occurrence of enteric pathogens in aquatic environment associated with waterborne disease transmission, and the phenotypic and the genotypic tracking of human versus animal sources of fecal bacteria with the detection and monitoring of caffeine in source water. Additionally, a detailed description of a novel analytical technique developed using gas chromatography coupled with ion-trap tandem mass spectrometry detection system (IT-MS/MS) for determination of caffeine in aquatic systems is presented.

2. Waterborne Pathogens

Different types of microbial pathogens, such as bacterial, viral and protozoan are excreted through feces and can be transmitted to humans through water (WHO, 1993). It has been identified that most of the water impairment worldwide has been caused by the fecal pathogens (USEPA, 2002a). With the increase in urbanization and drastic changes in climate, it is expected that the source waters are more vulnerable to known as well as emerging pathogens (WHO, 2003). Waterborne pathogens of greatest concerns to public and environmental health have five important characteristics (Rosen, 2000):1) they are shed into the environment in high numbers, 2) they are highly infectious to humans at low doses, 3) they have the ability to multiply outside of a host under favorable environmental conditions, 4) they can survive and remain infectious in the environment for long periods, and 5) they are highly resistant to water treatment. In this section, the descriptions of the microbial pathogens that are identified as the causative agents of recreational and drinking water-associated outbreaks are provided.

2.1. Pathogenic Bacteria

Bacteria are unicellular organisms of 0.2 μm to 2 μm in size and different shapes: spherical (coccus), rod (bacillus), comma (vibrio), corkscrew (spirochete) and spiral (spirillium). The waterborne pathogenic bacteria of concern and their disease outcomes are listed in Table 1. While most waterborne pathogenic bacteria are considered to be of fecal origin (animals and/or humans) the pathogenic species of *Aeromonas*, *Legionella*, *Mycobacterium* and *Vibrio* may be endemic to water. USEPA (2000) has identified that fecal pathogenic bacteria are the most leading causes of source water impairment. Diarrhea, abdominal cramps, vomiting, anorexia and nausea are the most common clinical symptoms of gastrointestinal illness caused by waterborne bacterial pathogens. Some pathogens, such as *Salmonella typhi* and *Salmonella paratyphi* strain A, B and C spread from the intestine into the blood stream and cause enteric typhoid and paratyphoid fevers (WHO, 2005).

Table 1. Waterborne bacterial pathogens and their associated diseases (AWWA, 2006)

Bacteria	Disease	Clinical symptoms
Aeromonas hydrophila	Gastroenteritis and wound infection	Diarrhea, nausea, septicemia and fevers
Campylobacter	Campylobacteriosis	Acute diarrhea, meningitis and GuillainBarré syndrome (paralysis)
Escherichia coli O157:H7 *(Enteropathogenic)*	Gastroenteritis	Diarrhea, nausea, septicemia and fevers
Legionella pneumophila	Legionellosis	Severe respiratory illness or Pontiac fever (non pneumonic and influenza-like illness)
Leptospira interrogans	Leptospirosis (Weil's disease)	Jaundice and fever
Mycobacterium avium	Gastroenteritis	Diarrhea, nausea, vomiting and Buruli ulcer (acute human skin disease)
Salmonella typhi and *Salmonella paratyphi*	Enteric fever	High fever, diarrhea, ulceration of small intestine, anorexia and septicemia
Salmonella (~ 2000 serotypes)	Salmonellosis	Diarrhea
Shigella (4 serogroups)	Shigellosis	Diarrhea, fever, nausea, vomiting and hemolytic uremic syndrome
Vibrio cholerae	Cholera	Acute diarrhea, dehydration and kidney failure
Yersinia enterocolitica	Yersinosis	Diarrhea, acute mesenteric lymphadenitis and joint pain

2.2. Pathogenic Viruses

Viruses are 0.02 μm to 0.3 μm in sizes and are considered as the smallest known agents of disease. More than 120 different types of enteric viruses are known to infect humans

(AWWA, 2006). These viruses are excreted in the feces of infected individuals and may directly or indirectly contaminate water intended for drinking, recreation and crop irrigation. The viruses must require a host cell for multiplication and proliferation. The common waterborne viruses that can infect humans are enteroviruses, hepatitis viruses, rotaviruses, reoviruses, caliciviruses (Norwalk and Sapporo viruses), astroviruses and adenoviruses (Table 2). Most of these viruses are responsible for the gastrointestinal and respiratory tract illness. Some viral pathogens can cause acute illness, such as meningitis, encephalitis, paralysis, myocarditis, hepatitis, pneumonia and conjunctivitis. Major waterborne viral disease outbreaks are attributed to sewage contamination of source water or inadequate treatment of private and semipublic water supplies (Warrington et al., 2001).

Table 2. Waterborne viral pathogens and their associated diseases (AWWA, 2006)

Virus	Disease	Clinical symptoms
Adenoviruses (~ 49 serotypes)	Gastroenteritis and respiratory disease	Severe respiratory illness, pneumonia, conjunctivitis and diarrhea
Astroviruses	Gastroenteritis	Watery diarrhea, vomiting, fever, anorexia and abdominal pain
Caliciviruses (Lordsdale-like, Norwalk-like and Sapporo-like)	Gastroenteritis	Diarrhea, vomiting, septicemia and fevers
Enteroviruses [5 groups: Poliovirus (3 types), enterovirus A (12 types), enterovirus B (37 types), enterovirus C (11 types) and enterovirus D (2 types)]	Gastroenteritis, meningitis, and heart anomalies	Acute respiratory illness, paralysis and encephalitis
Hepatitis A virus	Infectious hepatitis	Jaundice, acute liver inflammation and fever
Hepatitis E virus	Infectious hepatitis	Jaundice, acute liver inflammation and fever
Reoviruses	Gastroenteritis	Diarrhea, vomiting, septicemia and fevers in infants
Rotaviruses	Gastroenteritis	Acute diarrhea in infants

2.3. Pathogenic Protozoa

Protozoa are single cell organisms of sizes from 2 μm to 100 μm and morphologically altered inside the host during their complex life cycle (Rosen, 2000). Protozoa usually survive outside the host by formation of cyst. The cysts are resistant to environmental stresses, such as sunlight, temperature, moisture and pH, and can be transmitted from host to host via water. Table 3 lists waterborne pathogenic protozoa and the disease associated with them. The protozoa responsible for the most of the gastrointestinal outbreaks are *Cryptosporidium parvum* and *Giardia lamblia*. The persistence of the *Cryptosporidium* oocysts and *Giardia* cysts in water environment and their resistance to chemical disinfectant is a concern for public and environmental health (Fayer and Nerad, 1996).

Table 3. Waterborne protozoan pathogens and their associated diseases (AWWA, 2006)

Protozoa	Disease	Clinical symptoms
Cryptosporidium	Cryptosporidiosis	Acute watery diarrhea, nausea, fever and fatigue. Life-threatening for immuno- compromised patients.
Cyclospora	Cyclosporiasis	Watery diarrhea, mild nausea, anorexia, and abdominal cramping
Entamoeba histolytica	Amebiasis	Prolonged diarrhea with bleeding, abscesses of the liver and small intestine
Giardia lamblia	Giardiasis	Diarrhea, anorexia, bloody stool, vomiting and indigestion
Naegleria fowleri	Primary amebic meningoencephalitis (PAM)	Inflammation of brain and meniges cause severe headache, stiff neck, photophobia and coma leading to death.

It has been reported that 30 *Cryptosporidium* oocysts and 10 *Giardia* cysts are able to cause mild to severe diarrhea and potentially shorten the life span of infants and immune compromised individuals, such as AIDS patients (AWWA, 2006). The occurrence of the *Cryptosporidium* oocysts and *Giardia* cysts are found to be correlated with fecal pollution (Rosen, 2000). In industrialized nations, the cryptosporidiosis and giardiasis are associated with drinking and recreational water contaminated by combined and sanitary sewer overflows, storm water drainage, malfunctioning of septic systems, and/or sewer line leakage (WHO, 1993).

3. Fecal Indicator Bacteria

The public health concern for prevalence of pathogens in source water is diseases. Direct surveillance of pathogens can provide information about the risk associated with the consumption of water. However, the waterborne pathogens are phylogenetically diverse, difficult to cultivate, patchy in distribution, and highly infectious in low doses (AWWA, 2006). Additionally, sensitivity, fidelity and costs of the assay methods to monitor waterborne pathogens have not been standardized yet for reliable application. The practical limitations for direct surveillance of pathogens necessitate monitoring the fecal indicator bacteria, such as *Escherichia coli*, total and fecal coliform, fecal enterococci, and *Clostridium perfringens* to conduct microbial risk assessment of source water quality (Wade et al. 2003; Wiedenmann et al., 2006). Ideal fecal indicator bacteria should mimic the fate of the enteric pathogens in water and its detection and enumeration should be carried out in an easy and accurate manner. *E. coli* have been used as the regulatory indicator bacteria for assessing fecal pollution in waterways worldwide since it is a universal intestinal flora of warm-blooded animals, easy-to-cultivate and present at a concentration of 10^6 cells/gram of colon contents (Clesceri et al., 1998). Hence, most of the MST studies have been performed on *E. coli* and to some extent on enteroccoci for tracking the origins of fecal pollution.

4. MST Methods

The MST methods have been classified into two types, microbiological methods which target the microorganisms and chemical methods which target the pharmaceuticals, personal health care products and byproducts of human or animal metabolites. In this section, the microbiological and chemical methods used for fecal source tracking are discussed.

4.1. Microbiological Methods

The microbiological methods can be classified into three types: population-dependent methods, species-dependent phenotypic methods and species-dependent genotypic methods.

4.1.1. Population-Dependent Methods

The population-dependent methods have lower discriminatory ability compared to species-dependent methods for tracking the source(s) of fecal pollution. The population-dependent methods use the test for presence and/or absence of the host-specific microorganisms, such as *Bacteroidales*, sorbitol fermenting bifidobacteria, bacteriophages of *Bacteroides fragilis*, F+ RNA coliphages, and enteric viruses.

4.1.1.1. Assay of Host-Specific Bacteroidales

Anaerobic bacteria of the order *Bacteroidales* have been identified as the major groups of bacteria in the feces of warm-blooded animal. These groups of bacteria are difficult to cultivate. Recently with the advent of molecular techniques, PCR primers specific for the rRNA genes of the order *Bacteroidales* have been designed to distinguish the fecal sources ruminant, human, dog, pig, horse and elk (Bernhard and Field, 2000; Dick et al., 2005a, b; Layton et al., 2006; Okabe et al., 2007). These molecular markers persist for a long time in the aquatic environment. These host-specific markers are found to be spatio-temporally stable, and the limit of detection correlates significantly with sewage contamination as well as with the density of fecal indicator bacteria. In some cases the limit of detection also predicts the occurrence of zoonotic pathogens (Walters et al., 2007). Limitation of this method includes the transfer of rRNA genes through horizontal gene transfer among the fecal bacteria of the host-sources in close contact e.g., humans and their pets.

4.1.1.2. Assay of Sorbitol-Fermenting Bifidobacteria

Bifidobacteria are the principal groups of anaerobic bacteria present in the feces of warm-blooded animals. Sorbitol-fermenting bifidobacteria are mostly present in the feces of humans (to some extent in the pig feces), and therefore have been used to track the fecal input from human (Long et al., 2005; Rhodes and Kator, 1999). This method has been found to distinguish human from animal sources of fecal contamination in Europe (Blanch et al.,

2006), USA (Long et al., 2005) and South Africa (Jagals and Grabow, 1996). The short time survival of bifidobacteria in the environment, and several days of incubation for the enumeration of these bacteria restrict the application of the methods in MST studies (Rhodes and Kator, 1999).

4.1.1.3. Assay of Bacteriophages

Bacteroides fragilis is an anaerobic and Gram-negative rod-shaped bacteria present universally in the feces of humans as well as animals. The bacteriophages are viruses that infect the bacteria. Bacteriophages specific for *B. fragilis* strain HSP40 (Tartera et al., 1989), *B. fragilis* strain RYC4023 (Puig et al., 1999), and *B. fragilis* strain RYC2056 (Puig et al., 1999) have been found in the wastewater contaminated with human feces. Although some of the bacteriophages are detected in the animal feces, the occurrence of high number of phages in human fecal wastes makes it a potential indicator of human-derived fecal pollution. Those facts that the bacteriophages do not replicate in the aquatic environments and the presence of bacteriophages correlate significantly with the occurrence of enteric viruses (Jofre et al., 1989), are the advantages of this method. The complex procedures for enumeration of bacteriophages specific to *B. fragilis* restrict the application of this method in MST studies (Puig et al., 1999).

4.1.1.4. Assay of F+ RNA Coliphages

Coliphages are viruses that infect the cells of *Escherichia coli*. The coliphages are classified into two groups:somatic coliphages and male-specific (F+) coliphages. The somatic coliphages attach directly to the lipopolysaccharides of *E. coli*. The F+ coliphages attach only to *E. coli* that has F plasmid. The F plasmid encodes F pilus, a site attachment for virus. The F+ coliphages have been separated into two types F+ DNA and F+ RNA coliphages. The F+ RNA coliphages have been biochemically and genetically characterized well. Therefore, F+ RNA coliphages serotyping and genotyping methods have been used for MST studies (Cole et al., 2003; Schaper et al., 2002; Stewart-Pullaro et al., 2006). The F+ RNA coliphages are further divided into four subgroups according to their serotypes. Members of subgroup II and subgroup III are predominant in human feces and/or sewage. Member of subgroup IV are predominant in the wastes of animal and livestock. Member of subgroup I is present both in human and animal feces. The presence of a particular subgroup of F+ RNA coliphages indicates the source(s) of fecal pollution. The limitations of these methods include the presence of low numbers of F+ RNA coliphages than fecal indicator bacteria, and F+ RNA coliphages are found to replicate in water environments (Havelaar et al., 1990).

4.1.1.5. Assay of Enteric Viruses

Fecal viruses have been used as the indicator to track the source(s) of fecal contamination (Fong and Lipp, 2005; Griffin et al., 2003). Adenoviruses (Fong et al., 2005; Jiang et al., 2001; Puig et al., 2000), enteroviruses (Fong et al., 2005; Puig et al., 2000), and polyoma viruses (McQuaig et al., 2006) have been used as the indicator of human-derived fecal contamination. Similarly, enteric viruses specific to animals, such as porcine (Teschoviruses and adenoviruses) (Hundesa et al., 2006; Jimenez-Clavero et al., 2003) and bovine (adenoviruses, polyoma viruses and enteroviruses) (Hundesa et al., 2006; Ley et al.,

2002) have been identified. One of the limitations of using enteric viruses as the indicator for source tracking is the occurrence of low numbers of enteric viruses in environmental samples. Although nested-PCR and real-time-PCR assays significantly improve the detection limit of enteric viruses, these PCR methods can identify few enteric viruses (Jiang et al. 2001; McQuaig et al., 2006). In addition, these PCR-based methods cannot discriminate viable from nonviable viruses and sometimes lead to erroneous results.

4.1.2. Species-Dependent Phenotypic Methods

The low discriminatory power and limited application of population-dependent MST method, such as human versus animal fecal contamination have prompted the need to develop species-dependent phenotypic MST methods. The target microorganisms in species-dependent methods are fecal indicator bacteria, such as *Escherichia coli* and enterococci. Fecal indicator bacteria are present universally in all potential sources contributing to fecal pollution, and the bacteria are easy to cultivate. Several phenotypic methods: antibiotic resistance profiling (ARP), serotyping, carbon utilization profiling (CUP) and fatty acid profiling (FAP) have been used in MST studies. However, CUP (Blanch et al., 2006; Griffith et al., 2003; Hagedorn et al., 2003) and FAP (Parveen et al., 2001; Seurinck et al., 2006) have been applied in a limited number of MST studies. The spatio-temporal variation in the profiles of CUP and FAP is not able to identify the sources of fecal pollution. In contrast, ARP and serotyping methods are able to identify the sources correctly and these techniques are discussed in detail in this chapter.

4.1.2.1. Antibiotic Resistance Profiling (ARP)

ARP has been used to discriminate humans and various animal sources by testing the isolates of fecal *E. coli* and fecal enterococci against a panel of antibiotics (5 to 9 antibiotic agents) (Hagedorn et al., 1999; Harwood et al., 2000; Wiggins et al., 1999). ARP method is based on the underlying hypothesis that humans, domestic- and wild-animals have been exposed to different types of antibiotics, hence their fecal bacteria differ in types and levels of antibiotic resistance. As per the hypothesis, the antibiotic resistance types and levels expressed in the fecal indicator bacteria of humans should be more than of the wild animals. A reference library has been developed with known-sources of fecal *E. coli* and/or enterococci. The ARP of unknown *E. coli* and/or enterococci bacteria are usually compared with the reference library to identify its original source using statistical methods, such as cluster analysis and discriminant function analysis. ARP has been found to be successful in the identification of fecal sources in simple watersheds. However, this method has a lower discriminatory efficacy in the multifecal input watersheds. This lower discriminatory power of ARP in complex watersheds may be attributed to the exposures of human and domestic animal sources to the same class of antibiotics (Souza et al., 1999). The antibiotic resistance genes of fecal indicator bacteria are often plasmid encoded, and can be lost or altered in long term storage, and/or with changes in environmental conditions (Samadpour et al., 2005). Furthermore, ARP method is not effective in tracing the sources of animals which have not been exposed to antibiotics.

4.1.2.2. Serotyping

The underlying hypothesis for application of serotyping of *E. coli* in MST studies is that the *E. coli* strains obtained from the feces of humans and animals have different serotypes (Bettelheim et al., 1976; Hartley et al., 1975). The serotyping analysis used in various studies has found significant differences in the serotypes of *E. coli* between human and wildlife sources (Parveen et al., 2001). The application of serotyping method in MST is mainly restricted because of the requirement of large amount of antisera.

4.1.3. Species-Dependent Genotypic Methods

Genotypic species-dependent methods applied in fecal source tracking have been found to be more accurate and reliable than the species-dependent phenotypic methods. These methods include ribotyping, pulsed-field gel electrophoresis (PFGE), amplified fragment length polymorphism (AFLP) and repetitive extragenic palindromic (rep)-PCR. The genotypic species-dependent methods are based on the hypothesis that the fecal bacteria, such as *E. coli* and enterococci express the genotypic traits specific to their host. The characterization of the genotypic traits to establish a linkage between the fecal indicator bacteria (*E. coli* and enterococci) and its host source is the main task for the development of a robust genotypic method.

4.1.3.1. Ribotyping

Ribotyping is a DNA fingerprinting method where highly conserved rRNA genes are fingerprinted using oligonucleotide probe after treatment of genomic DNA with restriction endonucleases. The procedures for ribotyping methods involve cultures of *E. coli*, genomic DNA extraction, restriction enzyme digestion, gel electrophoresis, southern blotting and hybridization of oligonucleotide probes targeting the rRNA genes. The hypothesis for ribotyping method is that the *E. coli* strains obtained from human and animal sources are genotypically distinct and this genetic variability can be traced by genomic restriction fragment length polymorphism (RFLP) using rRNA genes as probes. A reference library of ribotype patterns from known-source fecal *E. coli* isolates is developed and the ribotype patterns of environmental *E. coli* isolates are matched with the reference library to identify their probable sources. The ribotyping method has mostly used *E. coli* as the target microorganism. Two types of restriction enzyme have been used to treat the genomic DNA in MST studies. The protocol developed by Samadpour (Griffith et al., 2003; Myoda et al., 2003; Samadpour and Chechowitz, 1995) uses two restriction enzymes (*EcoRI* and *PvuII*). The other investigators have used one restriction enzyme (*HindIII*) (Carson et al., 2001; Moore et al., 2005; Parveen et al., 1999; Scott et al., 2003). The two-enzyme protocol has been found to produce better results compared to one-enzyme protocol for differentiation of human and various animal sources (Moore et al., 2005; Myoda et al., 2003; Stoeckel et al., 2004).

4.1.3.2. PFGE

PFGE is a DNA fingerprinting method in which the DNA fingerprints are generated by digesting the genomic DNA with rare-cutting restriction endonucleases, followed by electrophoresis in an apparatus in which the polarity of the current is changed at predetermined intervals. The pulsed field allows clear separation of large molecular length DNA fragment ranging from 10 to 800 kb. PFGE has been considered as a gold-standard in epidemiological studies to differentiate the pathogenic strains. The application of PFGE in MST studies is limited. Simmons et al. (2000) used PFGE and observed that 51% of 439 *E. coli* isolates obtained from a stream in an urban watershed were classified correctly as wildlife and dogs. Kariuki et al., (1999) observed that PFGE DNA fingerprints is able to separate between children and chicken fecal *E. coli*. Parveen et al. (2001) reported that there was no significant relationship between PFGE patterns of fecal *E. coli* and their host sources.

4.1.3.3. AFLP

AFLP is a DNA fingerprinting method based on the selective amplification of a subset of DNA fragments generated by restriction enzyme digestion. The genomic restriction fragments are ligated with oligonucleotide adapters. A subset of restriction fragments are selectively amplified using PCR primers. The banding patterns of the genomic restriction fragments are considered as unique fingerprint for each strain. AFLP have been applied in the epidemiological studies for genotyping of pathogens because it has a good ability to differentiate clonally derived strains. AFLP analysis applied in MST studies have been found to produce high rate of correct classification with *E. coli* isolates obtained from human and various animal sources (Guan et al., 2002; Leung et al., 2004). Although AFLP has high discriminatory power and reproducibility, labor-intensive procedures and the cost associated with the analysis limit its application in large-scale MST studies.

4.1.3.4. Rep-PCR

Rep-PCR is a genotypic method that differentiates microorganisms by using primers complementary to interspersed repetitive consensus sequences. These noncoding sequences are present in multiple copies in the genomes of most Gram-negative and Gram-positive bacteria (Versalovic et al., 1991). Examples of these repetitive elements are the repetitive extragenic palindromic (REP) sequences, the enterobacterial repetitive intergenic consensus (ERIC) sequences, the BOX sequences and the polytrinucleotide $(GTG)_5$ sequences (Versalovic et al., 1994). These repetitive units are considered to be highly conserved because rep sites are crucial protein-DNA interaction sites and/or these sequences may disseminate themselves as selfish DNA by gene conversion. Amplification of the distinct rep sites produce diverse-sized DNA fragments that can be separated by agarose gel electrophoresis and the resulting banding patterns unique for specific bacterial strain can be compared (Versalovic et al., 1994). Rep-PCR has been widely used for bacterial taxonomy, diagnostic and epidemiological applications (Versalovic et al., 1994). It has also been emerging as a potential MST tool for the prediction of possible sources of fecal contamination of surface water owing to its success in classifying the correct host source, reproducibility, cost-effectiveness and easy operational procedures (Carson *et al.*, 2003; Dombek *et al.*, 2000; Johnson *et al.*, 2004; McLellan et al., 2003; Mohapatra *et al.*, 2007a; Seurinck et al., 2003). Five methods, namely REP-PCR (primer sets Rep1R-I and Rep2-I), ERIC-PCR (primer sets ERIC1R and ERIC2), ERIC2-PCR (primer ERIC2), BOX-PCR (primer BOX A1R), and $(GTG)_5$-PCR [primer $(GTG)_5$] are frequently used in rep-PCR fingerprinting analysis (Versalovic et al., 1994). Most of the MST studies for identification of the source of *E. coli* have utilized the rep-PCR primers listed above except $(GTG)_5$. Recently rep-PCR coupled with $(GTG)_5$ primer [$(GTG)_5$-PCR] has been found to produce more discriminative and complex fingerprint patterns than REP, ERIC, ERIC2 and BOX A1R primers for differentiation of fecal *E. coli* from humans, poultry and wild birds (Mohapatra et al., 2007b). Rep-PCR DNA fingerprinting is simple and easy to perform and, thus, may prove to be a cost-effective screening tool for rapid determination of *E. coli* isolates identity and tracking the non-point sources of fecal contamination of surface water.

4.2. Chemical Methods

There are a few chemical markers that have been used for tracking the sources of fecal pollution in water environment. These include fecal sterols and stanols (Bull et al., 2002; Edwards et al., 1998; Standley et al., 2000), bile acids (Bull et al., 2002; Elhmmali et al., 2000; Isobe et al., 2002) and long-chain alkyl benzene (laundry additives) (Eganhouse et al., 1983). All these chemical markers have several limitations including lack of specificity for fecal input, alteration by environmental microorganisms and requirements of expensive analytical techniques (Murray et al., 1987). These limitations restrict effective applications of chemical markers in MST studies.

Caffeine is considered as one of the major ingredients in a variety of beverages, food products, and over-the-counter medicines, including anticold, antipyretic and analgesic drugs (Mazzafera, 2002). Considering its uptake with beverages, foods and medicines, caffeine is probably the most widely consumed drugs in the world (Ogunseitan, 1996). Caffeine is added on the United States Environmental Protection Agency list of high production volume of chemical (USEPA, 2002b). The global average consumption of caffeine is between 80 and 400 mg per person per day (Gokulakrishnan et al., 2005). In humans, dietary caffeine is metabolized by hepatic cytochrome P450 1A2 pathways, and from 0.5% to 10% of unmetabolized caffeine is excreted through urine (Berthou et al., 1992). Because of its extensive use in food, beverages and medicines, caffeine has been detected in surface water, groundwater and wastewater effluents worldwide. As caffeine has been emerging as an important chemical tracer for tracking the human fecal waste input into source water, it is necessary to develop accurate, reliable and real-time monitoring methods (Mohapatra et al., 2006).

An integrated approach combining caffeine with other microbiological MST methods and water chemistry characteristics is believed to provide a better tool in interpretation of not only a source but also a level of contamination in aquatic system. Correlations between caffeine, fecal indicator bacteria and nutrients in rural freshwater and urban marine systems were a subject of the study carried out by Peeler et al., 2006. The results found in this study indicated that measurements of caffeine, nutrients, particularly nitrate, and fecal indicator bacteria can aid in distinguishing human versus non-human sources of surface water contamination. It was also noted that the relationships among the indicators measured was dependent on the extent to which different removal mechanisms influence the persistence of each indicator in a given environment.

4.2.1. Detection of Caffeine

Due to a wide range of concentrations of caffeine in source water, a few different analytical methodologies have been used for analysis of this anthropogenic input indicator. Buerge et al., (2003) and Peeler et al., (2006) employed triple-quadruple mass spectrometer in MS/MS and selective ion monitoring (SIM) modes using ^{13}C-labeled caffeine as an internal standard to analyze their wastewater and natural water samples. The method detection limits (MDL) achieved were 2 and 10 ng l^{-1} for GC-MS/MS and GC-SIM techniques, respectively with fortified quality control samples prepared in DI water showing the recoveries in the range of from 81 to 127%. The mean extraction efficiency of ^{13}C-caffeine from natural waters was somewhat lower than in DI water (84%) and showed a larger range (34 – 113%). The method detection limit achieved in other studies varied depending on a methodology employed: 40 μg l^{-1} for high performance liquid chromatography (HPLC) with photodiode array detection (Piocos et al., 2000); 40 ng l^{-1} and 5μg l^{-1} for GC-SIM and HPLC systems, respectively (Seiler et al., 1999). Siegener and Chen (2002) used GC-SIM analytical methodology with a surrogate internal standard to assess caffeine level in sea water samples. The MDL achieved was 5ng l^{-1}, but the recoveries of the surrogate standard were very low. For terphenyl-d^{14} it was on average 25-51% and for ^{13}C (trimethyl)-caffeine it was in the range of 27-57%. Liquid chromatography coupled with mass spectrometry detection system provided satisfactory sensitivity with MDL = 5-10 ng l^{-1} (Metcalfe et al., 2003) and 10-25 ng l^{-1} (Ternes et al., 2001) although the recoveries for caffeine in the fortified quality control samples of surface or ground waters were around 48-68%. The analytical methodology based on gas chromatography with ion-trap tandem mass spectrometry detection system developed by Verenitch et al. (2006) achieved MDL at 20 ng l^{-1} with no use of internal standard to verify the recovery of the target analyte.

In this chapter we presented in details the methodology developed by the authors and based on a use of gas chromatography with ion-trap tandem mass spectrometry detection system. Isotope dilution method with a use of ^{13}C-labeled (trimethyl)-caffeine was employed to assess and correct recoveries of native caffeine in water samples of various sources.

4.2.1.1. Materials and Sample Preparation

Caffeine was purchased from Sigma-Aldrich Canada (Oakville, Canada); trimethyl-^{13}C-labeled caffeine, used as surrogate internal standard (SIS), was from Cambridge Isotope Laboratories (Andover, MA, USA). Anhydrous sodium sulfate (Na_2SO_4) purchased from Fisher and used to remove moisture from a sample extract was baked at 400 °C for 4 hrs prior to use. All solvents (methanol [MeOH], methyl tert-butyl ether [MTBE], acetone, hexane and dichloromethane [DCM]) were HPLC grade and were purchased from Fisher Scientific (Ottawa, Canada). All glass ware including sampling amber bottles were rinsed with DCM, acetone, MeOH and as a last step, double distilled deionized water and baked at 300°C overnight. Solid phase extraction (SPE) cartridges used in the sample preparation procedure were Oasis HLB 6mL, 0.2 g from Waters Co. (Milford, Massachusetts, USA).

Standard (STD) stock solutions of native and ^{13}C-labeled caffeine were prepared in methanol. Calibration solutions of different concentrations 10, 20, 40, 60, 80, 100, 200, 500 and 1000 pg μl^{-1} for caffeine with constant, 200 pg μl^{-1} concentration of the surrogate internal standard in each of them were prepared in DCM. A standard solution of caffeine at the concentration of 100 pg μl^{-1} in DCM was used for the optimization of IT-MS/MS parameter.

One liter grab samples were collected by hand at the water surface at different locations on West coast of Vancouver Island, British Columbia, Canada. The locations of sample sites were characteristic to specific human activities in that area and included marine research station, river samples from up- and downstream of a source of sewage contamination, sewage treatment plant (STP), lakes of various size from 53 to 189,000 dam^3 with different density of residential development around. All samples were collected and placed in plastic bottles and immediately transported to the laboratory where they were frozen and kept at -20 °C until the extraction procedure took place. Samples were processed usually within a 30 days period after their collection.

The procedure for caffeine extraction from water samples was an adaptation of the method well presented in the literature. Briefly, 10 µl of 2000 pg μl^{-1} solution of surrogate internal standard of ^{13}C-labeled caffeine in methanol was added into 1 l of each sample so that its theoretical concentration in the final extract of 100 µl was 200 pg μl^{-1}. The sample was then filtered through 0.45 µm GF/C filter which had been pre-washed with hexane and DCM, oven dried and ashed for 1 hr at 500 °C. To the fortified samples of 1 l of distilled de-ionized water, 10, 20, 30, 50 and 100 µl of 200 pg μl^{-1} of the standard solution of caffeine in methanol was added. This corresponds to the concentrations of caffeine of 2.0, 4.0, 6.0, 10.0 and 20.0 ng l^{-1}. If necessary, the pH of the sample filtrate was adjusted with 1 M NaOH to pH 7.5. The SPE cartridge (Oasis HLB) was conditioned with 3 ml of MTBE, then 3 ml of MeOH followed by 6 ml of deionized water, and then the sample was passed through the cartridge at approximately 10 ml min^{-1}. All sample bottles were rinsed with 10 ml of pH=7.5 deionized water three times and the rinses were combined and passed through the SPE cartridge. After the extraction was completed, the cartridges were washed with 2 ml of 25% MeOH/water solution to remove the polar co-extractives and further dried under full vacuum for 5min. The elution of caffeine was performed using 1 ml of MeOH followed by 6 ml of MeOH/MTBE (1:9, v/v). The extract was dried to dryness and re-dissolved in 1 ml of DCM. The solution was treated with baked sodium sulfate to remove moisture and transferred to a Kuderna Danish evaporative concentrator using 0.5 ml x 3 of DCM. The volume of the final extract was reduced to 100 µl using a gentle stream of nitrogen. The sample was then analyzed on GC-IT-MS/MS by injecting 2 µl of the sample extract.

4.2.1.2. Instrumentation and IT-MS/MS Conditions

Analyses were conducted on Varian CP 3800 gas chromatograph equipped with a 30 m x 0.25 mm ID x 0.25 µm film thickness CP-SIL 8CB-MS capillary column. The gas chromatograph was directly interfaced to a Varian Saturn 2200 ion-trap mass spectrometer. All injections (2 µl) were made using a Varian CP-8200 autosampler. The flow of He through a GC column was constant and set at 1 ml min^{-1}. The programmable temperature of the vaporization injector was maintained at 250 °C, the transfer line at 300 °C, the ion-trap at 220 °C and the manifold at 80 °C. The injector was operated in splitless mode for 0.5min, then turned to the split mode at the ratio of 100:1. The column temperature program was as follows: initial temperature 70 °C, maintained for 1.0 min, then ramped at 25 °C min^{-1} to 180

°C and at 5 °C min^{-1} to 240 °C, then held at this temperature for 3 min. Total run time was 20.4 min.

The first step of the IT-MS/MS optimization procedure was a selection of an appropriate precursor ion of caffeine. The precursor ion selected from the full scan mass spectrum of the analyte for the sequential application of MS/MS conditions, was the most abundant ion. For caffeine it was its molecular ion, *m/z*=194. In order to improve IT-MS/MS specificity (e.g., decrease of potential interference from organic matter ions) the isolation width of the precursor ions for the surrogate internal standard and native caffeine with *m/z*=197 and 194, respectively was reduced to 1 *m/z*. After the application of the second ionization step (collision induced dissociation voltage) to the selected precursor ion, the MS/MS spectrum was obtained. Figure 1a and b present the mass spectra of native caffeine obtained in different modes: electron impact (EI) ionization mode followed by a full mass scan, a) and MS/MS mode, b). As expected, the isotope labeled caffeine gave the mass spectra similar to its native analog both in EI ionization full mass scan mode and MS/MS mode, Figure 1c, d. A mass segment range from *m/z*=80 to 200 was employed at the stage of optimization of MS/MS conditions. Five major product ions 108, 122, 149, 165, 193 were selected, on the basis of their high abundances, as the characteristic ions of the performance of the selected MS/MS conditions. Besides the common MS parameters such as axial modulation voltage: 4.0 V; electron multiplier voltage: 1950 V, some MS/MS parameters were set at their default values (GC-MS Manual, 1999). Those were Filament/Multiplier Delay: 10 min; Peak Threshold: 0; Mass Defect: 0 mmu/100 u; Background Mass: 45 *m/z*; RF Dump Value: 650 *m/z*; Filament Current: 80 μA; AGC Target: 2000; Prescan Ionization Time: 1500 μs; Scan Time: 0.50 s scan^{-1}; Multiplier Offset: +/-300 V. Some ion preparation mode (IPM) parameters set at their default values or once adjusted were kept constant both in the process of IT-MS/MS optimization and further analyses of water samples: Isolation Windows: 1 *m/z*; Low/High Offset: 6/2 DAC steps; Ionization Storage Level: 48 *m/z*; Ejection Amplitude: 20 V; Modulation Rate: 3000 μs step^{-1}; Modulation Range: 2 steps; number of frequencies 1, waveform type – resonant, CID Frequency Offset: 0 Hz, Electron Energy: 70 eV. The excitation storage level (ESL) was calculated based on the molecular weight of the analyte and "q_z" value equal to its default setting of 0.400.

Under MS/MS conditions product ions are formed from the precursor ions by collision induced dissociation. The amount of energy that is converted to internal energy in the precursor ion exposed to CID voltage and collisions with He atoms depends on the number of collisions (excitation time), the relative energy of the collisions (CID) and the rate that the internal energy is removed by the collisional deactivation. CID in the ion trap is always in competition with ion ejection. If the CID amplitude selected is too large, the precursor ion will be ejected to the trap electrodes before it can collide with background helium atoms. If the CID voltage is too small, the energy of the precursor ion will not exceed the internal energy threshold required to break the chemical bonds and form product ions. ET is the duration of the resonance excitation voltage applied at constant radio frequency (RF) to the endcap electrodes of the ion trap mass analyzer to affect the formation of product ions from an isolated precursor ion via CID with damping gas molecules.

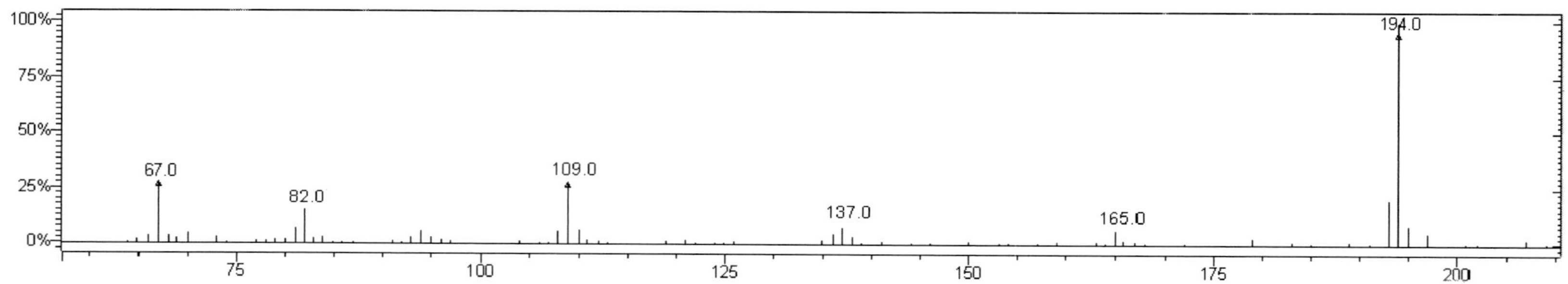
100%
75%
50%
25%
0%
194.0
67.0
82.0
109.0
137.0
165.0
75
100
125
150
175
200

a)

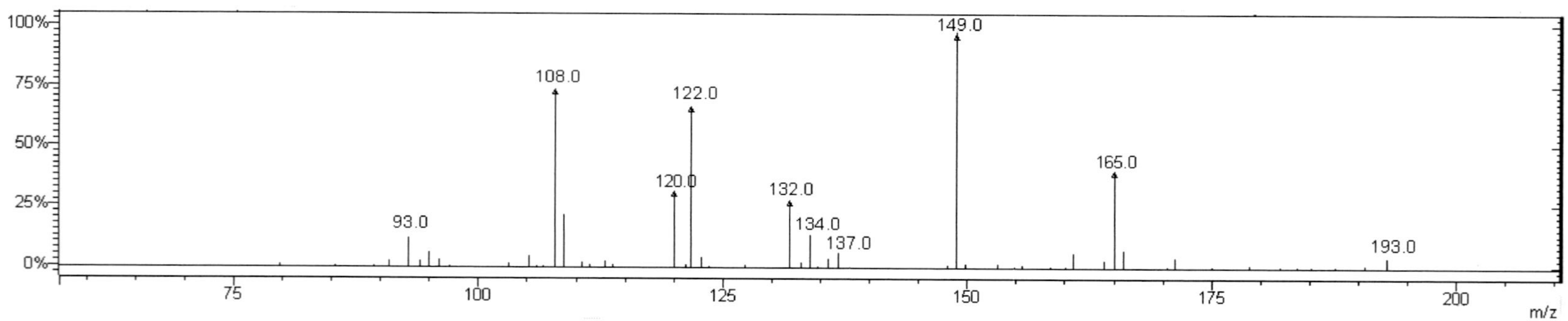
100%
75%
50%
25%
0%
149.0
108.0
122.0
120.0
132.0
134.0
137.0
93.0
165.0
193.0
75
100
125
150
175
200
m/z

b)

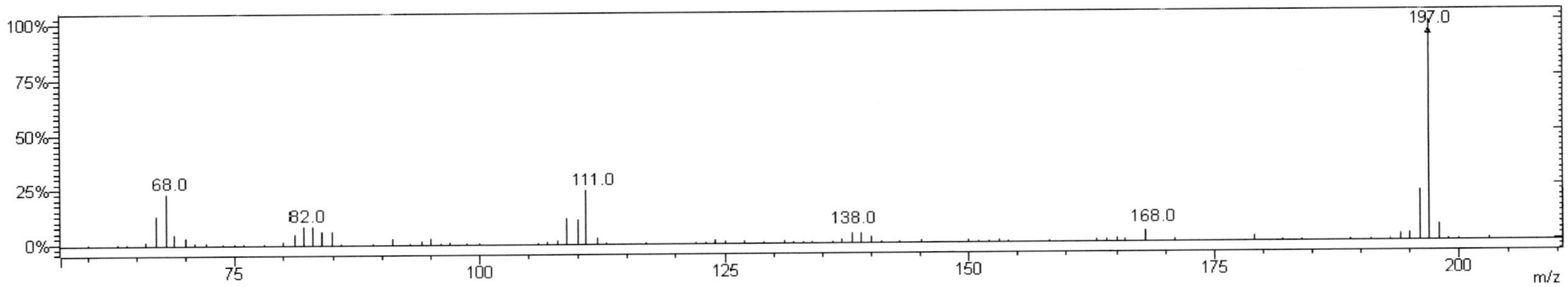

c)

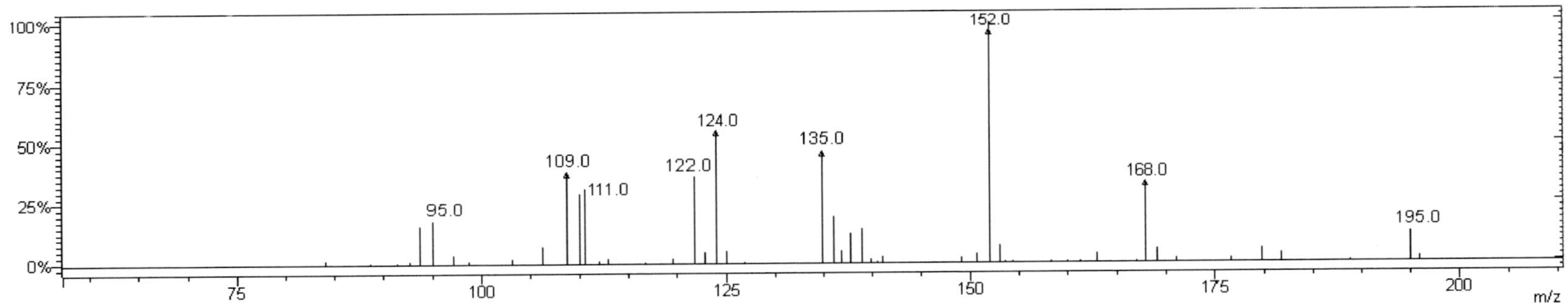

d)

Figure 1. Total ion counts mass spectra of caffeine (a, b) and its ^{13}C-labeled analogue (c, d) obtained in an ion-trap mass analyzer at the mode of EI (a, c) followed by a full mass scan and MS/MS mode performed at the optimized CID amplitude (b, d).

IT refers to the duration of the ion isolation waveform voltage, which is applied to the endcap electrodes of the ion trap during the isolation of the precursor ions into the ion trap. Shorter IT is used when the parent ion is considered unstable. Longer IT may be desirable when stability is not an issue and high mass cleanup is required (i.e. high background/column bleed). MIT is reserved for the main scan as an upper limit for the ionization time allowed to achieve the target number of ions during the ionization mode. The effect of each parameter in general has been described in details elsewhere (March, 1997; 1995; 2005).

So to achieve the highest sensitivity and accuracy in determination of caffeine in water samples, the authors conducted a detailed optimization of a set of instrumental IT-MS/MS parameters, CID, ET, IT and MIT. Four series of injections of standard solution of caffeine at the concentration of 100 pg μl^{-1} were made in order to investigate the signal intensities of the product ions of caffeine by varying each one of the four instrumental parameters, cited above. Initially, the operating parameters chosen for optimization were set at the default values and then were optimized one by one in the following order CID, ET, IT and MIT. For each series of injections, the instrumental parameter under investigation was gradually increased and the peak area of the product ions with *m/z*=108, 122, 149, 165 and 193 was integrated. Three replicate injections were performed and averaged for each data point obtained in this process of optimization so to evaluate the deviation caused by the instrument fluctuation.

The optimization of the CID voltage was performed at the resonant conditions in two steps (Verenitch et al., 2006). For the first step, the CID voltage was incrementally raised from 0 to 4.0 V and a full mass spectrum of product ions was acquired at each CID amplitude. The best CID was the one that gave the highest total area counts of the selected product ions (*m/z*=109, 122, 149 and 165) and very little of *m/z*=193 and the precursor ions (*m/z*=194). Once a rough estimate of the most suitable CID amplitude was determined, the voltage was optimized using lower increment. The results of the optimization experiments of IT-MS/MS parameters are presented on the Figure 2a-d.

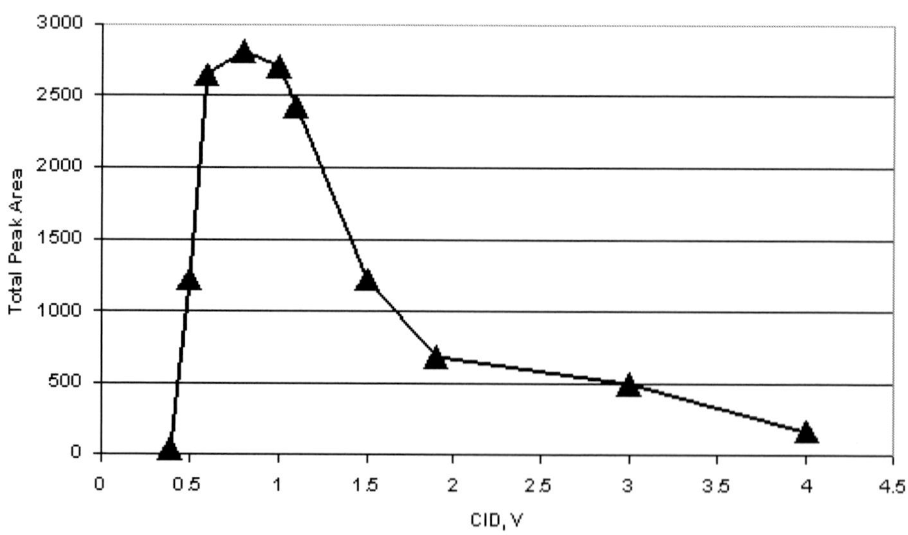

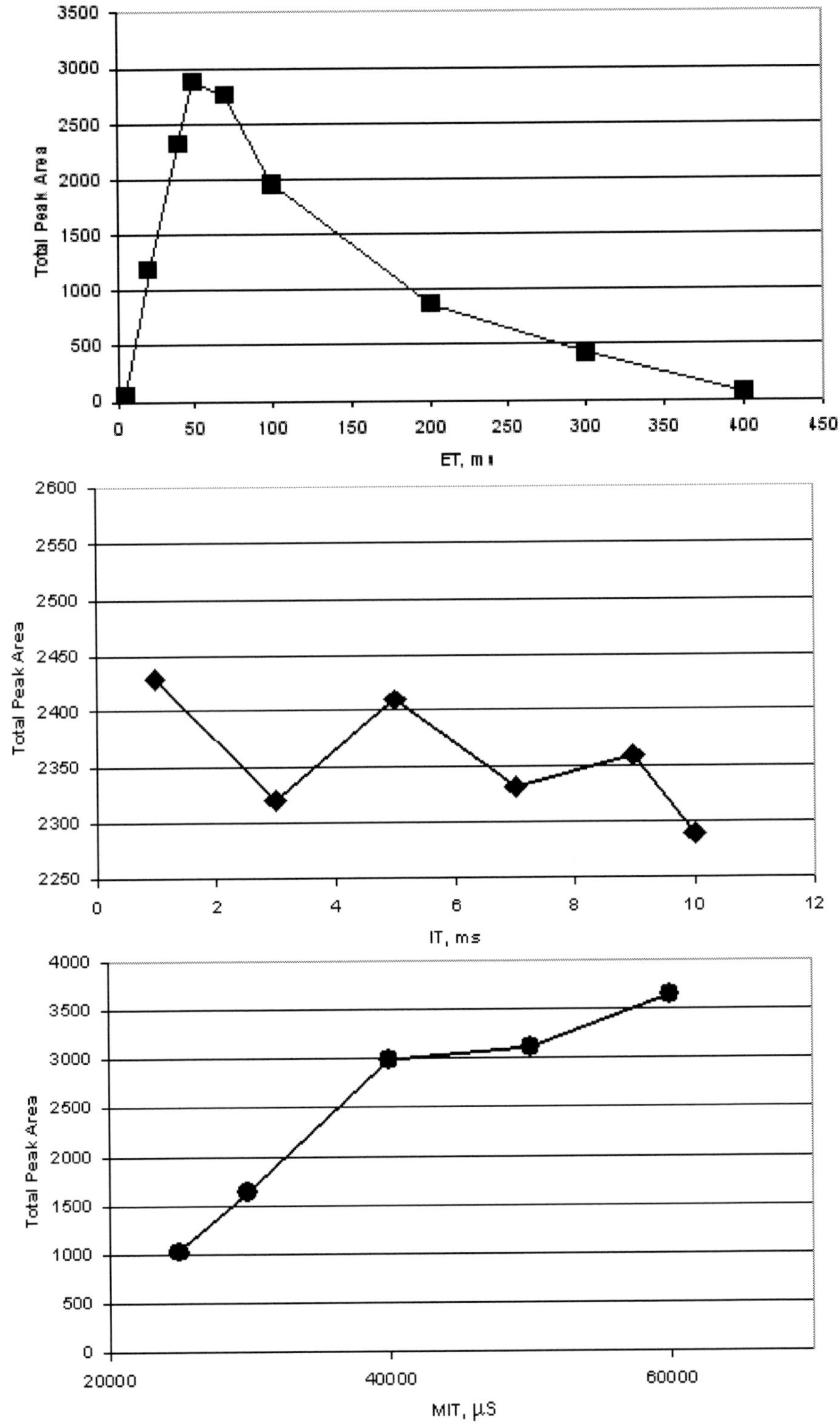

Figure 2. Plots of total area counts of the selected product ions obtained during the optimization process of MS/MS parameters versus (a) CID amplitude; (b) excitation time (ET); (c) isolation time (IT); and (d) maximum ionization time (MIT) for the molecules of native caffeine.

The variation patterns of CID amplitude, Figure 2a and excitation time (ET), Figure 2b were very similar. Both low and high values for these parameters resulted in a decrease on the total area counts of the product ions of caffeine. While no or very low signal of the selected product ions was observed when CID and ET approached 0.4 V or 4.0 V and 1 ms or 400 ms, respectively, a maximum area counts of the sum of these ions, *m/z*=109, 122, 149 and 165 occurred when CID was in the range 0.8 -1.1V and ET was around 50 ms.

The plot of isolation time (IT) Figure 2c varied in the range between 1 to 10 ms showed that the sum of the area counts of the selected product ions of caffeine in MS/MS mode was not substantially affected by the variation of this parameter.

The maximum ionization time (MIT) can substantially affect the sensitivity of the ion-trap mass spectrometer operated in MS/MS mode, as an increase of this parameter from 25,000 μs to its maximum value of 65,000 μs resulted in almost linear increase of the total area counts of the product ions. We have chosen 40,000 μs as the optimized value for MIT in this study. Although the higher values of MIT = 60,000 μs produces higher response in total area counts of the selected product ions, it may cause loss of correct isotope ratios or quantitative linearity especially when analyzing real samples with potential matrix effect.

Except for isolation time, all the parameters had a significant effect on the MS/MS determination of caffeine and thus their optimization was required. Based on the results achieved in these experiments, the optimum conditions for the determination of caffeine by IT-MS/MS were the following: CID=1.0 V; ET=50 ms; IT=5 ms and MIT=40,000 μs.

The obtained optimum conditions of IT-MS/MS were applied to check the sensitivity and linearity of the ion-trap tandem mass spectrometry detector. For this purpose a series of standard solution of caffeine with concentrations varying between 10 up to 1000 pg μl^{-1}, were analyzed. Due to the low background signal, high signal-to-noise (*S/N)* ratios were obtained even for the standard solution of the lowest concentration, S/N_{ave}=112. The limit of detection (LOD) determined using the formula LOD = 3 x SDV was 500 fg μl^{-1}, where SDV is standard deviation determined from seven replicate analyses of the standard solution of caffeine at the concentration of 5 pg μl^{-1}.

Linearity of the response of the ion-trap mass spectrometry detector in MS/MS mode for caffeine was studied by constructing a seven-point calibration curve using standard solutions covering concentrations from 10 to 1000 pg μl^{-1}. In these solutions, the concentration of ^{13}C-labeled caffeine used as the internal standard was kept constant at 200 pg μl^{-1}. We performed the injections by increasing gradually the concentration of caffeine. The range of the concentrations used, was sufficiently representative for the determination of caffeine in surface water. A good linearity with the correlation coefficient r^2 =0.986 was achieved, *Peak Size/PS IS* = *Amount/Amt.IS* x *1.2908 -0.0524*. Where *Peak Size* is the area counts of the analyte; *PS IS* is peak size of the internal standard; *Amount* is the amount of the analyte in pg; *Amt.IS* is the amount of the internal standard in pg.

4.2.1.3. Fragmentation and Interpretation of MS/MS Spectra

Ion-trap tandem mass spectrometry as well as its multistep MS^n (where $n > 2$) experiments have been gaining popularity not only in analysis of trace level of a variety of organic analytes (Verenitch et al., 2006, 2007; Kuchler et al., 2000; Hayward et al., 2001; Gomara et al., 2006; Malavia et al., 2004) but also as an essential technique for the structural analysis of a wide range of environmentally and biologically relevant compounds (Afonso et al., 2005; Nunez et al., 2004; Jensen et al., 2007). Such system gives quite a considerable increase of informing power in such areas as the fundamental study of ion structure, as well as for the detection and quantification of molecules in complex matrices. The technique of collision spectroscopy (or tandem mass spectroscopy, or MS/MS, or MS^2) at the presence of a collision gas in a suitable region(s) of the spectrometer increases both the number of ions and the abundance of naturally occurring decomposition products.

The energy deposition mechanism operating in collisional experiments has been the object of many studies which indicate that, aside from a relatively small quantity of ions which experience electronic excitation, most of the collisionally-induced decompositions originate from vibrationally-excited precursors. Quite a high internal energy distribution is observed; such a distribution allows the activation of different decomposition channels with different activation energies which can lead to a unique fragmentation pathway of a selected precursor ion.

A few papers (Liguori et al., 1991, Williams et al., 2006) were devoted to the elucidation of fragmentation patterns of caffeine in tandem mass spectrometry. Liguori et al., 1991 have developed a method based on gas chromatography/triple quadrupole mass spectrometry (tQ-MS/MS) for identification and characterization of caffeine and its metabolites in human urine. They used mass-analyzed ion kinetic energy (MIKE) and high energy collision induced dissociation spectra for elucidation of fragmentation pathways of the analytes of interest. Recently J.P. Williams et al., 2006 studied rapid desorption electrospray ionization (DESI) of caffeine as well as other drugs and their fragmentation using a triple-quadrupole and hybrid quadrupole time-of-flight mass spectrometry (Q-ToF). The mechanisms of ion activation employed by these techniques were different than the combination of EI and CID processes used by ion-trap tandem mass spectrometry (IT-MS/MS) instrument (Verenitch et al. 2006). This caused a formation of different fragmentation products: *m/z* 109, 136, 137, 165, 193 (Liguori et al., 1991) and *m/z* 110, 123, 138 and 195 (Williams et al., 2006) versus *m/z* 108, 109, 120, 122, 132, 137, 149, 165 and 193 obtained by the authors using conditions of tandem ion-trap mass spectrometry, Figure 1b.

Electrospray ionization (ESI) of caffeine employed by LC-MS/MS instruments (Metcalfe et al., 2003; Ternes et al., 2001; Thevis et al., 2004) is characterized as a soft ionization technique which primarily yields protonated or deprotonated species with little or no fragmentation occurring in the source. The most abundant product ions produced at these conditions are *m/z* 138 $[M - H_3C\text{-}N\text{-}CO + H]^+$ and *m/z* 110 $[M - CO\text{-}N(CH_3)\text{-}CO + H]^+$.

The authors investigated the fragmentation pathways of caffeine and its ^{13}C-labeled analogue at the conditions of low energy collisionally induced dissociation using ion-trap tandem mass spectrometry. Various mass spectrometric conditions using Varian 2200 ion-trap tandem mass spectrometer coupled with CP 3800 gas chromatograph were employed to elucidate fragmentation pathways for the product ions of caffeine observed in the collision-induced dissociation spectra. They included electron impact ionization at E=70 eV and mass spectral measurements performed in single, double and triple-stage mass spectrometry, MS^n ($n = 1$, 2 and 3). Product ion identification and fragmentation pathways of caffeine and its trimethyl-^{13}C labeled analogue along with ion structures and fragmentation pathway mechanisms determined based on both previously published data and the author's results are presented in this chapter.

MS^n experiments (where n = 3) were performed on both native and ^{13}C-labeled caffeine. Their molecular ions were used as the first precursors. CID amplitude of different magnitude depending on the desired product ions was applied to initiate the second ionization step (MS^2) producing the first CID mass spectra. Product ions of various *m/z* values were produced and selectively isolated for further dissociation (MS^3) at different CID voltages.

Due to the presence of heteroaromatic rings, purine compounds generally form highly stable molecular ions under the conditions of electron impact ionization. As a result, the most abundant peak in the EI mass spectra of caffeine in ion-trap mass spectrometer is represented by the molecular ion, from which a number of consecutive and competitive fragmentation pathways are populated, giving rise to peaks of weak to moderate relative intensity, Figure 1a, c. Since the molecular ion of caffeine with *m/z*=194 (*m/z*=197, for isotope labeled analyte) dominated all other ions produced during the electron ionization, the full scan mass spectrum of this compound may be characterized as non-dissociative, similar to polychlorinated biphenyl congeners (March et al., 1997). The energy of electrons, during their impaction onto caffeine molecules, while transformed into the internal energy of the molecular ion lead to the quantitative dissociation of methyl isocyanate group associated with a retro-Diels-Alder process (Liguori et al., 1991) with a consecutive loss of CO producing the product ion with *m/z*=137 and 109, respectively. Conversely, the process of collisionally induced dissociation in MS/MS mode was more dissociative (see Figure 1b, d) producing a number of product ions. The dissociative character of CID, when used in an ion-trap mass spectrometer, has been previously reported on the example of PCB congeners by Leonards et al. (1996).

The amount of internal energy deposited into the molecular ion during the CID process can be varied by changing either the amplitude or the duration of the resonant excitation potential (excitation time). CID breakdown study has been conducted by the authors by analyzing the relative intensities of the precursor and product ions as a function of the CID amplitude. The results of this study for the most abundant ions are presented in the Table 4. The intensities of the most abundant peaks with *m/z* 193, 165, 149, 137, 132, 122, 120, 109, 108 for caffeine and *m/z* 196, 168, 152, 139, 135, 124, 122, 111, 109 for ^{13}C-caffeine (not shown here) as a function of CID voltage experience similar patterns: while molecular ions of both analytes quickly disappear at CID = 0.5 V, the intensities of the product ions increase competitively with the raise of CID amplitude. The results presented in the Table 4 show that the relative intensity of the product ion with *m/z* 193 (the species resulted from the loss of a hydrogen atom from probably one of the methyl groups) increases up to 100% first, with the raise of CID voltage, and sharply goes down from CID = 0.8 V to 1.0 V. The relative intensities of the product ions with *m/z* 149 and 108 for native caffeine become dominant at different CID voltages. While the relative intensity of the species with *m/z* 149 is at 100%, the relative abundance of the ions at *m/z* 108 stays at around 70-80% for the CID range between 1.0 to 1.8 V. At the CID = 2.0 V the relative intensity of the species at *m/z* 108 raises to 100% and stays at that level up to CID = 2.6 V, while the relative abundance of the product ions with *m/z* 149 drops to the level of around 50-60%.

Table 4. Normalized relative abundances (%) of the product ions of Caffeine *m/z* 194 in MS/MS mode as a function of CID amplitude

	CID amplitude, V settings in MS/MS mode														
m/z	**0.0**	**0.2**	**0.4**	**0.5**	**0.7**	**0.8**	**1.0**	**1.2**	**1.4**	**1.6**	**1.8**	**2**	**2.2**	**2.2**	**2.4**	**2.6**
93					1.7	2.5	15.6	25.7	32.3	2.9	19.9	29.5	42.8	43.0	16.0	46.6
94						2.4	5.9	14.8	10.1	20.1	26.6	18.3	24.9	16.7	29.7	20.0
108			0.6	3.0	5.5	28.3	67.4	70.8	77.7	87.1	88.9	100.0	100.0	100.0	100.0	100.0
109			7.1	10.9	8.7	23.3	27.7	59.5	47.6	47.2	47.5	26.3	16.4	31.0	75.2	66.7
120					7.4	22.7	52.8	54.4	75.2	54.8	70.0	33.4	61.3	36.7	74.7	76.6
121			1.2	0.6		6.3		22.0	5.9			8.1		13.6	5.5	13.7
122					9.1	30.2	69.6	69.0	68.7	57.1	88.3	58.2	89.5	79.3	64.9	99.0
132					5.9	18.2	45.8	30.4	48.6	31.9	41.8	27.9	66.8	46.5	47.9	42.0
137			7.6	4.9	4.3	14.8	10.6	17.6	23.4	16.7	17.5	16.3	18.5	13.4	12.8	21.6
149			1.7	1.4	27.6	69.8	100.0	100.0	100.0	100.0	100.0	46.7	56.0	66.6	44.6	36.2
165			4.5	6.8	15.4	25.1	35.1	36.1	50.7	63.2	54.1	54.1	65.4	57.9	64.3	78.1
166			1.7	0.9	2.5	4.5	12.7	6.8	7.1			24.3	5.4	8.8	11.9	16.9
191								6.9	10.1	29.0					5.0	
192								3.7	1.7	0.0	4.7			7.7		
193		50.0	100.0	100.0	100.0	100.0				1.8		1.8	3.0	2.3		5.4
194	100.0	50.0	6.5	7.0								5.1	6.7			11.2

The optimized range of CID voltage is considered to be the one that gives the highest total area counts of the selected product ions and very little of molecular (precursor) ions. In our case, for analysis of caffeine, the ions with *m/z* 108, 122, 149 and 165 (*see the section above)* were selected as the product ions requiring maximization of the total relative abundance. The molecular ion of caffeine and its first product ion *m/z* 194 and *m/z* 193, respectively were the species requiring minimization of their relative abundances in the process of optimization of CID conditions. Based on these criteria, the optimized range of CID voltage in the MS/MS determination of caffeine was found to be between CID = 0.8 to 1.4 V, Table 4 (*see the section above*).

It must be noted that although the fragmentation of native caffeine and its ^{13}C-labeled analogue at various CID amplitude showed very similar patterns, there was a slight difference in the *fragmentation efficiencies*, E_f of these two compounds at a given set of CID resonant excitation conditions. This difference is presented on the Figure 3 a,b which shows MS/MS spectra of caffeine and its isotope labeled analogue obtained at the identical experimental conditions.

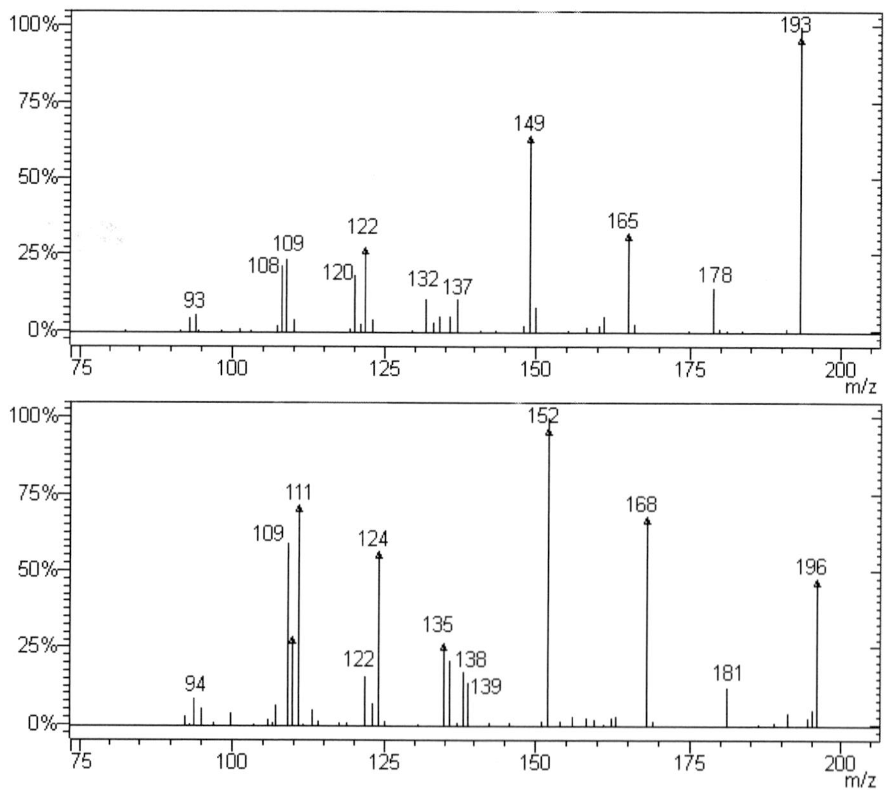

Figure 3. CID mass spectra of caffeine (a) and its ^{13}C-labeled standard (b) at the identical MS/MS conditions.

As demonstrated by Figure 3 a,b at the CID = 0.8 V the fragmentation efficiency expressed by the equation below, for ^{13}C-labeled caffeine standard is a bit higher than for its native analyte, which resulted in lower abundance of its first product ion at *m/z* 196 with higher intensities for more advanced fragmentation species such as *m/z* 168, 152, 135, 124,

122, 111 and 109 when compared to their respective fragmentation ions formed from the molecular ion of native caffeine:

$$E_f = \frac{\sum F_i}{(P + \sum F_i)}$$

where P is the sum of the ion intensities of the molecular and the first product ions, [M+] and [M+] - H at a given CID amplitude; F_i is a product ion intensity at a given CID.

Several investigations have been performed to gain data on fragmentation and dissociation of caffeine and its metabolites exposed to different types of initial and secondary ionizations: EI (Liguori et al., 1991; Dawson et al., 1976), DESI (Williams et al., 2006) and ESI (Thevis et al., 2004). At the conditions of EI as the primary ionization and collision induced dissociation as the secondary stage of ionization carried out on the molecular ion of caffeine in an ion-trap, a slight difference in a fragmentation pathway was observed (Figure 1b) when compared to the other techniques (Liguori et al., 1991; Williams et al., 2006 and Thevis et al., 2004). The relative abundances of the product ions obtained for caffeine and its ^{13}C-labeled analogue in the mass range between *m/z* 100 to 200 at the optimized IT-MS/MS conditions are presented in the Table 5 in comparison with the literature results. The differences between the fragmentation products of caffeine in a multisector instrument (triple quadrupole mass spectrometer or tQ-MS/MS "in space") and IT-MS/MS (MS/MS "in time") may be explained by the fact that the parent ions collisionally activated *via* resonant excitation in an ion-trap are excited between collisions; as such, the ions undergo stepwise activation coupled with collisional cooling by the He buffer gas. The resonant excitation potential or CID is applied here at the amplitude of 1.0 V for 50 ms compared to the 10 to 50 μs residence times of the ions in the center quadrupole of a triple quadrupole mass spectrometer (Dawson et al., 1976).

For tQ-MS/MS instruments, the pre-selected ions undergo a variety of interactions with the target gas leading to a formation of a family of excited species with quite a large energy distribution, which enhances the feasibility of accessing decomposition channels having large differences in activation energies, such as a loss of H$^\cdot$ atom due to the cleavage of C-H bond (product ion with *m/z* 193) and the fragmentation driven by a retro-Diels-Alder mechanism (Rao et al., 1972) resulting in a loss of methyl-isocyanate [CH_3N=C=O], (product ions with *m/z* 137) followed by the elimination of a molecule of carbon monoxide [C=O], (ion species with *m/z* 109) (Liguori et al., 1991).

The energy deposition mechanism in collision experiments performed by IT-MS/MS using a supplementary radio frequency (RF) voltage is considered a step-by-step one, in which low activation energy processes are favored. As a result, in the CID fragmentation spectra of caffeine produced at IT-MS/MS conditions, a number of new ion species were formed (Table 5) along with the product ions common for triple quadrupole MS/MS (Liguori et al., 1991) and LC-MS/MS (Thevis et al., 2004). Although at different relative abundances, the product ions of native caffeine with *m/z* 193, 165, 137 and 109 were identified in the MS/MS spectra of both tQ-MS/MS and IT-MS/MS (Table 5, 6) ionization techniques.

Table 5. Relative intensities (in brackets) of molecular and product ions obtained for caffeine and its ^{13}C-labeled analogue at MS^2 conditions by different mass analyzers

Analyte	Molecular Ion, m/z	Product Ions, m/z									Technique	Source
Caffeine	194(0)	193(0.6)	165(35.1)	149(100)	137(10.6)	132(45.8)	122(69.6)	120(52.8)	109(27.7)	108(67.4)	GC-IT-MS/MS	authors
13C-Caffeine	197(0)	196(1.5)	168(49.8)	152(100)	139(7.3)	135(27.7)	124(68.8)	122(31.3)	111(30.3)	109(30.1)	GC-IT-MS/MS	authors
Caffeine	195(0)	-	-	-	138(100)	-	123(14)	-	110(52)	-	LC-MS/MS	Thevis
Caffeine	194(0)	193(100)	165(2.6)	-	137(12.5)	-	-	-	109(6.0)	-	GC-tQ	Liguori

Table 6. IT-MS/MS data with proposed assignments for caffeine and its isotope labeled standard

								Product Ions, m/z								
Analyte	Molecular Ion, m/z	-H	-O	-H -O	-CO -H	-H, -CO2	-C*H3NCO	-C*H3NCO -H	-H -CO2 -C*H3	-CO -H -C*H3NC	-H -CO2 -HC*N	-C*H3NCO -C*H3	-H -CO2 -NC*H3	-C*H3NCO -CO	-CO -H – C*H3NCO	-C*H3NCO -NC*H3	-H -CO2 – CNC*H3
		[M+] -1	[M+] -16	[M+] -1 -16	[M+] -28 -1	[M+] -1 -44	[M+] -57	[M+] -57 -1	[M+] -1 -44 -15	[M+] -28 -1 -41	[M+] -1 -44 -27	[M+] -57 -15	[M+] -1 -44 -29	[M+] -57 -28	[M+] -28 -1 -57	[M+] -57 -29	[M+] -1 -44 -41
caffeine	194[M+]	193	178	177	165	149	137	136	134	124	122	122	120	109	108	108	108
13C-caffeine	197[M+]	196	181	180	168	152	139	138	136	126	124	123	122	111	110	109	110

The product ions with *m/z* 149, 132, 120 and 108 have been observed only in the spectra produced by IT-MS/MS instrument. The strategy used for the elucidation of the fragment ions of caffeine in an ion-trap mass spectrometer under collision-induced dissociation conditions was based on the spectral information from multi-step mass spectral data (MS^n) obtained on both analytes, caffeine and its ^{13}C-labeled analogue. The spectral data generated by the ion-trap analyzer were used to link compositions via genealogical relationships.

The starting point of the general strategy for fragmentation studies of caffeine under MS/MS conditions in an ion-trap was the CID spectra of both caffeine and its ^{13}C-labeled analogue obtained from their molecular ions under various CID amplitudes, Table 4 . The results obtained showed the dynamics of the product ions of both analytes in terms of their *m/z* and corresponding relative abundances at various CID conditions.

The next step helping the elucidation process was a formation of ions of third generation, MS^3 experiments. This procedure was carried out on both the molecular ion of caffeine *m/z* 194 (197) and the selected product ions with *m/z* 193 (196), 178 (181), 165 (168), 149 (152) obtained at the corresponding MS^2 conditions. The isolation window in all these experiments was *m/z* = 1. The CID amplitudes chosen to perform these experiments were based on the principles of maximizing the relative abundance of an investigated product ion produced under MS^2 conditions, and its moderate subsequent fragmentation under MS^3 conditions. For instance, for the identification of the origin of the fragment ion with *m/z* 149 (152) obtained under MS^2 conditions, a generation of MS^3 spectra was carried out on three different product ions *m/z* = 193, 178 and 165. As it turned out, a generation of the species with m/z = 149 was possible only when MS^3 conditions were applied to the MS^2 produced product ion *m/z* = 193. The conditions of this experiment were the following: CID = 0.4 V applied to the molecular ion *m/z* 194 (197) (MS^2 spectrum) and CID = 0.4 V applied to the product ion *m/z* 193 (196) (MS^3 spectrum), Figure 4a.

This experiment demonstrates the power of multi-step mass spectral data, MS^n in identification of the origin of ions produced under MS^{n-1} conditions. On the Figure 4a we also indicated *m/z* of the corresponding product ions obtained at the same conditions for ^{13}C-labeled caffeine without showing their relative abundances on the graph. A use of isotope labeled caffeine exposed to the same fragmentation conditions provides a valuable source of information in identification of a structure of a product ion of the native analyte.

MS^3 experiment was also applied for elucidation of the product ion with *m/z* 165 (168). The CID amplitudes of 2.2 V and 0.6 V were applied to the molecular ion at *m/z* 194 (197) and the product ion *m/z* 165 (168), respectively (*MS^3 scheme194>165>product ions*), Figure 4b. The corresponding product ions of MS^3 spectrum of ^{13}C-labeled caffeine without their relative intensities are also presented on the graph. Without the spectral information from multi-step mass spectral data obtained on trimethyl ^{13}C-labeled caffeine in parallel with its native compound, different assignments could be proposed for some fragments. The MS^2 data obtained on trimethyl ^{13}C-labeled caffeine showed that the product ion with *m/z* 149 in the CID fragmentation of the native caffeine corresponded to the fragment with *m/z* 152 of the isotope analogue produced under similar MS^2 conditions from the corresponding molecular ion, Figure 1b, d. The MS^3 spectral information obtained on *m/z* 194 followed by isolation and collisionally induced dissociation of *m/z* 193 confirmed that the fragmentation leading to a formation of *m/z* 149 (152) begins with the loss of a hydrogen atom from one of the methyl groups with the following loss of neutral CO_2 group producing the ions with *m/z* 149 (152) without a loss of any of the isotope labeled methyl groups ($^{13}CH_3$). Product ion *m/z* 149 (152) undergoes further fragmentation forming ions with *m/z* 108 (109), 120 (122), 122 (124), 132 (135) and 134 (136), Figure 4a, Scheme 1. Selective fragmentation of the ion at *m/z* 149 (152) was studied at MS^3 conditions by applying CID voltage of 1.0 V to the molecular ion of caffeine *m/z* 194 (197) with isolation and further fragmentation of the product ion at *m/z* 149 (152) at the CID amplitude of 0.6 V (*MS^3 scheme 194(197)>149(152)>product ions*), Figure 5a, b. The product ions generated at these conditions helped to elucidate the fragmentation pathway from *m/z* 194 (197) to *m/z* 149 (152) and further down, Scheme 1. It must be pointed out that the formation of MS^3 product ions with *m/z* 108 (109), 120 (122), 122 (124), 132 (135) and 134 (136) although at different relative abundances was observed at different MS^3 conditions: *MS^3scheme 194[1.0 V]>149[0.6 V]>products* and *MS^3scheme 194[0.4 v]>193[0.6 V]>products*, Figure 6a, b. The results of these experiments confirm that the fragmentation of the precursor ion with *m/z* 193 produces mostly the product ion *m/z* 149 which further decomposes with the formation of the ions with *m/z* 108 (109), 120 (122), 122 (124), 132 (135) and 134 (136), Figure 4a and 6a,b.

A presence of the ions with *m/z* 137 (139), 136 (138), 122 (124), 109 (111) and 108 (109) in the IT-MS/MS spectra of caffeine (Table 4, Figure 1b, d) can be explained by the retro-Diels-Alder mechanism resulting in a loss of methyl-isocyanate [$CH_3N{=}C{=}O$], (-57u, product ions with *m/z* 137) followed by the elimination of a molecule of carbon monoxide [C=O], (-28u, ion species with *m/z* 109), or expel of a hydrogen atom from one of the methyl groups (*m/z* 136). The product ions with *m/z* 137 can also lead to a formation of ions with *m/z* 122, 108 by means of a cleavage of one of the N – CH_3 bonds (-15u, *m/z* 122) or a loss of NCH_3 group (-29u, *m/z* 108), Scheme 1.

This elucidation has been well studied using such techniques as tQ-MS/MS (Liguori et al., 1991; Williams et al., 2006), LC-MS/MS (Thevis et al., 2004) and direct mass spectrometry method (Rao et al., 1972). A formation of *m/z* 165 (168) ions (Figure 1b, d) under the conditions of resonant excitation of collisionally induced dissociation of the molecular ion of caffeine *m/z* 194 (197) in an ion-trap (MS^2) can be rationalized as shown in Scheme 2. This fragmentation involves a loss of CO with a subsequent expel of hydrogen atom from one of the methyl groups. The first step of this pathway is accomplished by α-cleavage next to the carbonyl group, with stabilization of the charge on the carbonyl O atom. Although CO could arguably be lost at this point, generation of a potentially more stable ion in a ring seems more appealing. To accomplish this, the double bond nearest the carbonyl group donates one electron to form a new N – C single bond, the five-membered ring closes. The charge remains on the carbonyl O. Finally, heterolytic cleavage of C – C bond between the ring and the carbonyl group moves the electron pair onto the carbonyl C atom, expelling a neutral molecule of CO and forming the ion at *m/z* 166 (169) with a subsequent loss of H atom producing the ion residue at *m/z* 165 (168). MS^3 experiments conducted on the ions *m/z* 194 at CID = 2.2 V followed by CID = 0.6 V on *m/z* 165 (Figure 4b) demonstrated that the fragment at *m/z* 165 subsequently expels methyl-isocyanate (CH_3NCO, -57u) or methyl isocyanide (CH_3NC, -41u) generating the ions at *m/z* 108 (110) and 124 (126), respectively, Scheme 1.

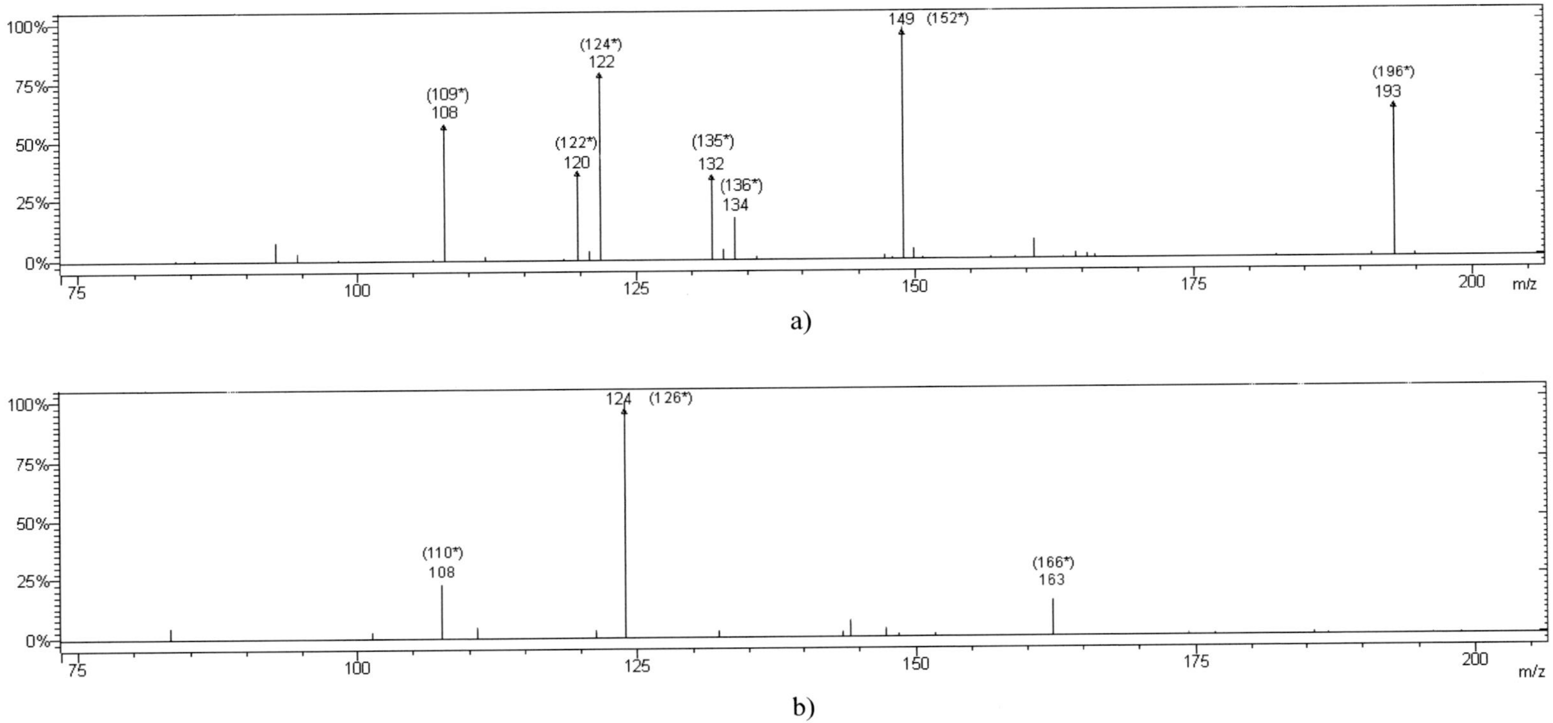

Figure 4. Ion-trap MS^3 mass spectra of caffeine with molecular ion used as the precursor ion at different sequential breakdowns: (a) m/z 194(197) > 193(196) > product ions and (b) m/z 194 (197) > 165(168) > product ions.

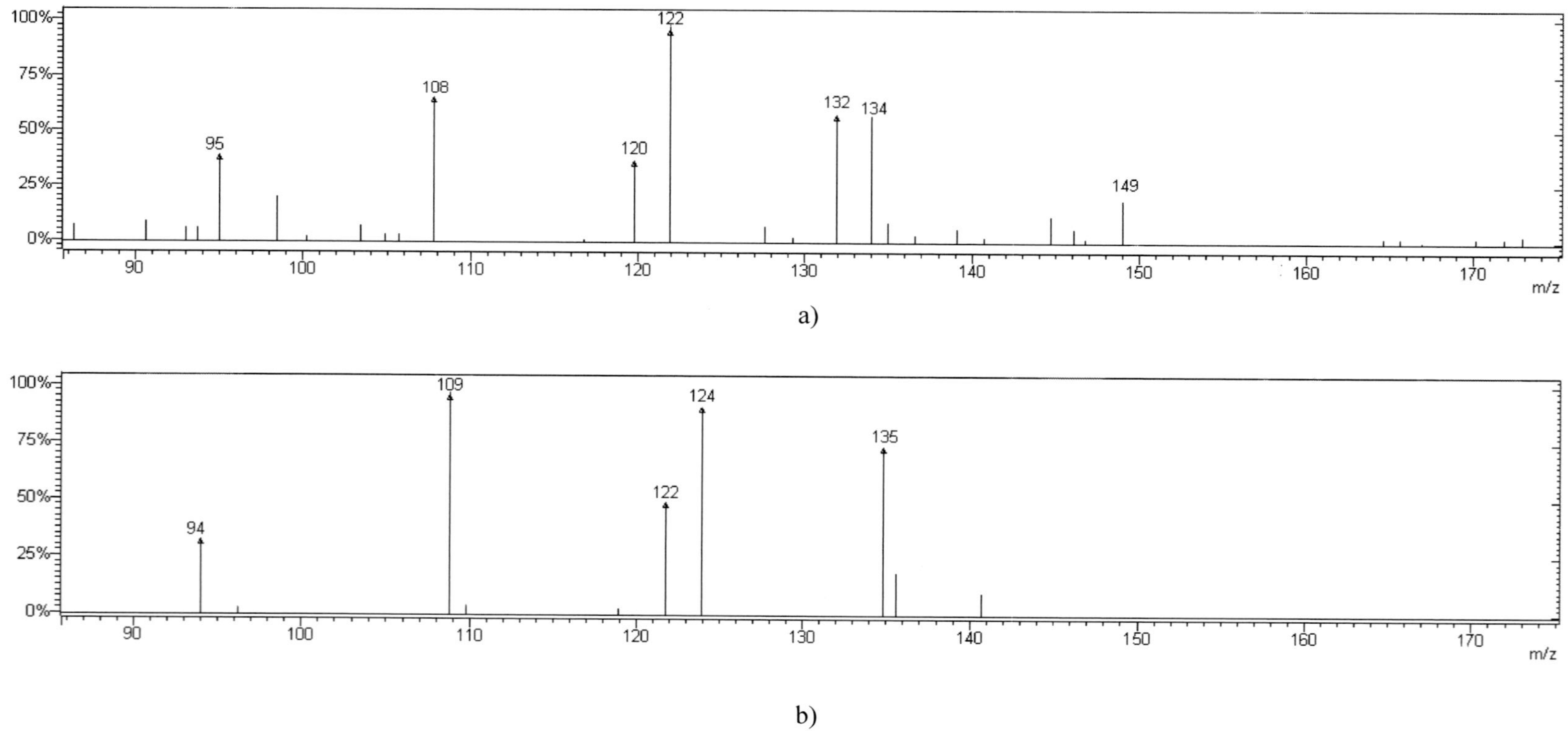

Figure 5. MS^3 mass spectra of caffeine (a) and its ^{13}C-labeled analogue (b) at the following dissociation conditions: CID = 1.0 V applied to the molecular ion followed by isolation and CID fragmentation of the product ion with *m/z* 149 and *m/z* 152, respectively at the CID amplitude of 0.6 V.

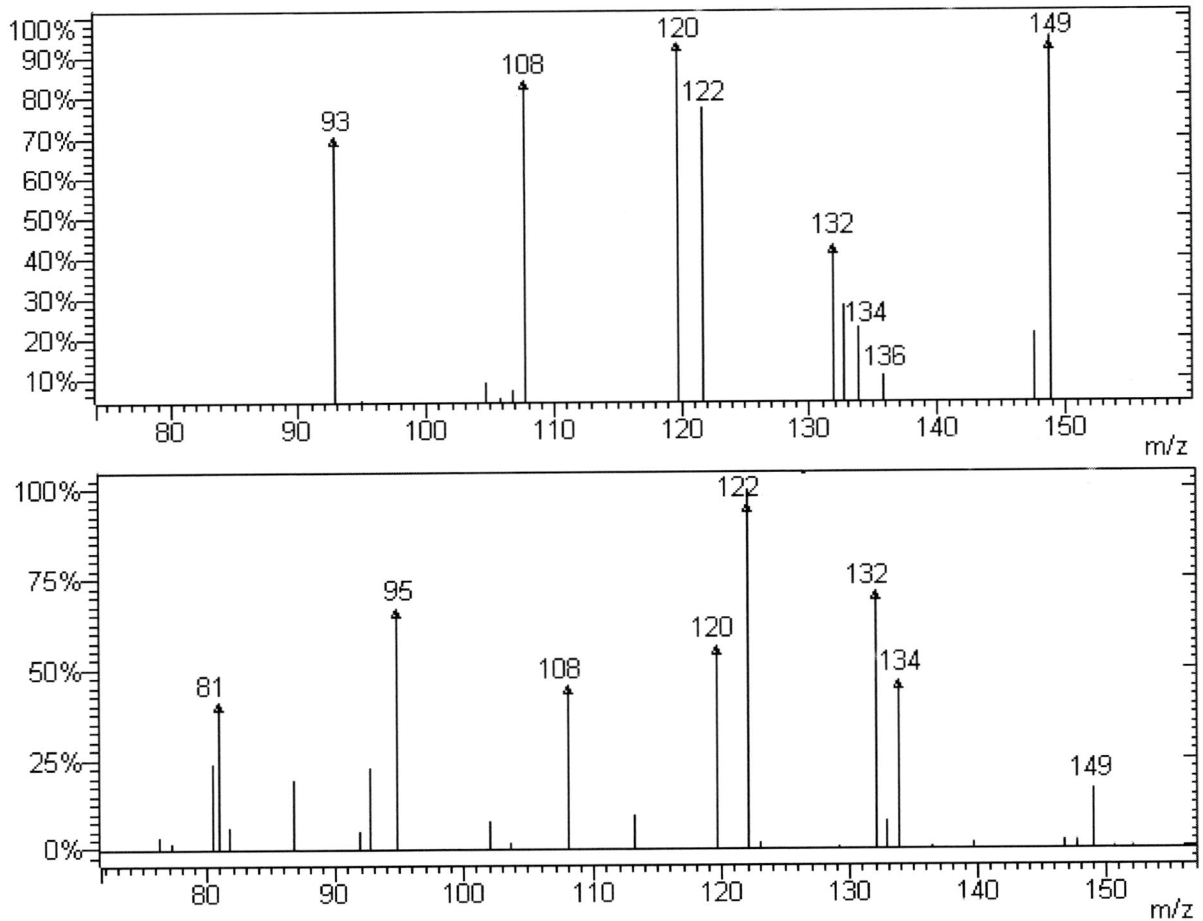

Figure 6. Ion-trap MS^3 mass spectra of caffeine at: (a) CID = 1.0 V applied to the molecular ion *m/z* 194 followed by isolation and CID fragmentation of *m/z* 149 at the amplitude of 0.6 V; (b) CID = 0.4 V applied to the molecular ion *m/z* 194 and isolation and dissociation at CID =0.6 V of the product ion *m/z* 193.

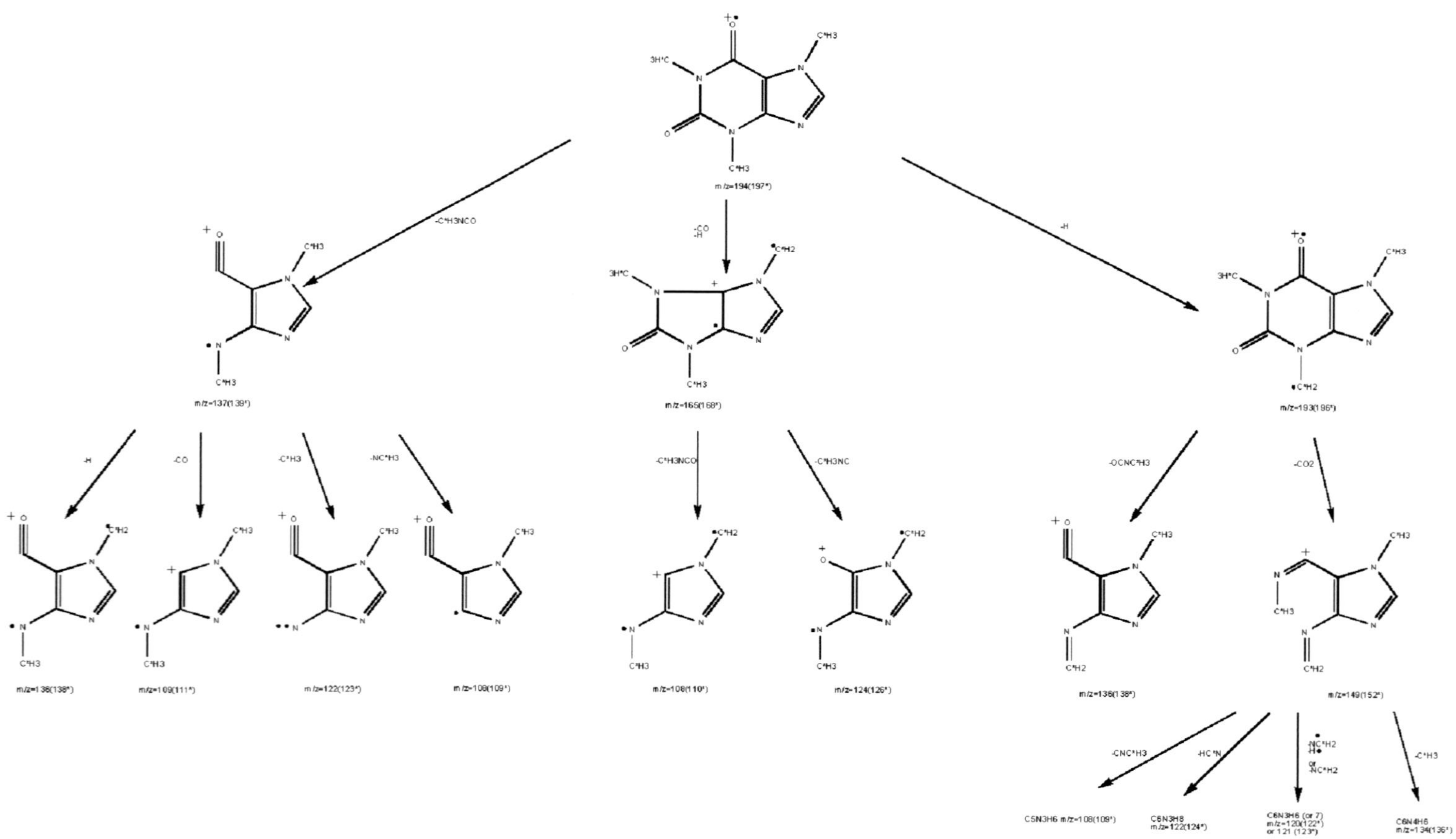

Scheme 1. Fragmentation pathways of caffeine in an ion-trap at the optimized MS/MS conditions.

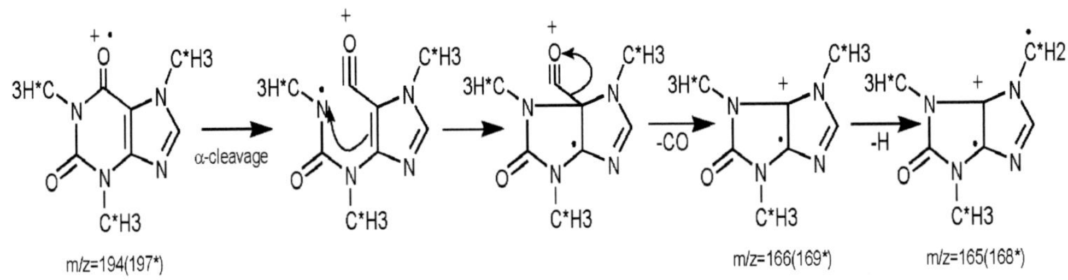

Scheme 2. Representation of the fragmentation resulting in formation of the product ions with *m/z* 165(168).

The fact that for the latter a removal of the residue CH_3NC is involved, is based on the analysis of the trimethyl ^{13}C-labeled caffeine. A shift of the ion at *m/z* 124 to *m/z* 126 in the MS^3 spectrum of the molecular ion of the labeled caffeine *m/z* 197 with a subsequent isolation and CID fragmentation of the ion at *m/z* 168 Figure 4b indicates to the loss of one of the labeled methyl groups with the presence of the remaining other two on the final product ion.

As demonstrated above, a combination of a single and multi-step MS^n (where n = 1-3) fragmentations of caffeine and its ^{13}C-labeled analogue provided sufficient information for constructing the genealogical relationship (Scheme 1) between the precursors and their product ions. For elucidation of some fragment ions for which several compositions were possible, MS^2 and MS^3 dissociation of an isotope labeled analogue was used to confirm the structures assigned to the ions of the native analyte obtained by ion-trap in MS^2 mode.

4.3. Monitoring of Caffeine

4.3.1. QA/QC in Monitoring

The developed method based on gas chromatography with IT-MS/MS detection system was routinely applied by the authors for analysis of caffeine in various sources of marine and fresh water. The identification of the analytes, caffeine and its ^{13}C-labeled standard was based on the chromatographic retention time and MS/MS spectrum of each compound obtained individually using standard solutions containing just one analyte. A molecular ion of each analyte was selected as the precursor ion for the sequential application of MS/MS conditions. Five of the most abundant product ions were selected for the identification of each compound. One of the criteria of the analyte identification in the samples under MS/MS conditions was that the ratios of the five chosen product ions had to be within +/- 20% of that established from the analysis of the corresponding authentic standards, Table 7.

To insure ultimate instrument performance, for GC-IT-MS/MS system, a number of tests were performed on a routine basis. The tests were designed to assess: GC column performance, retention time windows, ultimate sensitivity, multipoint calibration and linearity, instrument detection limits, sample carryover, continuous calibration verification. IT-MS/MS detector was also optimized for resolution, transmission and mass calibration using perfluorotributylamine (PFTBA).

The target compounds were identified as native caffeine or its ^{13}C-labeled surrogate internal standard, only when the chromatographic peaks obtained satisfied all of the following criteria. 1) The retention time of a specific analyte must be within +/-0.2 min window of that obtained during analysis of the authentic compounds in the calibration standards. All native and surrogate ion peak maxima must be coincident within 3 seconds. 2) The threshold of the MS/MS spectral match of a specific compound in a sample and its analogue in a standard mixture was set at 700 out of max 1000. Only the ions with intensities higher than 40% of the Reference Spectrum base peak were considered when calculating the spectral match. 3) All five product ions of each analyte (see Table 4) must be present, and must be detected at their exact m/z. 4) The signal-to-noise ratio in each compound must be > 3 for a sample extract, and > 10 for a calibration standard. 5) The ratios between the integrated signals of the product ions chosen for identification of native caffeine and its isotope labeled standard must be within +/- 20% of the values outlined in the Table 7.

Table 7. Some characteristics of the product ions selected

Analyte	Precursor ion, m/z	MS/MS Identification Product ions, *m/z*	Ratios of Product Ions
Caffeine	194	108/122/149/165/193	74.8/68.4/100.0/42.6/4.6
^{13}C-Caffeine	197	109/124/152/168/195	38.2/54.6/100.0/33.4/12.4

Each batch of samples consisted of nine samples, plus three QA/QC samples: a sample duplicate, a replicate sample spiked with known amount of native caffeine, 20 ng l^{-1} (200 pg μl^{-1} in the final sample extract) and a procedural blank. The replicate sample spiked with known amount of caffeine was used as a laboratory reference material (LRM). ^{13}C-labeled caffeine spiked into each sample at the concentration in the final extract of 200 pg $\mu l^{-1}$was used to determine the recovery efficiency. It was added to each sample before filtration. Corrections for recoveries of the native caffeine were made against the ^{13}C-labeled surrogate internal standards.

The recovery of SIS in a sample was determined against a "standard check" containing ^{13}C-labeled caffeine at the concentration of 200 pg μl^{-1}. High recoveries of SIS in all the samples analyzed (Table 8) indicate onto high efficiencies of both the sample preparation procedure and the analytical determination of the analytes of interest.

In order for the data to be acceptable, the following QA/QC criteria had to be met. The reproducibility of duplicate analysis had to be between 60 and 130 % and the % recovery of surrogate internal standard had to be between 50 to 130%.

Concentrations of caffeine in distilled de-ionized (DDI) water samples used as a blank were in the range between 0.6 and 1.4 ng l^{-1} which translated into the method detection limit (MDL) of 1.0 – 2.0 ng l^{-1} { $MDL = mean_{blank} + 3SD_{blank}$). Fortified samples of DDI water spiked with the known amounts of caffeine covering the range between 2.0 to 20.0 ng l^{-1} showed acceptable recoveries of 80.2 to 103.4%.

Table 8. The concentrations of caffeine found in sea and fresh water samples collected from the sites with different human impact levels. ND = not detected, where MDL = 2 ng l^{-1}

Sample Type	Number of samples analyzed	Concentration range of caffeine found, ng l^{-1}	Recovery of SIS, %
Seawater	76	4.5 – 149.0	76.0 – 104.1
River 100 up/s STP	2	2.1-3.2	66.0 – 67.0
River 400 down/s STP	2	7.2 – 15.4	74.4 – 97.7
Lake of high human impact	13	6.1 – 21.7	61.0 – 91.6
Lake of moderate human impact	10	1.8 – 10.4	92.3 – 116.4
Lake of low human impact	10	ND – 6.5	73.4 – 106.7

4.3.2. Tracking Anthropogenic Input

Over hundred samples of marine and fresh water origins have been analyzed by the authors using the optimized GC-IT-MS/MS methodology. The level of caffeine found in a blank sample was subtracted from the results obtained for surface water samples. All results were grouped into four categories showing good correlation with the anthropogenic burden associated with domestic wastewater contamination. Group one included 76 marine water samples collected around Bamfield research station. Group two, three and four presented the results obtained on fresh water samples collected from the lakes with various density of residential developments characterized as high, moderate and low, respectively, Table8. The results for four fresh water samples from up and down stream of STP were presented separately. The results obtained on the marine water samples indicated a wide variation of the level of caffeine ranging from 4.5 to 149.0 ng l^{-1}, depending on the location of a sampling site in the marine inlet studied. The concentration of caffeine in the samples from the lakes with high density of residential development around (group two) was in the range between 6.1 to 21.7 ng l^{-1}. The lakes with moderate density of residential development around showed lower level of caffeine in their surface water, between 1.8 to 10.4 ng l^{-1}. The samples collected from the lakes with low density or no residential development around were characterized with low concentration of caffeine present. The level of caffeine in this group of samples was ranging from non detectable (ND) to 6.5 ng l^{-1}. Caffeine was present in all surface water samples near sewage treatment plants (STP). In comparison to previously published data on the range of concentrations of caffeine in sea water (Siegener et al., 2002; Weigel et al., 2002) and streams of Canada (Metcalfe et al., 2003), the United States (Kolpin et al., 2002) and Germany (Ternes et al., 2001), the levels of this compound detected in our study were in good agreement with Siegener et al., 2002, Weigel et al., 2002 and Metcalfe et al., 2003, while two order of magnitude lower than by Ternes et al., 2001 and Kolpin et al., 2002. The recoveries of surrogate internal standard spiked in marine water samples were in the range of 76.0 – 104.1%. Fresh water samples spiked with ^{13}C-caffeine showed 61.0 – 91.6%, 73.4 –

106.7% and 92.3 – 116.4% recoveries for the groups with high, moderate and low density of residential developments around the lakes, respectively. The river samples collected up and down stream of STPs presented the recoveries for SIS of 66.0 – 67.0% and 74.4 – 97.75%, respectively.

Buerge et al., 2003 have shown that caffeine loads in untreated wastewater when normalized for the population have very small variations (15.8 +/- 3.8 mg $person^{-1}$ day^{-1}), reflecting a rather constant consumption. Due to substantial elimination in the water treatment process, the effluent loads of caffeine from wastewater treatment plants (WWTP) were significantly lower (0.06 +/- 0.03 mg $person^{-1}$ day^{-1}). Although being efficiently (up to 81 – 99%) eliminated in most WWTPs, caffeine was persistently found in all Swiss lakes and rivers (6 – 250ng l^{-1}), except for remote mountain lakes (<2 ng l^{-1}). A good correlation was found between the levels of caffeine in lakes and anthropogenic burden created by domestic wastewater. Based on the results obtained on the Swiss lakes studied by Buerge et al., 2003 a numerical model taking into account such variables as flushing, biodegradation, and indirect photodegradation via HO* radicals as elimination processes and caffeine inputs was developed. The model successfully described the depth- and seasonal-dependent concentrations of caffeine in the lakes studied.

Standley et al., 2000 developed a molecular tracer method identifying organic matter sources to surface waters. Wastewater treatment plant effluent, agricultural and feedlot runoff, urban and suburban runoff, and wildlife were targeted in the study. The tracers included fecal steroids, caffeine, consumer product fragrance materials (FMs), and petroleum and combustion byproducts. The analyses of water samples collected from 19 watersheds were compared with land-use of those watersheds. The following significant correlations were found between watershed scale land-use and tracers: WWTPs with caffeine and fragrance materials, agriculture with epicoprostanol content of steroids, and urban land-uses with the polycyclic aromatic hydrocarbons. The range of concentration of caffeine detected in the water samples was between <20 and 115 ng l^{-1}.

Siegener et al., 2002 monitored caffeine in Boston Harbor and Massachusetts Bay seawater. The level of the analyte detected in those samples was from 140 to 1600 ng l^{-1} and from 5.2 to 71 ng l^{-1}, respectively. Sources of caffeine appear to be anthropogenic inversely correlating with salinity, indicating that it may be used as a tracer of wastewater contamination inputs to marine systems.

Glassmeyer et al., 2005 targeted 110 chemical analytes in the samples collected at 10 different locations including upstream and two successive downstream from a WWTP, and treated WWTP effluent. The results of this work indicated that 35 out of 110 chemicals may be useful as indicators of human fecal contamination in source water. For most of these compounds, there is an increase in the frequency of detection and concentration in the WWTP effluent sample and two successive downstream samples as compared to the water sample collected upstream. Also, the chemical concentrations and occurrences decrease downstream with distance from the WWTPs. It was concluded also that compounds that are typically only used by humans, such as some pharmaceuticals and caffeine would be more desirable indicator candidates than wastewater compounds because they are ingested and excreted from human body.

Peeler et al., 2006 focused in their study on the hypothesis that measurements of caffeine, nutrients, and indicator bacteria can distinguish human versus non-human sources of contamination in rural freshwater and urban marine systems. Based on the results obtained on a number of samples collected in rural areas, good correlations were found between the level of caffeine (from <5 to 196 ng l^{-1}) and nitrate (from 0.1 to 53.9 μM) to population centers and their associated wastewater treatment plants. Indicator bacteria in these systems were not correlated with these chemical parameters and were not associated with human population. As a matter of fact, the greatest bacterial abundance was detected in an isolated wetland free from human impact but heavily populated by wildlife. Caffeine in the samples from urban area (from <5 to 204 ng l^{-1}) positively correlated with fecal coliform abundance and with nitrate. The results of this study confirmed the hypothesis that measurements of caffeine, nutrients, particularly nitrate, and indicator bacteria can aid in distinguishing human versus non-human sources of contamination in surface water.

Conclusion

Freshwater resources are increasingly stressed by environmental loading of pathogens attributed to urban development, human population growth, agricultural practices and overdrawing of aquifers. Additionally, the changes in climate have also a significant impact on the viability, survivability and dynamics of pathogens in aquatic environments. Direct monitoring and detection of pathogens in aquatic environment is a great challenge owing to their phylogenetical diversity and their presence in low numbers. A freshwater management approach has been developed by the regulatory authorities to protect the source water quality by surveillance of fecal indicator bacteria. A key requirement to implement best management practices to reduce the loading of pathogens responsible for waterborne enteric illness is the identification of fecal pollution sources, and subsequently eliminates and/or abates them. The microbiological population-dependent, and species-dependent phenotypic and species-dependent genotypic methods developed to track the origin of sources of fecal contamination have some practical limitations (spatio-temporal varability, instability of the phenotypic and genotypic markers under different environmental stresses, and the size of the reference library) and need to be resolved before their reliable field application.

Caffeine recently has been used as an important chemical tracer for surveillance of human fecal waste input into source water. As a marker, caffeine was found to have significant correlation with fecal indicator bacteria and other aquatic nutrients. It also possesses important properties, such as stability, source-specificity and long term persistence in water environment. One of the challenges for monitoring caffeine in aquatic environments is its presence in trace quantities. The analytical method presented in this chapter demonstrated that trace levels of caffeine can be detected and monitored in different aquatic systems (surface water, wastewater and seawater) using gas chromatography (GC) coupled with IT-MS/MS detection system. After optimization of GC-IT-MS/MS parameters, a limit of detection of 500 fg μl^{-1} with $S/N = 3$ was achieved. A method of isotope dilution using ^{13}C-labeled caffeine as a surrogate internal standard was employed to determine and correct the recovery of native caffeine in water samples. Collision-induced fragmentation pathways of caffeine in an ion-trap tandem mass spectrometer have been investigated. New product ions not previously reported in the literature have been identified in the CID fragmentation of caffeine. Various mass spectrometric conditions have been employed to elucidate fragmentation pathways for the product ions observed in the CID spectra. Ion structures and fragmentation pathway mechanisms have been presented and compared with the literature.

Surface marine and fresh water samples collected in various watersheds were analyzed for caffeine as an indicator of domestic wastewater contamination. Caffeine concentrations in lakes and rivers, as well as in seawater correlated with the anthropogenic burden introduced by domestic wastewater or human activities of the surrounding area. The results presented by the authors are in good agreement with the literature data.

Further studies are required to evaluate the efficacy of caffeine as a robust surrogate of human fecal waste. The issues, such as biological and chemical persistency of caffeine in various environments (Bradley et al., 2007), correlation of caffeine concentration with the prevalence of human-specific enteric pathogens, as well as with nutrients and other characteristic parameters of aquatic ecosystems should be addressed.

References

Afonso C., Riu A., Xu Y., Fournier F., Tabet J-C. Structural characterization of fatty acids cationized with copper by electrospray ionization mass spectrometry under low energy collision-induced dissociation. *J. Mass Spectrom.* 2005; 40: 342.

AWWA. (2006) Waterborne pathogens, 2nd edn., *American Water Works Association*, Wasington D.C.

Bernhardt, A.E., Field, K.G., A PCR assay to discriminate human and ruminant feces on the basis of host differences *Bacteroides-Prevotella* genes encoding 16S rRNA. *Appl. Environ. Microbiol.* 2000; 72: 5915-5926.

Berthou, F., Guillois, B., Riche, C., Dreano, Y., Jacqz-Aigrain, E., Beaune, P. Interspecies variations in caffeine metabolism related to cytochrome P450 1A enzymes. *Xenobiotica* 1992; 22: 671-680.

Bettelheim, K. A., Ismail, N., Shinebaum, R., Shooter, R. A., Moorhouse, E., Farrell, W. The distribution of serotypes of *Escherichia coli* in cow-pats and other animal material compared with serotypes of *E. coli* isolated from human sources. *J. Hygiene (London)*, 1976; 76: 403–406.

Blanch, A.R., Belanche-Muñoz, L., Bonjoch, X, Ebdon, J., Gantzer, C, Lucena, F., Ottoson, J., Kourtis, C., Iversen, A., Kühn, I., Mocé, L., Muniesa, M., Schwartzbrod, J., Skraber, S., Papageorgiou, G.T., Taylor, H., Wallis, J., Jofre, J. Integrated analysis of established and novel microbial and chemical methods for microbial source tracking. *Appl. Environ. Microbiol.* 2006; 72: 5915-5926.

Bradley, P.M., Barber, L.B., Kolpin, D.W., McMahon, P.B., Chapelle, F.H. Biotransformation of caffeine, and cotinine, and nicotine in stream sediments: implications for use as wastewater indicators. *Env. Toxicol. Chem.* 2007; 6: 1116-1121.

Buerge, I.J., Poinger, T., Nuller, M.D., Buser, Hans-Rudolf. Caffeine, and Anthropogenic Marker for Wastewater Contamination of Surface Waters. *Environ. Sci. Technol.* 2003; 37: 691-700.

Bull, I.D., Lockheart, M.J., Elhmmali, M.M., Roberts, D.J., Evershed, R.P. The origin of faeces by means of biomarker detection. *Environ. Int.* 2002; 27: 647–654.

Carson, C.A., Shear, B.L., Ellershiek, M.R., Asfaw, A. Identification of fecal *Escherichia coli* from humans and animals by ribotyping. *Appl. Environ. Microbiol.* 2001; 67: 1503–1507.

Carson, C. A., Shear, B.L., Ellersieck, M.R., and Schnell, J.D. Comparison of ribotyping and repetitive extragenic palindromic-PCR for identification of fecal *Escherichia coli* from humans and animals. *Appl. Environ. Microbiol.* 2003; 69: 1836-1839.

Clesceri LS, Greenberg AE and Eaton AD (1998) Standard methods for the examination of water and wastewater, 20th edition, American Public Health Association, Washington, D.C.

Cole, D., Long, S.C., Sobsey, M.D. Evaluation of F+ RNA and DNA coliphages as source-specific indicators of fecal contamination in surface waters. *Appl. Environ. Microbiol.* 2003; 69: 6507-6514.

Craun, G.F., Calderon, R.L., Craun, M.F., 2004. In: Cotruvo, J.A., Dufour, A., Rees,G., Bartram, J., Carr, R., Cliver, D.O., Craun, G.F., Fayer, R., Gannon, V.P.G. (Eds.), Waterborne outbreaks caused by zoonotic pathogens in the USA. World Health Organization, IWA Publishing, London, pp. 120-135.

Davies, J.M., Mazumder, A. Health and environmental policy issues in Canada: the role of watershed management in sustaining clean drinking water quality at surface sources. *J. Environ. Manage.* 2003; 68: 273-286.

Dawson P.H. *Quadrupole Mass Spectrometry and Its Applications.* Elsevier Scientific, Amsterdam, 1976. GC-MS Manual, Varian, Walnut Creek, CA, 1999.

Dick, L.K., Bernhardt, A.E., Brodeur, T.J., Santo Domingo, J.W., Simpson, J.M., Walters, S.P., Field, K.G. Host distributions of uncultivated fecal *Bacteroidales* reveal genetic markers for fecal source identification. *Appl. Environ. Microbiol.* 2005a; 71: 3184-3191.

Dick, L.K., Simonich, M.T., Field, K.G. Microplate subtractive hybridization to enrich for source-specific *Bacteroidales* fecal pollution indicators. *Appl. Environ. Microbiol.* 2005b; 71: 3179-3183.

Dombek, P.E., Johnson, L.K., Zimmerley, S.T., Sadowsky, M.J. Use of repetitive DNA sequences and the PCR to differentiate *Escherichia coli* isolates from human and animal sources. *Appl. Environ. Microbiol.* 2000; 66: 2572-2577.

Eaganhouse, R. P. (Ed.), Molecular markers in environmental geochemistry. ACS symposium series 671; American Chemical Society: Washington, D.C. 1997; 426 pp.

Eganhouse, R.P., Blumfield, D.L., Kaplan, I.R. Long-chain alkylbenzenes as molecular tracers of domestic wastes in the marine environment. *Environ. Sci. Technol.* 1983 ; 17: 523–530.

Edwards, D.D., McFeters, G.A., Venkatesan, M.I. Distribution of *Clostridium perfringens* and fecal sterols in a Benthic coastal marine environment influenced by the sewage outfall from McMurdo Station. *Appl. Environ. Microbiol.* 1998; 41: 1139–1143.

Elhmmali, M.M., Roberts, D.J., Evershed, R.P. Combined analysis of bile acids and sterols/stanols from riverine particulates to assess sewage discharges and other fecal sources. *Envrion. Sci. Technol.* 2000; 34: 39–46.

Fayer, R., Nerad, T. Effects of low temperatures of viability of *Cryptosporidium parvum* oocysts. *Appl. Environ. Microbiol.* 1996; 62: 1431-1433.

Fong, T.T., Lipp, E.K. Enteric viruses of humans and animals in aquatic environments: health risks, detection, and potential water quality assessment tools. *Microbiol. Mol. Biol. Rev.* 2005; 69: 357–371.

Fong, T.T., Griffin, D.W., Lipp, E.K. Molecular assays for targeting human and bovine enteric viruses in coastal waters and their application for library-independent source tracking. *Appl. Environ. Microbiol.* 2005; 71: 2070–2078.

Gomara B., Fernandez M.A., Gonzalez M.-Jose, Ramos L. Feasibility of gas chromatography – ion trap tandem mass spectrometry for the determination of polychlorinated biphenyls in food. *J. Sep. Sci.* 2006; 29: 123.

Glassmeyer S.T., Furlong E.T., Kolpin D.W., Cahill J.D., Zaugg S.D., Werner S.L., Meyer M.T., Kryak D.D. Transport of chemical and microbial compounds from known wastewater discharges: potential for use as indicators of human fecal contamination. *Environ. Sci. Technol.* 2005; 39: 5157-5169.

Gokulakrishnan, S., Chandraraj, K., Gummadi, S.N. Microbial and enzymatic methods for the removal of caffeine. *Enzyme Microb. Technol.* 2005; 37: 225-232.

Griffin, D.W., Donaldson, K.A., Paul 3rd, J.H., Rose, J.B. Pathogenic human viruses in coastal waters. *Clin. Microbiol. Rev.* 2003; 16: 129–143.

Griffith, J.F., Weisburg, S.B., McGee, C.D. Evaluation of microbial source tracking methods using mixed fecal sources in aqueous test samples. *J. Water Health* 2003; 1: 141–152.

Guan, S., Xu, R., Chen, S., Odumeru, J., Gyles, C.L. Development of a procedure for discriminating among *Escherichia coli* isolates from animal and human sources. *Appl. Environ. Microbiol.* 2002; 68: 2690–2698.

Hagedorn, C., Crozier, J.B., Mentz, K.A., Booth, A.M., Graves, A.K., Nelson, N.J., Reneau Jr., R.B. Carbon source utilization profiles as a method to identify sources of fecal pollution in water. *J. Appl. Microbiol.* 2003; 94: 792–799.

Hagedorn, C., Robinson, S.L., Filtz, J.R., Grubbs, S.M., Angier, T.A., Reneau Jr., R.B. Determining sources of fecal pollution in a rural Virginia watershed with antibiotic resistance patterns in fecal streptococci. *Appl. Environ. Microbiol.* 1999; 65: 5522–5531.

Hartly, C.L., Howne, K., Linton, A.H., Linton, K.B., Richmond, M.H. Distribution of R plasmids among O-antigen types of *Escherichia coli* isolated from human and animal sources. *Antimicrob. Agents Chemother.* 1975; 8: 122–131.

Harwood, V.J., Whitlock, J., Withington, V. Classification of antibiotic resistance patterns of indicator bacteria by discriminant analysis: use in predicting the source of fecal contamination in subtropical waters. *Appl. Environ. Microbiol.* 2000; 66: 3698–3704.

Havelaar, A.H., Pot-Hogeboom, W.M., Furuse, K., Pot, R., Hormann, M.P. F-specific RNA bacteriophages and sensitive host strains in feces and wastewater of human and animal origin. *J. Appl. Microbiol.* 1990; 69: 30-37.

Hayward D.G., Holcomb J., Glidden R., Wilson P., Harris M., Spencer V. Quadrupole ion storage tandem mass spectrometry and high-resolution mass spectrometry:

complementary application in the measurement of 2,3,7,8-chlorine substituted dibenzo-*p* dioxins and dibenzofurans in US foods. *Chemosphere.* 2001; 43: 407.

Hundesa, A., Maluquer de Motes, C., Bofill-Mas, S., Albinana-Gimenez, N., Girones, R. Identification of human and animal adenoviruses and polyomaviruses for determination of sources of fecal contamination in the environment. *Appl. Environ. Microbiol.* 2006; 72: 7886–7893.

Isobe, K.O., Tarao, M., Zakaria, M.P., Chiem, N.H., Minh, L.Y., Takada, H. Quantitative application of fecal sterols using gas-chromatography-mass spectrometry to investigate fecal pollution in tropical waters: western Malaysia and Mekong Delta, Vietnam. *Environ. Sci. Technol.* 2002 ; 36: 4497–4507.

Jagals, P., Grabow, W.O.K. An evaluation of sorbitol-feremnting Bifidobacteria as specific indicators of human fecal pollution of environmental water. *Water SA (Pretoria)* 1996; 22: 35-238.

Jensen S.S., Ariza X., Nielsen P., Vilarrasa J., Kirpekar F. Collision-induced dissociation of cytidine and its derivatives. *J. Mass Spectrom.* 2007; 42: 49.

Jiang, S., Noble, R., Chu, W. Human adenoviruses and coliphages in urban runoff-impacted coastal waters of Southern California. *Appl. Environ. Microbiol.* 2001; 67: 179–184.

Jimenez-Clavero,M.A., Fernandez, C., Ortiz, J.A., Pro, J., Carbonell, G., Tarazona, J.V., Roblas, N., Ley, V. Teschoviruses as indicators of porcine fecal contamination of surface water. *Appl. Environ. Microbiol.* 2003; 69: 6311–6315.

Jofre, J., Blasi, M, Bosch, A., Lucena, F. Occurrence of bacteriophages infecting *Bacteroides fragilis* and other viruses in polluted marine sediments. *Water Sci. Technol.* 1989; 21: 15-19.

Johnson, L.K., Brown, M.B., Carruthers, E.A., Ferguson, J.A., Dombek, P.E., Sadowsky, M.J. Sample size, library composition, and genotypic diversity among natural populations of *Escherichia coli* from different animals influence accuracy of determining sources of fecal pollution. *Appl. Environ. Microbiol.* 2004; 70: 4478-4485.

Kariuki, S., Gilks, C., Kimari, J., Obanda, A., Muyodi, J., Waiyaki, P., Hart, C. A. Genotype analysis of *Escherichia coli* strains isolated from children and chickens living in close contact. *Appl. Environ. Microbiol.* 1999; 65: 472–476.

Kolpin D.W., Furlong, E.T., Meyer, M.T., Thurman, E.M., Zaugg, S.D., Barber, L.B., Buxton, H.T. Pharmaceuticals, Hormones, and Other Organic Wastewater Contaminants in U.S. Streams, 1999-2000: A National Reconnaissance. *Environ. Sci. Technol.* 2002; 36: 1202-1211.

Kolpin D.W., Skopec M., Meyer M.T., Furlong E.T., Zaugg S.D. Urban contribution of pharmaceuticals and other organic wastewater contaminants to streams during differing flow conditions. *Sci. of the Total Environ.* 2004; 328: 119-130.

Kuchler Th, Brsezinski H. Application of GC-MS/MS for the analysis of PCDD/Fs in sewage effluents. *Chemosphere.* 2000; 40: 213.

Layton, A., McKay, L., Williams, D., Garrett, V., Gentry, R., Sayler, G. Development of *Bacteroides* 16S rRNA gene TaqMan-based real-time PCR assays for estimation of total, human, and bovine fecal pollution in water. *Bacteroidales* fecal pollution. *Appl. Environ. Microbiol.* 2006; 72: 4214-4224.

Leonards, P.E.G., Brinkman, U.A.Th., Cofino, W.P. The use of gas chromatography with ion-trap MS/MS detection for the determination of planar PCBs in biota and sediment. *Chemosphere*. 1996; 32: 2381-2387.

Leung, K.T., Mackereth, R., Tien, Y.-C., Topp, E. A comparison of AFLP and ERIC-PCR analyses for discriminating *Escherichia coli* from cattle, pig and human sources. *FEMS Microbiol. Ecol.* 2004; 47: 111–119.

Levy, D.A., M.S. Bens, G.F. Craun, R.L. Calderon, Herwaldt, B.L. Surveillance for Waterborne-Disease Outbreaks—United States, 1995-1996. Center for Disease Control Morbidity and Mortality Weekly Report 1998; 47 (SS-5):1-34.

Ley, V., Higgins, J., Fayer, R. Bovine enteroviruses as indicators of fecal contamination. *Appl. Environ. Microbiol.* 2002; 68: 3455–3461.

Liguori A., Mascaro P., Porcelli B., Sindona G., Uccella N. Identification of caffeine and its metabolites in human urine extracts by electron impact ionization tandem mass spectrometry. *Org. Mass Spectrom.* 1991; 26: 608.

Liguori, A., Mascaro, P., Porcelli, B., Sindona, G., Uccella, N. Identification of caffeine and its metabolites in human urine extracts by electron impact ionization tandem mass spectrometry. *Org. Mass Spectrom*. 1991; 26: 608-612.

Long, S.C., Arango, P.C., Plummer, J.D. An optimized enumeration method for sorbitol-fermenting Bifidobacteria. *Can. J. Microbiol*. 2005; 51: 413-422.

Malavia J., Santos F.J., Galceran M.T. Gas chromatography – ion trap tandem mass spectrometry versus GC-high-resolution mass spectrometry for the determination of non-*ortho*-polychlorinated biphenyls in fish. *J. Chromatogr. A.* 2004; 1056: 171.

March, R.E, 1997. An Introduction to Quadrupole Ion-trap Mass Spectrometry. *J. Mass Spectrom.* 1997; 32: 351-369.

March, R.E., Todd, J.F.J., 1995. Practical aspects of ion-trap mass spectrometry, Vol. I, II and III. CRC Press, Boca Raton.

March, R.E., Todd, J.F.J., 2005. Quadrupole ion-trap mass spectrometry, 2nd ed., Wiley, New Jersey.

Mazzafera, P. Degradation of caffeine by microorganisms and potential use of decaffeinated coffee husk and pulp in animal feeding. *Scientia Agricola* 2002; 59: 815-821.

McLellan, S.L., Daniels, A.D., Salmore, A.K. Genetic characterization of *Escherichia coli* populations from host sources of fecal pollution by using DNA fingerprinting. *Appl. Environ. Microbiol.* 2003; 69: 2587-2594.

McQuaig, S.M., Scott, T.M., Harwood, V.J., Farrah, S.R., Lukasik, J.O. Detection of human-derived fecal pollution in environmental waters by use of a PCR-based human polyomavirus assay. *Appl. Environ. Microbiol.* 2006; 72: 7567–7574.

Meays, C.L., Broersma, K., Nordin, R., Mazumder, A. Source tracking fecal bacteria in water: a critical review of current methods. *J Environ. Manage.* 2004; 73: 71-79.

Metcalfe C.D., Koenig B.G., Bennie D.T., Servos M., Ternes T.A., Hirsch R. Distribution of acidic and neutral drugs in surface waters near sewage treatment plants in the lower great lakes, Canada. *Env. Toxicol. Chem*. 2003; 22: 2872.

Metcalfe, C.D., Koenig, B.G., Bennie, D.T., Servos, M., Ternes, T.A., Hirsch, R. Distribution of acidic and neutral drugs in surface waters near sewage treatment plants in the lower great lakes, Canada. *Env. Toxicol. Chem*. 2003; 22: 2881-2889.

Mohapatra, B.R., Broersma, K., Nordin, R., Mazumder, A. Evaluation of repetitive extragenic palindromic-PCR for discrimination of fecal *Escherichia coli* from humans, and different domestic- and wild-animals. *Microbiol. Immunol.* 2007a; 51: 733-740.

Mohapatra, B.R., Broersma, K., Mazumder, A. Comparison of five rep-PCR genomic fingerprinting methods for differentiation of fecal *Escherichia coli* from humans, poultry wild birds. *FEMS Microbiol. Lett.* 2007b; 277: 98-106.

Mohapatra, B.R., Harris, N., Nordin, R., Mazumder, A. Purification and characterization of a novel caffeine oxidase from *Alcaligenes* species. *J. Biotechnol.* 2006; 125: 319-327.

Moore, D.F., Harwood, V.J., Ferguson, D.M., Lukasik, J., Hannah, P., Getrich, M., Brownell, M. Evaluation of antibiotic resistance analysis and ribotyping for identification of fecal pollution sources in an urban watershed. J. Appl. Microbiol. 2005; 99: 618–628.

Murray, A.P., Gibss, C.F., Kavanagh, P.E. Linear alkylbenzenes (LABs) in sediments of Port Philip Bay (Australia). *Mar. Environ. Res.* 1987; 23: 65-76.

Myoda, S.P., Carson, C.A., Fuhrmann, J.J., Hahm, B.-K., Hartel, P.G., Kuntz, R.L., Nakatsu, C.H., Sadowsky, M.J., Samadpour, M., Yampara-Iquise, H. Comparing genotypic bacterial source tracking methods that require a host origin database. *J. Water Health* 2003; 1: 167–180.

Nunez O., Moyano E., Galceran M.T. High mass accuracy in-source collision-induced dissociation tandem mass spectrometry and multi-step mass spectrometry as complementary tools for fragmentation studies of quaternary ammonium herbicides. *J. Mass Spectrom.* 2004; 39: 873.

Ogunseitan, O.A. Removal of caffeine from wastewater by *Pseudomonas putida* Biotype A: implications for water pollution index. *World J. Microbiol. Biotechnol.* 1996; 12: 251-256.

Okabe, S., Okayama, N., Savichtcheva, O., Ito, T. Identification and quantification of host-specific *Bacteroides-Prevotella* 16S rRNA genetic markers for assessment of fecal pollution in freshwaters TaqMan-based real-time PCR assays for estimation of total, human, and bovine fecal pollution in water. *Bacteroidales* fecal pollution. *Appl. Microbiol. Biotechnol.* 2007; 74: 890-901.

Parveen, S., Hodge, N.C., Stall, R.E., Farrah, S.R., Tamplin, M.L. Genotypic and phenotypic characterization of human and non-human Escherichia coli. *Water Res.* 2001; 35: 379–386.

Parveen, S., Portier, K.M., Robinson, K., Edmiston, L., Tamplin, M. Discriminate analysis of ribotype profiles of *Escherichia coli* for differentiating human and nonhuman sources of fecal pollution. *Appl. Environ. Microbiol.* 1999; 65: 3142–3147.

Peeler, K.A., Opsahl, S.P., Chanton, J.P. Tracking anthropogenic inputs using caffeine, indicator bacteria, and nutrients in rural freshwater and urban marine systems. *Environ. Sci. Technol.* 2006; 40: 7616-7622.

Piocos, E.A., de la Cruz, A.A. Solid phase extraction and high performance liquid chromatography with photodiode array detection of chemical indicators of human fecal contamination in water. *J. Liq. Chromatogr. Relat. Technol.* 2000; 23: 1281-1291.

Puig, A., Queralt, N., Jofre, J., Araujo, R. Diversity of *Bacteroides fragilis* strains in their capacity to recover phages from human and animal wastes and from faecally polluted waste water . *J. Appl. Microbiol.* 1999; 65: 1772-1776.

Puig, M., Jofre, J., Lucena, F., Allaard, A., Wadell, G., Girones, R. Detection of adenoviruses and enteroviruses in polluted waters by nested PCR amplification. *Appl. Environ. Microbiol.* 2000; 60: 2963–2970.

Rao G.S., Khanna K.L., Cornish H.H. Mass spectrometric identification of methylxanthines and methyluric acids, the possible metabolites of caffeine. *J. Pharm. Sci.* 1972; 61: 11, 1822.

Rhodes, M.W., Kator, H. Sorbitol-feremnting bifidobacteria as indicators of diffuse human fecal pollution in estuarine watersheds. *J. Appl. Microbiol.* 1999; 87: 528-535.

Rosen, B. 2000. Waterborne pathogens in agricultural watersheds. US Department of Agricultural, Natural Resources Conservation Service, Watershed Science Instutute, School of Natural Resources, University of Vermont, Burlington, Vermont.

Samadpour, M., Chechowitz, N., 1995. Little Soos Creek Microbial Source Tracking. Kings County Department of Public Works, Seattle.

Samadpour, M., Roberts, M.C., Kitts, C.L., Mulugeta, W., Alfi, D. The use of ribotyping and antibiotic resistance patterns for identification of host sources of *Escherichia coli* strains. *Lett. Appl. Microbiol.* 2005; 40: 63–68.

Schaper, M., Jofre, J., Uys, M., Grabow, W.O. Distribution of genotypes of F-specific RNA bacteriophages in human and non-human sources of fecal pollution in South Africa and Spain. *J. Appl. Microbiol.* 2002; 92: 657-667.

Scott, T.M., Parveen, S., Portier, K.M., Rose, J.B., Tamplin, M.L., Farrah, S.A., Koo, A., Lukasik, J. Geographical variation in ribotype profiles of *Escherichia coli* isolates from humans, swine, poultry, beef, and dairy cattle in Florida. *Appl. Environ. Microbiol.* 2003; 69: 1089–1092.

Scott, T.M., Rose, J.B., Jenkins, T.M., Farrah, S.R., Lukasik, J. Microbial source tracking: current methodology and future directions. *Appl. Environ. Microbiol.* 2002; 68: 5796-5803.

Seiler, R.L., Zaugg, S.D., Thomas, J.M., Howcroft, D.L. Caffeine and Pharmaceuticals as Indicators of Waste Water Contamination in Wells. *Ground Water*. 1999; 37: 405-410.

Seurinck, S., Deschepper, E., Deboch, B., Verstraete,W., Siciliano, S. Characterization of *Escherichia coli* isolates from different fecal sources by means of classification tree analysis of fatty acid methyl ester (FAME) profiles. *Environ. Monit. Assess.* 2006; 114: 433–445.

Seurinck, S., Verstraete, W., and Siciliano, S.D. Use of 16S-23S rRNA intergenic spacer region PCR and repetitive extragenic palindromic PCR analyses of *Escherichia coli* isolates to identify nonpoint fecal sources. *Appl. Environ. Microbiol.* 2003; 69: 4942-4950.

Siegener, R., Chen, R.F. Caffeine in Boston Harbor seawater. *Mar. Pollut. Bull.* 2002; 44: 383-387.

Simmons, G. M., Waye, D. F., Herbein, S., Myers, S., Walker, E. Estimating nonpoint fecal coliform sources in Northern Virginia's Four Mile Run watershed, p. 248–267. *In* T. Younos and J. Poff (ed.), Proceedings of the Virginia Water Research Symposium 2000, VWRRC Special Report SR-19–2000, Blacksburg.

Simpson, J.M., Domingo, J.W.S., Reasoner, D.J. Microbial source tracking: state of the science. *Environ. Sci. Technol.* 2002; 36: 5279-5288.

Souza, V., Rocha, M., Valera, A., Eguiarte, L.E. Genetic structure of natural populations of *Escherichia coli* in wild hosts on different continents. *Appl. Environ. Microbiol.* 1999; 65: 3373–3385.

Standley, L.J., Kaplan, L.A., Smith, D. Molecular Tracers of Organic Matter Sources to Surface Water Resources. *Environ. Sci. Technol.* 2000; 34: 3124-3130.

Stewart-Pullaro, J., Daugomah, J.W., Chestnut, D.E., Graves, D.A., Sobsey, M.D., Scott, G.I. F+ RNA coliphage typing for microbial source tracking in surface waters. *J. Appl. Microbiol.* 2006; 101: 1015–1026.

Stoeckel, D.M., Mathes, M.V., Hyer, K.E., Hagedorn, C., Kator, H., Lukasik, J., O'Brien, T.L., Fenger, T.W., Samadpour, M., Strickler, K.M., Wiggins, B.A. Comparison of seven protocols to identify fecal contamination sources using *Escherichia coli*. *Environ. Sci. Technol.* 2004 ; 38: 6109–6117.

Tartera, C., Lucena, F., Jofre, J. Human origin of *Bacteroides fragilis* bacteriophages present in the environment. *Appl. Environ. Microbiol.* 1989; 55: 2696-2701.

Ternes T., Bonerz M., Schmidt T. Determination of neutral pharmaceuticals in wastewater and rivers by liquid chromatography-electrospray tandem mass spectrometry. *J. Chromatogr. A.* 2001; 938: 175.

Ternes, T., Bonerz, M., Schmidt, T. Determination of neutral pharmaceuticals in wastewater and rivers by liquid chromatography-electrospray tandem mass spectrometry. *J. Chromatogr. A*, 2001; 938: 175-185.

Thevis M., Opfermann G., Krug O., Schanzer W. Electrospray ionization mass spectrometric characterization and quantitation of xanthine derivatives using isotopically labeled analogues: an application for equine doping control analysis. *Rapid Commun. Mass Spectrom.* 2004; 18: 1553.

Togola A., Budzinski H. Analytical development for analysis of pharmaceuticals in water samples by SPE and GC-MS. *Anal. Bioanal. Chem.* 2007; 388: 627-635.

Upton, S.J. 1999. Waterborne/foodborne outbreaks of *Cryptosporidium parvum*. http://www.ksu.edu/parasitology/water. Accessed on 19 November, 2007.

USEPA. (2000) National water quality inventory-1998 report to congress. Office of water, United States Environmental Protection Agency, Washington, D. C., EPA 841-R-00-001. pp. 1-12.

USEPA. (2002a) Wastewater technology fact sheet, bacterial source tracking. Office of water, United States Environmental Protection Agency, Washington, D. C., EPA 832-F-02-010. pp. 1-12.

USEPA. (2002b) U. S. Environmental Protection Agency, Office of Pollution Prevention and Toxics. OPPT High Production Volume Chemicals. http://www.epa.gov (September 2002).

USEPA. (2005) Microbial source tracking guide. Office of Research and Development, United States Environmental Protection Agency, Cincinnati, Ohio, EPA/600-R-05-064. pp. 150.

Verenitch S.S., deBruyn A.M.H., Ikonomou M.G., Mazumder A. Ion-trap tandem mass spectrometry-based analytical methodology for the determination of polychlorinated biphenyls in fish and shellfish. Performance comparison against electron-capture detection and high-resolution mass spectrometry detection. *J. Chromatogr. A*. 2007; 1142: 199.

Verenitch, S.S., Lowe, C.J., Mazumder, A. Determination of acidic drugs and caffeine in municipal wastewaters and receiving waters by gas chromatography ion-trap tandem mass spectrometry. *J. Chromatogr. A*. 2006; 1116: 193-203.

Versalovic, J., Koeuth, T., Lupski, J.R. Distribution of repetitive DNA-sequences in eubacteria and application to fingerprinting of bacterial genomes. *Nucleic Acids Res* 1991; 19: 6823-6831.

Versalovic, J., Schneider, M., de Bruijn, F.J., Lupski, J.R. Genomic fingerprinting of bacteria with repetitive sequence-based polymerase chain reaction. *Methods Mol. Cell Biol.* 1994; 5: 25-40.

Vitousek, P.M., Mooney, H.A., Lubchenko, J., Mellilo, J.M. Human domination of Earth's ecosystem. *Science* 1997; 277: 494-499.

Wade, T.J., Pai, N., Eisenberg, J.N.S., Colford, J.M.J. Do US EPA water quality guidelines for recreational water prevent gastrointestinal illness? *Env. Health Perspect.* 2003; 111: 1102-1109.

Walters, S.P., Ganon, V.P.G., Field, K.G. Detection of *Bacteroidales* fecal indicators fecal indicators and the zoonotic pathogens *E. coli* O157:H7, *Salmonella*, and *Campylobacter* in river water. *Environ. Sci. Technol.* 2007; 41: 1856-1862.

Warrington, P. (2001) Aquatic pathogens, Viruses. Department of Environmental Quality, Victoria, British Columbia, Canada. http:env.gov.bc.cs/wat/wq/ref/viruses.html, accessed 17 November 2007.

WHO (1993) Waterborne infections, gudelines for drinking water quality. World Health Organization, Geneva (online), http://www.studiengang-wasser.de/ VorlHygieneTeil5.pdf, accessed 13 December 2006.

WHO (2003) Emerging issues in water and infectious diseases. World Health Organization, Geneva (online), http://www.who.int/water_sanitation_health/ emerging/en/emerging. pdf, accessed 13 December 2006.

WHO (2005) Water-related diseases. World Health Organization, Geneva (online), http://www.who.int/water_sanitation_health/diseases/typhoid/en/, accessed 17 November 2007.

Wiedenmann, A., Kruger, P., Dietz, K., Lopez-Pila, J.M., Szewzyk, R., Botzenhart, K. A randomized controlled trial assessing infectious disease risks from bathing in fresh recreational waters in relation to the concentration of *Escherichia coli*, intestinal enterococci, *Clostridium perfringens*, and somatic coliphages. *Env. Health Perspect.* 2006; 114: 228-236.

Williams J.P., Nibbering N.M.M., Green B.N., Patel V.J., Scrivens J.H. Collision-induced fragmentation pathways including odd-electron ion formation from desorption electrospray ionization generated protonated and deprotonated drugs derived from tandem accurate mass spectrometry. *J. Mass Spectrom.* 2006; 41: 1277.

Weigel S., Kuhlmann J., Húhnerfuss H. Drugs and personal care products as ubiquitous pollutants: occurrence and distribution of clofibric acid, caffeine and DEET in the North Sea. *Sci. of the Total Environ.* 2002; 295: 131-141.

Wiggins, B.A., Andrews, R.W., Conway, R.A., Corr, C.L., Dobratz, E.J., Dougherty, D.P., Eppard, J.R., Knupp, S.R., Limjoco, M.C., Mettenburg, J.M., Rinehardt, J.M., Sonsino, J., Torrijos, R.L., Zimmerman, M.E. Use of antibiotic resistance analysis to identify nonpoint sources of fecal pollution. *Appl. Environ. Microbiol.* 1999; 65: 3483–3486.

In: Caffeine and Health Research
Editor: Kenneth P. Chambers

ISBN 978-1-60456-437-2

Chapter II

Topical and Transdermal Delivery of Caffeine

Charles M. Heard*
Welsh School of Pharmacy, Cardiff University

Abstract

There are distinct advantages for clinicians to have at their disposal products for the effective delivery of caffeine into and across skin and some 200 research articles having been published on the subject to date. For example, topical application of caffeine has been shown to confer protection from photodamage and inhibit UVB-induced skin carcinogenesis. Furthermore, delivery of therapeutic levels of caffeine into the systemic circulation via the transdermal route from a patch device has advantages including the ability to provide controlled, sustained release of drug through the skin, directly into the bloodstream and limiting the probability of caffeine intoxication occurrence. Another advantage of the transdermal route is that it bypasses first pass hepatic metabolism, whereby caffeine is caffeine is metabolized to three primary metabolites: paraxanthine (84%), theobromine (12%), and theophylline (4%). This article seeks to review the current status of topical and transdermal delivery for caffeine and other xanthine derivatives in terms of potential for the development of therapeutic systems and their scope of applicability.

1. Introduction

Drug delivery aspects are very important in the development of pharmaceuticals. There are distinct advantages for clinicians to have at their disposal products for the effective delivery of drugs into and across skin. Caffeine is a xanthine alkaloid compound that has

* Tel: +44 (0)29 20875819, Fax: +44 (0)29 20874149, Email: heard@cf.ac.uk

numerous pharmacological actions in humans and some 200 research articles having been published to date on its topical delivery. In the forthcoming pages we will see numerous applications for topically applied caffeine. This article seeks to review the current literature for the topical and transdermal delivery for caffeine and, where appropriate, other xanthines in terms of potential for the development of therapeutic systems and their scope of applicability.

2. Skin Structure

The skin is comprised of three major histologically distinct zones: the epidermis, (comprised of stratified epithelial tissue), the dermis and the hypodermis. The epidermis can be further sub-divided into regions of viable tissue, commencing with the stratum basale, and outer non-viable stratum corneum. The dermis is comprised essentially of elastic collagen bundles and is host the dermal microvasculature that supplies the stratum basale by passive efflux. The hypodermis is comprised of adipocytes that contain fat deposits. Very broadly Dermatologicals generally act upon viable epidermis and transdermal systems target the micro blood vessels of the dermis.

3. Modes of Topical Delivery to the Skin

Caffeine is one of the most studied compounds in terms of topical and transdermal delivery, typically as a pure substance but sometimes as part of a complex mixture, eg a natural product extract. One of the earliest papers on the subject was published by Feldman and Maibach (1970). When considering the application of an entity such as caffeine to the skin there are three main modes which essentially differ depending on the target. The umbrella term is ‘topical delivery’, as this can be defined as the application of drug or drug loaded device to a surface. Dermal, or dermatological drug delivery concerns application of a formulation, usually cream or gel based, to an area of involved skin for action within that tissue. ‘Cosmaceutical’ is a recently contrived term, the meaning of which is intended to convey the fact that the distinction between dermatological formulations and those intended to simply confer enhanced aesthetic properties to the skin is not well defined. Transdermal systems are generally intended to deliver drugs to the system following transport across the epidermis and uptake by the microvasculature of the dermis and transcutaneous delivery refers to the diffusion of a drug across the entire skin to underlying tissues. Both transdermal and transcutanous systems often involve patch-based devices, although gels that are capable of delivering such are known. These distinctions, although often vague, are important as they affect the dosage form, the amounts administered and methods of determining delivery. However, both the transdermal and transcutaneous routes of drug delivery offer a convenient, painless, and non-invasive method of therapy without the difficulties, discomfort, and scope for error of intravenous or oral administration. Cosmetic products are intended for localisation on and in the stratum corneum only, although some are intended to act within the hypodermis. For a comprehensive introduction to the subject area, the reader is referred to a recent book (Williams, 2003).

It is worth mentioning at this stage that orally dosed caffeine (eg consumed as coffee or tea) is known to lead to changes within the skin, in particular increases in skin temperature have been documented (Tagliabue et al, 1994). However, others found a low correlation between the change in metabolic rate during the 3 h after the caffeine consumption and the mean change in skin temperature (Koot and Deurenberg, 1995). More alarmingly, one study into lifestyle factors and their importance in the aetiology of basal cell carcinoma by (Sahl et al, 1995) indicated that caffeine consumption was higher in those presenting with basal cell carcinoma.

In the following sections the topical application of caffeine is considered in its mode and then in terms of specific areas of interest within that mode.

4. Caffeine and Dermatological/Dermal Delivery

Dermatological or dermal delivery aims to deliver pharmacologically actives to involved areas of the skin. However, there is a subtle difference in that dermal formulations are always administered to the skin, whereas dermatologicals include both drugs applied to the skin and those administered by other routes in order to elicit their pharmacological activity within the skin.

4.1. Quantitation - Depth Profiling

Depth profiling is the most appropriate method for the quantitative determination of drug localised within the skin, where drug typically drug concentration is pictured as a function of relative or actual skin depth. The conventional way to achieve this is by use of the Franz diffusion cell, or variant, where the skin membrane is mounted between donor and receptor compartments and the dose applied to the skin. After the required time the skin is recovered from the cell and the depth profile obtained. 'Tape stripping' achieves this by the repeated application of an adhesive disc or tape to an area previously dosed with drug; the amount of drug on the discs are then determined. ^{14}C-labelled caffeine was found to penetrate rapidly into human epidermis and corium from ointment bases following a 90 s rubbing procedure (Zesch et al, 1979). Depth profiling was attained by removal of the horny layer using Scotch tape followed by 16 x 10 μ horizontal sections using a 'freeze-dry microtome' (cryostat). Over a period of 10-1000 min amounts of caffeine localised were vehicle dependent (Table 1). It was further concluded that in the absence of blood and lymph vessels, the levels of caffeine in skin in vitro were 450 x higher than in vivo.

More recently, the percutaneous absorption of caffeine from two vehicles, an emulsion and an acetone solution, was quantified by in vivo techniques in humans (Chambinremoussenard et al, 1993). A surface recovery technique over a 6 h application and a stripping method after a 30 min application were performed on the volar aspect of the forearm on 12 volunteers. Two phases were distinguished in the percutaneous absorption of caffeine: a higher filling up of the stratum corneum with the oil-in-water emulsion than with the acetone solution, which was then followed by a steady-state flux corresponding to the penetration in the living tissues. The permeability constants k_p with emulsion and acetone were 1.59×10^{-4} and 9.53×10^{-8} cm h^{-1} respectively. The stripping method showed concentrations of caffeine in stratum corneum that were five times higher with emulsion (212 ng cm^2) than with acetone 37 ng cm^2. With acetone as a vehicle, approximately 40% of caffeine of the cornified layer was found around the treated area. This sizeable lateral spread within the stratum corneum was not observed with the emulsion.

Table 1. In vitro levels, expressed as mg substance/cm² skin surface applied in relation to the ointment base and period of penetration (Zesch et al, 1979)

Skin Layer	Penetration time (min)	Vaseline	Aqueous woolwax alcohol ointment	Aqueous hydrophilic ointment	Polyethylene glycol ointment
Horny layer	10	0.659	0.643	1.491	0.845
	30	1.358	1.464	1.978	0.832
	100	1.527	2.182	1.542	0.632
	300	2.362	1.592	2.362	0.797
	1000	1.550	2.326	1.550	0.081
Epidermis	10	0.012	0.019	0.133	0.001
	30	0.016	0.008	0.042	0.052
	100	0.204	0.137	0.508	0.216
	300	0.023	0.064	0.023	0.039
	1000	0.105	0.246	0.105	0.049
Corium	10	0.005	0.010	0.022	0.001
	30	0.028	0.009	0.215	0.007
	100	0.090	0.056	0.667	0.109
	300	0.072	0.144	0.072	0.037
	1000	0.306	0.45	0.306	0.072

4.2. Metabolism in the Skin

Like other methylxanthines, caffeine influences metabolic processes such as glycolysis and lipolysis. The concentration of cAMP is raised by the inhibition of phosphodiesterase, suggesting that caffeine is capable of influencing epidermal metabolic processes in addition to acting upon the peripheral vessels following topical application (Stüttgen and Neumann, 1972).

Caffeine is converted in the liver to three primary metabolites: paraxanthine (84%), theobromine (12%), and theophylline (4%) (PharmGkb). One advantage of topical delivery by any mode, is that first-pass hepatic metabolism is circumvented, essentially meaning that a significantly greater proportion of the applied dose remains bioavailable at the target site within the skin. However, the viable epidermis is host to an array of endogenous enzyme systems within the keratinocytes, and any topically administered drug is liable to undergo some degree of first pass metabolism before it reaches its target (Hikima et al, 2005).

The literature contains little on the cutaneous metabolism of caffeine, although the closely related xanthine theophylline is mentioned. The percutaneous absorption of theophylline in human skin from five sources was examined by use of a flow-through in vitro diffusion system (Ademola et al, 1992). The metabolites and unchanged drug were estimated by thin-layer chromatography. Correlation was evident in the percentage of the applied dose that diffused through the five skin samples (range 2.8 +/- 0.5% -7.7 +/- 0.8%); however, the percentage of applied dose absorbed varied between different skin samples (range 3.6 +/- 0.9%-33.4 +/- 2.4%). Between 0.2 +/- 0.1%-4.6 +/- 0.2% of the doses applied were metabolized, and over 60% of the total metabolites formed diffused through the skin.

The uptake and metabolism of theophylline by microsomes obtained from four of the human skin samples were measured. All preparations showed detectable activities for the metabolism of theophylline. Microsomal preparations from skin sources A, B, and E, and B, C, and E biotransformed theophylline to 1,3,7-trimethyluric acid and 1,3-dimethyluric acid, respectively. The activities of microsomes from skin samples C and E on the drug produced the pharmacologically active metabolite 3-methylxanthine. The specific activities of the microsomes from skin sources A-E for the formation of 1,3-dimethyluric acid and 3-methylxanthine varied fivefold. However, the variation in specific activities of the microsomes for the formation of 1,3,7-trimethyluric acid was twofold (range 2.8 +/- 0.1-6.2 +/- 0.5 pmol min^{-1} mg^{-1} protein). These metabolic data may be of value in the development of transdermal theophylline systems. The results indicate that a high level of absorption enhancement will be required before transdermal theophylline preparations could produce therapeutic plasma concentrations.

4.3. Skin Irritation

An irritant is defined by the Occupational Health and Safety Administration (OSHA) according to Appendix A 29 CFR 1910.1200, the Hazard Communication Standard as: a chemical, which is not corrosive, but which causes a reversible inflammatory effect on living tissue by chemical action at the site of contact. A chemical is a skin irritant if, when tested on the intact skin of albino rabbits by the methods of 16 CFR 1500.41 for four hours exposure or by other appropriate techniques, it results in an empirical score of five or more.

The effects of the application of skin irritants, norephedrine and imipramine, on the in vitro percutaneous absorption of three model compounds of diverse physicochemical properties, caffeine, indomethacin, and hydrocortisone (Nangia et al, 1993). Treatment with norephedrine increased the permeation of caffeine and hydrocortisone by two- to fourfold, while absorption of indomethacin declined an order of magnitude. A similar result was obtained for the effect of treatment with imipramine on transport of caffeine.

4.4. Psoriasis

Psoriasis is a chronic inflammatory disorder of the skin, affecting around 2% of the population. There are several different forms of the disease, the most common being psoriasis vulgaris, whereby epidermal hyperproliferation in the skin forms plaques which are thick and scaly.

It is believed that xanthines can inhibit cell proliferation by elevating intracellular cAMP. Therefore, these compounds can potentially be useful in hyperproliferative disorders. The efficacy of theophylline, caffeine and dyphylline on 3T3 fibroblast proliferation was recently assessed (Levischaffer and Touitou, 1991). 3T3 subconfluent cultures were incubated for 3 days with the xanthine derivatives (1 mM-1 μM). At 1 and 0.1 mM the three derivatives exhibited marked inhibition of fibroblast proliferation. Theophylline and caffeine were more potent than dyphylline. At a concentration of 1 mM, the three xanthine derivatives also inhibited proliferation of psoriatic dermal fibroblast, albeit to a lower extent. Caffeine was the most active compound followed by theophylline and dyphylline. It was concluded that xanthine derivatives are good candidates for use as fibroblast antiproliferative drugs. It was also concluded that 3T3 fibroblasts appear to be a valid system for the pharmacological screening of fibroblast antiproliferative drugs.

Animal and human studies suggested that the therapeutic benefit of the potent drug methotrexate in the treatment of rheumatoid arthritis might be substantially reduced in patients who are concomitantly consuming caffeine. One paper investigated the effect of caffeine consumption on the methotrexate dosing requirements in patients with psoriasis and psoriatic arthritis (Swanson et al, 2007). Results suggested that caffeine does not affect methotrexate dosage requirements in patients with psoriasis and psoriatic arthritis. However, their results did not rule out an effect of caffeine in other inflammatory diseases treated with methotrexate.

4.5. Photodamage

Photodamage can be defined as changes that occur within skin as a consequence of exposure to the sun or, more strictly, irradiation by ultraviolet (UV) radiation. Several groups have studied the beneficial effects of topically applied caffeine.

Oral administration of green tea or caffeine to SKH-1 mice for 2 weeks prior to a single application of UVB enhanced UVB-induced increases in the number of p53-positive cells, p21(WAF1/CIP1)-positive cells, and apoptotic sunburn cells in the epidermis (Lu et al 2000). Topical application of caffeine the dorsal skin of SKH-1 mice immediately after irradiation with UVB (30 mJ cm^2) enhanced UVB-induced apoptosis as measured by the number of morphologically distinct epidermal apoptotic sunburn cells and the number of caspase 3-positive cells (Lu et al, 2001). Time course studies indicated that UVB-induced increases in apoptotic sunburn cells were correlated with elevated levels of caspase 3, a key protease that becomes activated during an early stage of apoptosis. Topical application of caffeine immediately after UVB enhanced UVB-induced increases in caspase 3 (active form)-immunoreactive-positive cells and in caspase 3 enzyme activity in the epidermis. Topical application of caffeine had only a small stimulatory effect on UVB-induced increases in the level of wild-type p53 protein and these changes were not related temporally to caffeine-induced increases in apoptotic cells. There was little or no effect of topical applications of caffeine on epidermal cell proliferation as determined by bromodeoxyuridine (BrdU) incorporation into DNA. A pro-apoptotic effect of topical application of caffeine on UVB-irradiated mouse skin was thus proposed. It was later reported that UVB-induced increases in apoptosis in the epidermis of wild-type mice are predominantly (but not entirely) by p53- and Bax-dependent pathways and that topical application of caffeine can enhance UVB-induced increases in apoptosis by p53- and Bax-independent pathways (Lu et al, 2004).

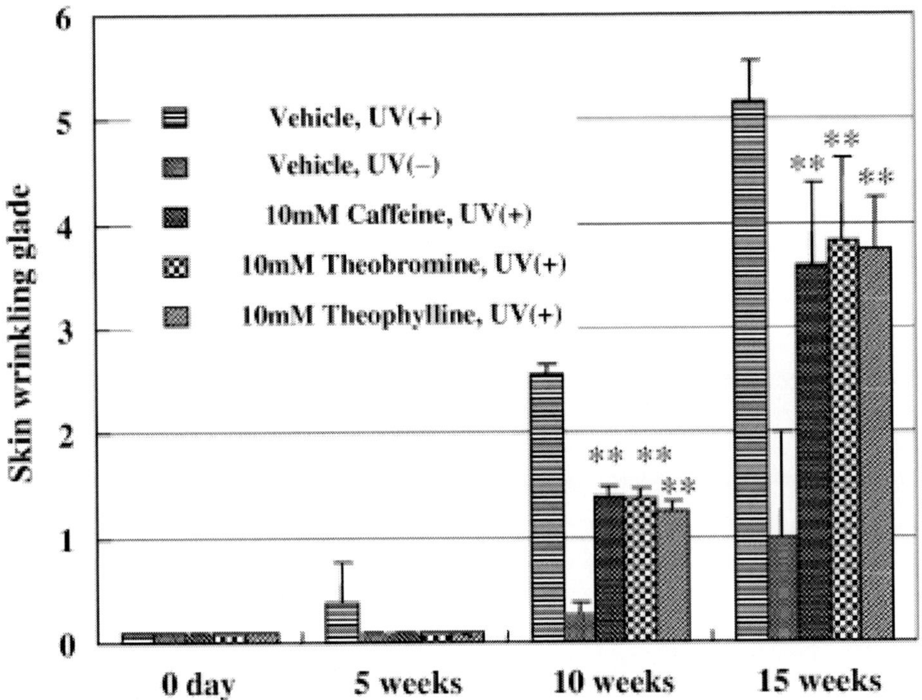

Figure 1. Suppression of skin-wrinkling grade by xanthine derivatives in hairless mouse dorsal skin exposed to irradiation. Each value represents the mean±SD (n=8). Wilcoxon's test. **P<0.01 vs. vehicle UV[+] (Mitani et al, 2007).

Topically applied caffeine was more recently found to confer protection to skin after UV irradiation (Koo et al, 2007). Hairless mice (SKH-1) were treated with UVB then 100 μL of 1-2% caffeine in acetone (or acetone only) three times weekly for 11 weeks then evaluated for roughness and presence of transverse rhytides. Results demonstrated that even after a single dose of UVB, topically applied caffeine more than doubled the number of apoptotic keratinocytes. A trend towards decreased solar elastosis was noted in the caffeine-treated group although this was not statistically significant. Other histological parameters including epidermal hyperplasia, solar elastosis and angiogenesis were increased in mice treated with UV but topical application of caffeine did not alter these particular UV effects.

Topical application of cacao beans, cola nuts extracts and caffeine, theobromine, and theophylline markedly prevented photodamage including wrinkle formation and histological alterations (Mitani et al, 2007) (Figure 1) A significant increase in total hydroxyproline content caused by UV irradiation was observed. In contrast, topical application of plant extracts and xanthine derivatives reduced total hydroxyproline and pepsin-resistant hydroxyproline content in comparison with that of the control (vehicle, UV-irradiation group). Moreover, naphthol AS-D chloroacetate esterase staining and diaminobenzidine staining suggested that leukocytes including neutrophils increased in the UV-exposed skin. In contrast, weak staining was observed in skin treated with xanthine derivatives.

Topical application of caffeine sodium benzoate (caffeine-SB) immediately after UVB irradiation of SKH-1 mice enhanced UVB-induced apoptosis by a 2- to 3-fold greater extent than occurred after the topical application of an equimolar amount of caffeine (Lu et al, 2007a). Although topical application of caffeine-SB or caffeine enhanced UVB-induced apoptosis, both substances were inactive on non-UVB-treated normal skin. Topical application of caffeine-SB or caffeine (each has UVB absorption properties) 0.5 h before irradiation with a high dose of UVB decreased UVB-induced thymine dimer formation and sunburn lesions (sunscreen effect). Caffeine-SB was more active than an equimolar amount of caffeine in exerting a sunscreen effect. In additional studies, caffeine-SB strongly inhibited the formation of tumours in UVB-pre-treated 'high-risk mice' and in tumour-bearing mice, and the growth of UVB-induced tumours was also inhibited. Caffeine-SB and caffeine are the first examples of compounds that have both a sunscreen effect and enhance UVB-induced apoptosis. The conclusion was that caffeine-SB and caffeine may be good agents for inhibiting the formation of sunlight-induced skin cancer.

Narayanan et al (1997) examined the comparative effects of staurosporine or caffeine on G_2-phase arrest and cyclin B1 expression in human skin fibroblasts (HSF) and transformed HeLa cells following gamma-irradiation were examined by flow cytometry. These results suggest that staurosporine and caffeine treatments act on different pathways of cell cycle control in normal and transformed cells, in terms of attenuation of G_2 block and diminution of elevated levels of cyclin B1 expression, in response to radiation. Subsequently, Deplanque et al (2000) suggested that caffeine primarily inhibits replicative DNA synthesis and suggest that, at least in normal cells, caffeine potentiates the cytotoxicity of radiation by intervening in DNA repair rather than by overriding the G2/M block.

Irradiation of female SKH-1 hairless mice with UVB (30 mJ cm^{-2}) twice a week for 10-20 weeks resulted in the formation of a large number of cellular patches (Lu et al 2005). Considered putative early cellular markers of the beginning of tumour formation, these started appearing after 4-6 weeks of UVB treatment, and multiple patches were observed after treatment for 10 weeks. Topical applications of caffeine to the dorsal skin of mice pre-treated with UVB for 20 weeks resulted in enhanced apoptosis selectively in focal basal cell hyperplastic areas of the epidermis (putative precancerous lesions), but not in areas of the epidermis that only had diffuse hyperplasia. The conclusion was that the chemopreventive effect of caffeine or green tea may occur by a pro-apoptotic effect preferentially in early precancerous lesions. In a subsequent study, SKH-1 mice were orally dosed with caffeine (0.1 mg $_{mL}^{-1}$ in the drinking water), with voluntary running wheel exercise, or a combination of caffeine and exercise for 2 weeks (Lu et al, 2007b). In addition to reducing bodily fat, this was found to stimulate the formation of UVB-induced apoptotic sunburn cells in the epidermis by 96, 120, and 376%, respectively; and stimulate the formation of UVB-induced caspase 3 (active form)-positive cells in the epidermis by 92, 120, and 389%, respectively (average of two experiments).

Kramata et al (2005) reported on the irradiation of SKH-1 mice with UVB light for 20 weeks resulted in a large number of patches of epidermal cells, which was visualized with an antibody that recognizes mutated p53 protein. Oral treatment of mice with caffeine (0.4 mg mL^{-1}) or green tea (6 mg tea solids mL^{-1}) as the drinking fluid during UVB irradiation decreased the number of patches by similar to 40%. Sequencing analysis of the p53 gene (exons 3 to 9) detected 88, 82 or 39 point mutations in 67, 70 or 29 patches from water, caffeine or tea treated mice, respectively. A major hotspot at codon 270 (Arg -> Cys) accounted for 47.7% (water), 70.7% (caffeine) or 46.2% (tea) of all mutations. Patches from caffeine treated mice had fewer types of mutations than patches from mice treated with water or tea. Administration of caffeine or tea during 20 weeks of UVB irradiation eliminated mutations at codons 149 (Pro -> Ser) and 210 (Arg -> Cys) but increased the frequency of mutations at codon 238 (Ser -> Phe). Topical applications of caffeine (1.2 mg in 100 μL acetone) once a day, five times a week for 6 weeks after stopping UVB decreased the number of patches by 63% when compared with mice treated with acetone. DNA sequencing analysis detected 63 and 68 mutations in 48 and 57 patches from acetone or caffeine treated mice, respectively. Although no differences in the frequency, position or types of mutations were observed, the caffeine group harboured less homozygous mutations (12.3% of the total) than the acetone group (31.3% of the total, $P = 0.029$). In summary, oral treatment of mice with caffeine or green tea during chronic UVB irradiation changed the mutation profile of the p53 gene in early mutant p53 positive epidermal patches, and topical applications of caffeine after discontinuation of chronic UVB irradiation specifically eliminated patches harbouring homozygous p53 mutations.

4.6. Xeroderma Pigmentosum

Xeroderma pigmentosum, is a relatively rare autosomal recessive genetic disorder of DNA repair in which the body's normal ability to remove damage caused by ultraviolet (UV) light is deficient. Patients with xeroderma pigmentosum variant (XP-V) have a higher risk to skin cancer and XP-V cells are extremely mutable by UV radiation. This can lead to multiple basaliomas and other skin malignancies at a young age and total avoidance of sunlight. Damage to DNA in epidermal cells occurs during exposure to UV light. The absorption of the high-energy light leads to the formation of pyrimidine dimers, namely CPDs (Cyclobutane-Pyrimidine-Dimers) and 6-4PP (pyrimidine-6-4-pyrimidone photoproducts). The normal repair process is called nucleotide excision repair. The damage is excised by endonucleases, then the gap is filled by a DNA polymerase and sealed by a ligase. The most common defect in xeroderma pigmentosum is a genetic defect whereby nucleotide excision repair (NER) enzymes are mutated, leading to a reduction in or elimination of NER. Unrepaired damage can lead to mutations, altering the information of the DNA. If mutations affect important genes, like tumour suppressor genes (e.g. p53) or proto oncogenes then this may lead to cancer. Since in XP patients the frequencies of mutations is much elevated, these patients have a predisposition for cancer.

Lehmann and Kirkbell (1974) reported in XP-V; (i) smaller replication products were accumulated after UV irradiation; (ii) the elongation of these products was delayed; (iii) the elongation was markedly inhibited by caffeine. XP-V cells UV-irradiated at mid-S phase were normally S-arrested, and no "override" by caffeine (i.e. abrogation of the S-chec$_{kp}$oint) was observed by flow cytometry, suggesting that caffeine does not act via cdc kinase here; (iv) butylphenyldeoxyguanosine (BuPGdR) inhibited elongation of replication products only in UV-irradiated XP-V cells; (v) dideoxycytidine or dideoxyinosine had no effect on this process in either normal or XP-V cells. Yamada et al (2003) reported that translesion replication in cisplatin-treated xeroderma pigmentosum variant cells is also caffeine-sensitive: features of the error-prone DNA polymerase(s) involved in UV-mutagenesis.

Patients with xeroderma pigmentosum variant show clinical photosensitivity, skin neoplasias induced by ultraviolet light, and defective post-replication repair, but normal nucleotide excision repair (Itoh et al, 2000). Among hereditary photosensitive disorders, including other xeroderma pigmentosum groups, Cockayne syndrome, and a newly established ultraviolet-sensitive syndrome, only xeroderma pigmentosum variant cells exhibited normal unscheduled DNA synthesis, normal recovery of RNA synthesis, but reduced recovery of replicative DNA synthesis (51 +/- 6% the rate relative to normal controls). This reduction of recovery of replicative DNA synthesis was enhanced in the presence of a non-toxic level of caffeine to 36 +/- 5%. In this study we assess the cellular markers in two independent families that included two photosensitive patients that were identified as xeroderma pigmentosum variant. Cells from heterozygotic parents showed normal levels of unscheduled DNA synthesis, recovery of RNA synthesis, and recovery of replicative DNA synthesis, but reduced rates of recovery of replicative DNA synthesis in the presence of 1 mM caffeine (53 +/- 8% relative to the normal control). Furthermore, with a colony-forming assay, the cells showed normal survival by ultraviolet without caffeine, but slightly reduced survival by ultraviolet with 1 mM caffeine present. In one family, we confirmed inheritance of two heterozygous mis-sense mutations. One mutation is an A -->G transition at nucleotide 1840 that generates a K535E mis-sense mutation. Another mutation is an A -->C transversion at nucleotide 2003 that generates a K589 mis-sense mutation. Each of these mutations were absent in 52 unrelated Japanese individuals. These results suggest that xeroderma pigmentosum variant heterozygotes can be identified by their sensitivity to ultraviolet irradiation in the presence of non-toxic levels of caffeine.

4.7. Skin Cancer

Skin cancer is a malignant growth on the skin which can have many causes, but is often a consequence of photodamage. Skin cancer generally develops in the epidermis (the outermost layer of skin), so a tumour is usually clearly visible and makes most skin cancers detectable in the early stages. Skin cancers are the fastest growing type of cancer in the United States. Skin cancer represents the most commonly diagnosed malignancy, surpassing lung, breast, colorectal and prostate cancer.

Generally, there is substantial evidence to support caffeine as an anti skin cancer drug. The earliest report appears to have been by Zajdela and Latarjet (1973) in their paper describing the inhibiting effect of caffeine on induction of skin cancers by ultraviolet radiation in mice. This was closely followed by an article in Nature by Rothwell (1974) who described the dose-related inhibition of chemical carcinogenesis in mouse skin by caffeine. However, a subsequent paper took a different view, suggesting that caffeine enhances skin tumour-induction in mice (Hoshino and Tanooka, 1979).

A number of more recent papers have examined the anti-cancer properties of caffeine as a component of a natural product, usually (green) tea, an aqueous infusion of dried unfermented leaves of *Camellia sinensis* (family Theaceae) from which numerous biological activities have been reported including antimutagenic, antibacterial, hypocholesterolemic, antioxidant, anti-tumour and cancer preventive activities. In addition to caffeine, green tea extract contains numerous polyphenolic compounds, the catechins. Using cell culture techniques, Valcic et al (1996) investigated the inhibitory effect of six green tea catechins and caffeine on the growth of four selected human tumour cell lines (MCF-7 breast carcinoma, HT-29 colon carcinoma, A-427 lung carcinoma and UACC-375 melanoma), although caffeine was found to be less active than the catechins.

However, oral administration of a high-dose level of the decaffeinated teas to high-risk SKH-1 mice was found to enhance the tumorigenic effect of UVB (Huang et al 1997). Oral administration of caffeine alone had a substantial inhibitory effect on UVB-induced carcinogenesis, and adding caffeine to the decaffeinated teas restored the inhibitory effects of these teas on UVB-induced carcinogenesis. In additional studies, topical application of a green tea polyphenol fraction after each UVB application inhibited UVB-induced tumorigenesis. The results indicated that caffeine contributes in an important way to the inhibitory effects of green and black tea on UVB-induced complete carcinogenesis.

In a subsequent study by the same group, oral administration of tea to SKH-1 mice inhibited the formation and decreased the size of non-malignant squamous cell papillomas and keratoacanthomas as well as the formation and size of malignant squamous cell carcinomas (Lou et al 1999). Furthermore, *decaffeinated* tea was inactive or less effective inhibitors of tumour formation than the regular teas, and adding caffeine back to the decaffeinated teas restored biological activity. Oral administration of caffeine alone (0.44 mg mL^{-1}) as the sole source of drinking fluid for 18-23 weeks inhibited the formation of non-malignant and malignant tumours, and this treatment also decreased tumour size in these high-risk mice. However, the contributory anti cancer effects of caffeine were downplayed in a recent article by Fujiki et al (1999).

Lu et al (2004) reported that the stimulatory effect of green tea and caffeine on UV-induced increases in the number of p53-positive cells, p21(WAF1/CIP1)-positive cells and apoptotic sunburn cells may play a role in the inhibitory effects of tea and caffeine on UV-induced carcinogenesis. The same group found that topical applications of caffeine or (-)-epigallocatechin gallate (EGCG) inhibited carcinogenesis and selectively increase apoptosis in UVB-induced skin tumours in mice (Lu et al, 2002). SKH-1 hairless mice were irradiated with ultraviolet B (UVB) twice weekly for 20 weeks. These tumour-free mice, which had a high risk of developing skin tumours during the next several months, were then treated topically with caffeine 6.2 μmol or EGCG 6.5 μmol once a day 5 days a week for 18 weeks in the absence of further treatment with UVB. Topical applications of caffeine to these mice decreased the number of non-malignant and malignant skin tumours per mouse by 44% and

72%, respectively. Topical applications of EGCG decreased the number of non-malignant and malignant tumours per mouse by 55% and 66%, respectively. Immunohistochemical analysis showed that topical applications of caffeine or EGCG increased apoptosis as measured by the number of caspase 3-positive cells in non-malignant skin tumours by 87% or 72%, respectively, and in squamous cell carcinomas by 92% or 56%, respectively, but there was no effect on apoptosis in non-tumour areas of the epidermis. Topical applications of caffeine or EGCG had a small inhibitory effect on proliferation in non-malignant tumours as measured by BrdUrd labelling (16-22%), and there was also a similar, but no significant, inhibitory effect on proliferation in malignant tumours.

Most recently Conney et al (2007) found that topical applications of caffeine to mice previously treated with UVB for 20 weeks (high risk mice without tumours) inhibited the formation of tumours (Table 2) and stimulated apoptosis in the tumours but not in areas of the epidermis away from tumours (Table 3). The selective effects of caffeine administration to stimulate UVB-induced apoptosis or apoptosis in tumours but not in normal epidermis or in areas of the epidermis away from tumours is of considerable interest, but the reasons for the selective effects of caffeine on apoptosis in DNA damaged tissues are unknown.

Table 2. Effect of topical applications of caffeine on carcinogenesis in high risk mice (Conney et al, 2007)

Treatment	Non-malignant tumours			Squamous cell carcinomas		
	% mice with tumours	Tumours per mouse	Tumour volume per mouse (mm^3)	% mice with tumours	Tumours per mouse	Tumour volume per mouse (mm^3)
Acetone	82	7.21±1.28	23.2±5.5	64	1.18±0.25	190±95
Caffeine	77	4.03±0.76	6.4±1.7	23	0.33±0.12	39±28
% decrease	(6)	(44)	(72)	(64)	(72)	(79)

4.8. Anti -Viral

Caffeine is known to possess anti-microbial properties (Shiraki and Rapp, 1988). In terms of skin-based infections, most published work involves its ability to inhibit the replication of herpes simplex virus (HSV) (Vonka el al, 1995). Caffeine is structurally similar to adenosine and will bind to adenosine receptors. It is possible that the caffeine binds to virus receptors used by the HSV and thereby inhibits the replication of HSV. The use of caffeine has been the subject of several patent applications, either as the single active ingredient (Potts, 1990) or co-formulated, eg with a bee product (Gee, 2003).

Table 3. Effect of topical applications of caffeine on apoptosis in tumours in high-risk mice (Conney et al., 2007)

Treatment	No of non-tumour areas, or tumours examined	Number of cells examined	Percent caspase-3 positive cells	% increase
Non tumour area Acetone Caffeine	370 271	123,000 92,000	0.159±0.015 0.165±0.027	- 4
Non-malignant tumours Acetone Caffeine	202 121	882,000 426,000	0.229±0.022 0.428±0.033	- 87
Carcinomas Acetone Caffeine	33 10	555,000 110,000	0.196±0.022 0.376±0.056	- 92

Caffeine was found to exert a synergistic effect with interferon on the replication of HSV (Vonka el al, 1995). The therapeutic efficacy of a caffeine gel (Cafon) has been shown against HSV-1 by Yoshida et al (1996) and Yamamura et al (1996). The midflanks of 6-week-old BALB/c mice were infected with HSV cutaneously after application of 10% caffeine (Cafon) gel, and was reapplied to the midflank 5 limes daily thereafter. Treatment with Cafon gel significantly retarded the development of skin lesions. Both midflanks were cutaneously infected, and a placebo and active gel were applied to the right and left midflanks, respectively. Cafon gel significantly retarded the appearance of vesiculation and reduced the number of vesicles compared with the placebo gel. Cafon gel was as effective as 5%, acyclovir ointment, and no significant difference was observed in the development of local lesions between these two topical preparations. The efficacy of Cafon gel also corresponded to that of oral treatment with 5 mg kg^{-1} or more of acyclovir in our cutaneous infection system. These results suggest that Cafon gel can be useful for the topical treatment of cutaneous HSV infection.

Interestingly, paresthesia, the sensation of tingling, induced by herpes simplex virus was found to be inhibited by topically applied caffeine through action on primary sensory neurons in rats (Shiraki et al, 1998).

4.9. Cosmaceutical

Caffeine appears in 'Health and Beauty' products for its purported antioxidant, dehydrating, and vaso-constricting properties. These include face creams/serum (eg Topix Peplenix Cream and Revale Skin which contains coffee-berry), body scrubs (eg Nyakio), eye gels (eg Origins No Puffery), where caffeine is claimed to help deflate puffy skin because it constricts blood vessels. It purportedly helps drain excess blood and lymph fluid to help temporarily deflate puffy eyes and reduce the appearance of dark circles.

Cellulite is defined as skin relief alterations that give the skin an orange peel or mattress appearance. The lesions tend to be asymptomatic and may be considered the anatomic expressions of the structures in the affected area, such as the fat and subcutaneous septa. Caffeine was the most common active ingredient found in a recent study of 32 cellulite products (Sainio et al 2000), where it's mode of action has been linked to the temporary dehydration of fluid from fat cells, making them appear smaller. L'Oreal Sublime gel is supported by data where 150 women lost an average of a half-inch off their thighs in four weeks and Elancyl Stretch Mark Cream (Galenic) – see 5.2.

Several commercially available topical formulations caffeine have been compared in terms of the permeation of caffeine across excised human upper leg epidermis (Dias et al, 1999). The products were Somma lotion (Natura, Brazil), Elancyl gel (Vichy, France) and Cellactia lotion (Pierre Fabre, France), all containing 3% caffeine. Although a skin-based condition, cellulite affects the adipose tissue beneath the dermis, thus the appropriate experimental model is transdermal/transcutaneous.

From Figure 2 it is apparent that there is a significant difference between Elancyl and the other two preparations, with the k_p data determined as follows: Elancyl gel (Vichy, France), Cellactia lotion (Pierre Fabre, France), Somma lotion (Natura, Brazil): 1.07 x 10^{-3}, 1.98 x 10^{-4}, 1.15 x 10^{-4} cm h^{-1}. The difference were attributed to conjectured absence of enhancing excipient in Cellactia and Somma.

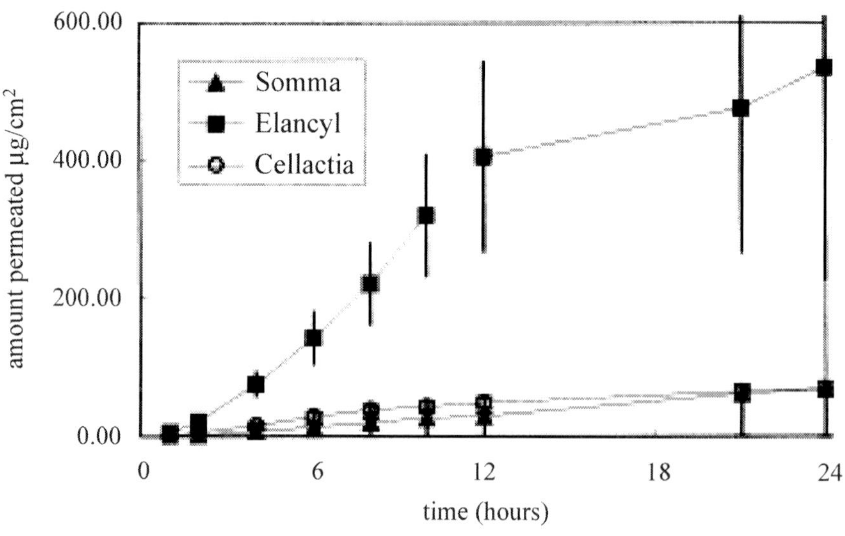

Figure 2. The permeation of caffeine from three commercial formulations through human epidermal membranes (n=4).

Laboratory data to support the use of caffeine against cellulite exists, for example the treatment of SKH-1 mice orally with caffeine significantly decreased the thickness of the dermal fat layer (Lu et al, 2007b). A double-blind, randomized, placebo-controlled study was recently conducted with 46 healthy female volunteers in order to test an anti-cellulite product containing retinol, caffeine and ruscogenine (Bertin et al, 2001). An evaluation of different parameters related to cellulite appearance, i.e., the skin macrorelief, the dermal and hypodermal structures, the skin mechanical characteristics, and the cutaneous flowmetry was assessed using several non-invasive methods. This combination of different evaluation methods resulted in the demonstration of significant activity of the anti-cellulite product versus baseline and showed its superiority versus the placebo in skin macrorelief (decrease of the "orange peel" effect) and an increase in cutaneous microcirculation. By using a combination of methods, it was possible to detail the activity of an anti-cellulite product and to show superiority of the product in comparison with the placebo.

Dermatographic urticaria (also known as *dermographism*, dermatographism or skin writing) is a skin disorder seen in 4-5% of the population, in which the skin becomes raised and inflamed when stroked or rubbed with a dull object. A study by Stuttgen and Neumann (1972) found that dermographism was inhibited in human skin after topical application of caffeine.

Hair follicles are surrounded by a close network of capillaries dendritic cells and stem cells, they represent an important target for drug delivery. Touitou et al (1994) noted significant accumulation of caffeine in the skin appendages using liposome carriers; also, when comparing the delivery of caffeine to appendage-free rat skin with that to normal skin, Illel et al (1991) found that the steady-state flux and the total diffusion in 24 h were 5x lower in follicle-free skin, supporting the importance of follicles in percutaneous absorption.

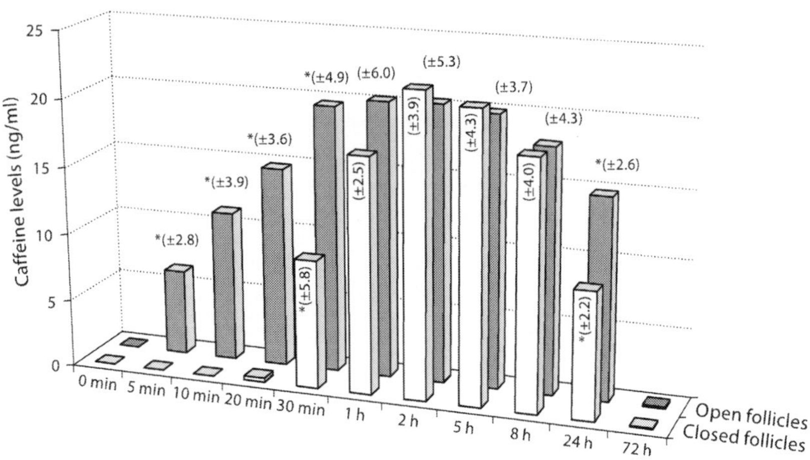

Figure 3 Caffeine levels in the blood after topical application with and without artificial blocking of the hair follicles. Data are expressed as mean±SD, with *p<0.05 considered significant (Teichmann et al, 2007).

The ability of a shampoo formulation containing caffeine as well as the fluorescent dye fluorescein to penetrate into hair follicles was investigated by in vivo laser scanning microscopy (Teichmann et al, 2007). A contact time of two minutes between the shampoo and the skin surface was sufficient for the formation to penetrate deeply into the hair follicles and to remain there for up to 48 hours, even after washing (Figure 3).

5. Transdermal and Transcutaneous Delivery of Caffeine

Delivery of therapeutic levels of caffeine into the systemic circulation via the transdermal route from a patch device has advantages including the ability to provide controlled, sustained release of drug through the skin, directly into the bloodstream and limiting the probability of caffeine intoxication occurrence. Another advantage of the transdermal route is that it bypasses first pass hepatic metabolism, whereby caffeine is caffeine is metabolized to three primary metabolites: paraxanthine (84%), theobromine (12%), and theophylline (4%). An acute overdose of caffeine, usually in excess of 400 milligrams (more than 3–4 cups of brewed coffee), can result in a state of central nervous system overstimulation or caffeine intoxication; however, significantly lower doses are generally delivered using the transdermal route. This could help circumvent overdosing and lead to fewer cases of caffeine addiction.

Although there is a rationale for the development of transdermal systems for delivering caffeine across skin, most of the published work carried out on the transdermal delivery of caffeine in fact involves its use as a model permeant and has become is a well-established benchmark for testing membranes, formulations and devices. Caffeine has a relatively high rate of permeation across skin despite its relatively high polarity which has been proposed as evidence that its route across skin cannot be entirely via the lipophilic transcellular route. Consequently, caffeine is often employed as a model permeant where mechanistic processes are under investigation. For example, appendage-free rat skin was compared to normal skin, using caffeine a model permeant (Illel et al, 1991). The steady-state flux and the total diffusion in 24 h were 5x lower in follicle-free skin, supporting the view that follicles have importance in percutaneous absorption.

5.1. Determination

The considerations for determining transdermal and transcutaneous delivery of compounds across skin are somewhat different to those in dermatological delivery, although the Franz diffusion cell (or variant thereof) is the standard apparatus. The objective is to achieve 0-order kinetics in the diffusion of a compound across skin. This is determined in terms of steady state flux (J_{ss}), which is related to its applied concentration and its inherent permeability (k_p) through the skin. The permeability of a material from an aqueous environment can be estimated from its octanol/water partition coefficient and its molecular weight. Based partially on data concerning caffeine, Rougier et al (1990) found that for a given thickness of stratum corneum and a given anatomical site, the penetration flux value of a substance depends only on its stratum corneum/vehicle partition coefficient. The log [octanol water partition coefficient] can be measured empirically or predicted from numerous software algorithms. Advanced Chemistry Development Labs. (Toronto, Canada) software gives a predicted value of -0.07 and, in its Sangster literature database, provides a measured value also of -0.07 - a rather hydrophilic molecule. The Potts and Guy equation gives a calculated value for k_p of 1.16×10^{-4} cm h^{-1} (Potts and Guy, 1992). Rougier et al (1990) reported that in vivo steady-state flux of penetration of a compound could be predicted from the simple measurement of the amount present in the stratum corneum after a contact time of 30 min.

5.2. Passive Diffusion

As a biological barrier the skin is notoriously variable. Akomeah et al (2007) reported high variability in CF permeation compared to the parabens may suggest the in vitro skin permeation of solutes becomes more sensitive to intra- and/or inter-subject variation in skin lipid content, appendageal density, and imperfections (pores, cracks) as the hydrophilic nature of the solute increases. Such variability in skin permeability suggests a difference in CF permeation kinetics relative to the parabens.

The permeation of caffeine across excised human upper leg skin, heat separated using conventional techniques to produce epidermal membranes was determined (Dias et al, 1999). In the experiments with saturated solutions, 1 mL was applied to the donor compartment. Where the products were tested 100 mg was applied to the surface of the membrane. The steady state flux for epidermal tissue can be estimated by linear regression through the data points obtained from 8 to 24 h was 6.65 ± 0.16 μg cm^{-2} h^{-1}. Based on a solubility of 25.8 mg mL^{-1} the permeability coefficient is 2.58 x 10^{-4} cm h^{-1}, comparing favourably with the value predicted by the Potts and Guy of 1.16 x 10^{-4} cm h^{-1}.

To obtain insight into the robustness of in vitro percutaneous absorption methodology, the intra- and inter-laboratory variation in this type of study was investigated in 10 European laboratories using caffeine, in addition to testosterone and benzoic acid as model permeants (van de Sandt et al, 2004). The mean maximum absorption rate of caffeine through human skin membranes was 2.24 ± 1.43 μg cm^{-2} h^{-1}, while the amount in the receptor fluid after 24 h was 24.5 ± 11.6% of the dose applied (9 laboratories). The mean maximum absorption rate of caffeine through rat skin (1 laboratory) was 6.82 μg cm^{-2} h^{-1} and the amount in the receptor fluid after 24 h was 53.7%. For both human and rat skin, the ratio TP:RF was only slightly higher than 1.0, indicating that only a small amount caffeine remained in the skin membrane after washing the application area. The total recovery of the radioactivity ranged between 66.4 and 100.6% (7 laboratories). Each laboratory performed 3–5 independent experiments. The CV value of the maximum absorption rate varied from 12.0% (lab 5) to 91.4% (lab 1). For the percentage in the receptor fluid (at 24 h), the CV values ranged between 5.4% (lab 5) and 66.0% (lab 1).

As a natural product, caffeine can be found in combination with other pharmacologically active agent within a plant or plant extract. When administered or consumed, a range of synergistic or complementary activities are experienced depending on the type and source of the plant. It was discussed earlier that, whether administered topically or orally, extract of *Camellia sinensis* exerts beneficial effects within the skin, inc cancer, and this seems to be at least partially attributable to the caffeine content. Delivering caffeine transdermally simultaneously with catechins was reported by Batchelder et al (2004).

Table 4. Solubility, steady state flux, permeability coefficient and cumulative permeation at 24h data for caffeine from different formulations saturated with green tea extract or guarana extract across full thickness porcine ear skin (n = 6, ± SEM)

Source	Vehicle	Solubility (mg cm^{-3})	J_{ss} (μg cm^{-2} h^{-1})	k_p (cm h^{-1})	Q_{24} (μg cm^{-2})
Green Tea *Camellia Sinensis*	Citrate phosphate buffer pH 6.5	15.96	5.5±0.5 x 10^{-3}	3.47±0.3 x 10^{-7}	0.32±0.05
	PEG 400	50.74	1.61±0.23	3.24±0.45 x 10^{-6}	46.8±3.4
	50:50 buffer: PEG400	31.09	7.78±1.39	2.50±0.45 x 10^{-4}	173±25
	DuroTak 387-2516 (1.35 mg cm^{-2})		1.05±1.1	-	28.4
Guarana *Paullinia Cupana*	Water	726.9	19.13±3.8	2.63±0.5 x 10^{-5}	419±103
	PEG 400	324.5	0.69±0.11	2.13±0.34 x 10^{-6}	8.34±1.33
	PG	320.4	3.13±0.52	9.8±1.6 x 10^{-6}	40.64±13.2
	DuroTak 387-2516 (5.55 mg cm^{-2})	-	1.83±0.7	-	73.4±15.6

PEG400 = polyethylene glycol 400.
PG = propylene glycol.

Transdermal delivery was determined across full thickness pig ear skin from saturated solutions of green tea extract in pH 5.5 citrate-phosphate buffer, polyethylene glycol 400 and a 50:50 mixture of the citrate phosphate buffer and polyethylene glycol. Caffeine was also delivered at concentrations above those previously reported, particularly from a model drug-in-adhesive patch (Table 4).

Caffeine is the major xanthine present in *Paullinia cupana*, commonly known as Guarana. Based on guarana featuring in putatively stimulating ingredients in a number of foods, drinks and dietary/herbal supplements, a recent paper investigated in vitro the transdermal delivery of the major pharmacologically active compounds (xanthines) contained in guarana extract (Heard et al, 2006). Saturated solutions of guarana were prepared in polyethylene glycol 400 (PEG400), propylene glycol (PG) and H_2O at 32°C. Transdermal delivery across full thickness pig ear skin was investigated in vitro using Franz-type diffusion cells, with reverse-phase HPLC being used for the quantification of the permeation of theobromine, theophylline, (+)-catechin and caffeine. For caffeine the greatest steady state flux was obtained from the water vehicle: 19 μg cm^{-2} h^{-1}, with 420 μg cm^{-2} permeating after 24 h. This was some 6 x times more than from a drug-in-adhesive patch and 10x greater than PG, a well-known penetration enhancer, and 50x that of the 'regular' excipient PEG400 (Table 4). A water vehicle also provided the greatest delivery of theobromine (μg cm^{-2} h^{-1}) and theophylline (0.022 μg cm^{-2} h^{-1}). An inverse relationship was noted between lipophilicity and k_p in each vehicle.

5.3. Commercial Formulations, Films and Devices

Other than cosmaceutical formulations (section 4.9), the products that are commercially available for the transdermal delivery of caffeine tend to be supplements based upon combinations of natural products, typically Guarana, which has a high content of caffeine and is incorporated in weight loss patches. Numerous examples are available, including: New Revolutionary Fat Patch (http://www.fatpatches.com), LePatch Diet Patch (http://www.vbyx.com/weight-loss-patch.htm), Premium Diet Patch (http:// www.slimstore.com/premiumdietpatch.htm). Typically, such web sites make extraordinary and unsubstantiated claims regarding the ability of such products to achieve significant weight loss.

However, the proposal that guarana extract (largely comprised of caffeine) is efficacious in weight loss is in fact borne out by recent findings by Andersen and Fogh (2001) and Lu et al (2007b), whereby caffeine was founds to significantly reduce fat cells. Treatment of SKH-1 mice orally with caffeine (0.1 mg mL^{-1} in the drinking water), voluntary running wheel exercise, or a combination of caffeine and exercise for 2 weeks (i) decreased the weight of the parametrial fat pads by 35, 62, and 77%, respectively; (ii) decreased the thickness of the dermal fat layer by 38,42, and 68%, respectively.

Caffeine absorption/desorption properties of cross-linked membranes prepared from poly(ethylene oxide-co-epichlorohydrin) P(EO/EP) copolymers were determined in order to study the possibility to apply these elastomeric membranes as reservoir in transdermal therapeutic systems (Mourges et al, 2004). The transport properties were simulated by using a series resistances model and considering the partition coefficient between the membrane and skin and a constant diffusion coefficient in both thin layers. From experimental and simulation results it was concluded that the main transport resistance is given by the skin but that the drug mass transfer could be enhanced by increasing the partition coefficient and the initial active molecule concentration in the membrane.

Nicoli et al (2004) investigated in vitro the transdermal permeation of caffeine from a bioadhesive film, using rabbit ear skin as a barrier. The effects of film composition and of the presence of penetration enhancers in the formulation were studied. The obtained fluxes were compared with those shown by commercial formulations. The results obtained indicate that the bioadhesive film gave rise to a higher transdermal permeation compared to a commercial gel and to a saturated solution of caffeine in water. Additionally, the film did not present the typical time lag of solution and gel. Another peculiar feature of the film is that the percentage of permeated active substance is much higher than that obtained from commercial formulations. It was possible to modulate caffeine permeation from the film by adding different enhancers/solvents.

5.4. Apnea in Neonates

Caffeine is commonly used in the treatment of preterm apnea, which can be defined as cessation of breathing resulting in pathological changes in heart rate and oxygen saturation, is a common occurrence in sick neonates. The skin of preterm neonates is more permeable compared to adults suggesting that transdermal drug delivery may offer advantages compared with the traditional intravenous or oral routes of drug administration used in neonatal intensive care. However, the skin of preterm infants varies considerably in its level of maturity.

To understand skin absorption in low birthweight infants (less than 1500 gm) with gestational age between 26 and 34 weeks, a group of 56 preterm babies was studied after percutaneous application of 7.5 mg twice daily of caffeine for babies with birthweight less than 1000 gm and 10 mg twice daily for babies with birthweight more than 1000 g (Amato et al, 1992; Amato et al, 1991). This study indicates an inverse relationship between gestational age and skin absorption of caffeine. Successful transdermal therapy in the neonate has been achieved with caffeine (and theophylline), with therapeutic blood drug concentrations being achieved for up to 7 days after topical application (Barrett and Rutter, 1994). However, the need for further development of neonatal transdermal delivery systems to provide a controlled rate of drug delivery was evident.

Premature neonates are often subjected to intensive clinical care and multiple drug therapy, which must be monitored carefully and continuously. The difficult and painful nature of repetitive blood sampling, particularly in this population, has provided considerable impetus for the development of non-invasive methods for monitoring blood analytes. The underdevelopment of the premature infant's epidermis, and more specifically the stratum corneum (SC), results in an increased permeability to molecular transport. A study by Sekkat et al (2002) investigated the feasibility of reverse iontophoretic monitoring of two model drugs, caffeine and theophylline. which are often administered to premature neonates. For this purpose, tape-stripped porcine skin, in vitro, which has been previously demonstrated to be an excellent model for premature neonatal skin, was employed. Reverse iontophoresis across intact membranes enabled a quantifiable extraction of both drugs predominantly at the cathode compartment. The mechanism of extraction of these essentially neutral drugs (caffeine and theophylline being uncharged at pH 7.4) was electroosmosis. However, when the SC was removed by progressive tape-stripping the amounts of drugs extracted by reverse iontophoresis were equivalent to those obtained by passive diffusion. In these circumstances, therefore, the benefit and usefulness of the applied electric field had been lost. In summary, the absence of an at least partially functional skin barrier obviates, in the case of neutral molecules, the control (and directional transport) offered by iontophoresis: in contrast, for ionized species, where the principal iontophoretic transport mechanism is electromigration, the approach should be valid.

Sekkat et al (2004) examined the passive permeation of caffeine, phenobarbital, and lidocaine across tape-stripped porcine skin barriers was measured in order to: (i) to validate differentially tape-stripped, porcine skin as an in vitro model for the evaluation of transdermal drug delivery to premature neonates, (ii) to determine whether the model could estimate neonatal skin permeability as a function of postconceptional age (PCA), and (iii) to demonstrate that iontophoretic delivery permits precise control of drug input independent of skin barrier function. For all drugs, passive permeation correlated with skin barrier function; that is, with transepidermal water loss (TEWL): $J_{ss} = A . \exp[B . TEWL]$. Combining this result with a previously derived dependence of TEWL upon the PCA of premature neonates in vivo allowed a relative value of J_{ss} to be predicted for a given PCA.

5.5. Vehicle/Formulation Effects

In the development of transdermal systems, much attention has focussed on the influence of the vehicle and formulation. Caffeine has been used widely as model compound. Frantz et al (1990) used acetone-deposited organic-solids of each chemical applied in 5-10 μg cm^{-2} amounts as C-14-labeled chemicals in 10 μL volumes of acetone. A rank order for the extent of penetration (percentage of dose absorbed over a uniform time period) was established using Fischer rat skin: caffeine > BA > SA > urea > ASA.

The interaction of a series of donor solvents including water, propylene glycol, two alcohols, four hydrocarbons, and light mineral oil with hairless mouse skin was studied in vitro by following the dermal absorption of caffeine as a reference compound (Rahman et al, 1992). Steady-state flux at saturation of caffeine was calculated for different donor solvents using solubility, donor concentration, and steady-state flux. The value of J_{ss} varied markedly with the donor solvent, indicating that caffeine permeation was significantly affected by vehicle/skin interactions. n-Propanol provided the highest value of J_{ss} among the various solvents. In the hydrocarbon series, the value of J_{ss} decreased exponentially as the chain length was increased. Propylene glycol yielded a lower value of J_{ss} compared to water. Light mineral oil provided the lowest value of flux at saturation, suggesting minimal interaction between this vehicle and mouse skin.

Liposomal vesicles was found to lead to deposition of 2260 μg cm^{-2} in the skin, some 3 times greater than from aqueous solution containing enhancers, the system which exhibited the second largest accumulation of drug in the skin (Touitou et al, 1994a). Using quantitative skin autoradiography, it was found that after 24 h, the greatest concentration of caffeine (280 μg g^{-1} tissue) was localized in the epidermis and the lowest amount (50 μg g^{-1} tissue) in the dermis. In addition, a relatively high concentration of caffeine was found in the appendages.

A series of copolymeric hydrogels were prepared from various molar ratios of N-isopropylacrylamide (NIPAAm), trimethyl acrylamidopropyl ammonium iodide (TMAAI), and 3-dimethyl (methacryloyloxyethyl) ammonium propane sulfonate (DMAPS) (Lee and Chiu, 2002a). Results showed that the swelling ratios of these copolymeric hydrogels increased with an increase of TMAAI content. The drug release behaviour of the ionic thermosensitive hydrogels related to their ionicity and drug types. Results indicated that the release ratio of caffeine in the hydrogels was not affected by the ionicity of hydrogels, but increased with increasing of the swelling ratio. The anionic solute (phenol red) strongly interacted with cationic hydrogel (very large K-d), so the phenol red release ratio in cationic gels was very low. On the other hand, CV was adsorbed only on the skin layer of the cationic hydrogel because of the charge repulsion, and released rapidly. Therefore the release ratio was highest for cationic hydrogel to cationic drug. In addition, the partition coefficients and the drug delivery behaviour of the present gels were also investigated.

The influence of various drugs with different charges on the drug release behaviour in porous ionic thermosensitive hydrogels was investigated (Lee and Chiu, 2002b). The present hydrogels were prepared from N-isopropylacrylamide (NIPAAm) and cationic monomer, trimethyl (acrylamido propyl) ammonium iodide (TMAAI), or anionic monomer, acrylic acid (AA), or zwitterionic monomer, N',N-dimethyl (acrylamido propyl) ammonium propane sulfonate (DMAAPS), or nonionic monomer, poly(ethylene glycol) methylether acrylate

(PEGMEA), and pore-forming agent, poly(ethylene glycol) (PEG) with different molecular weights.

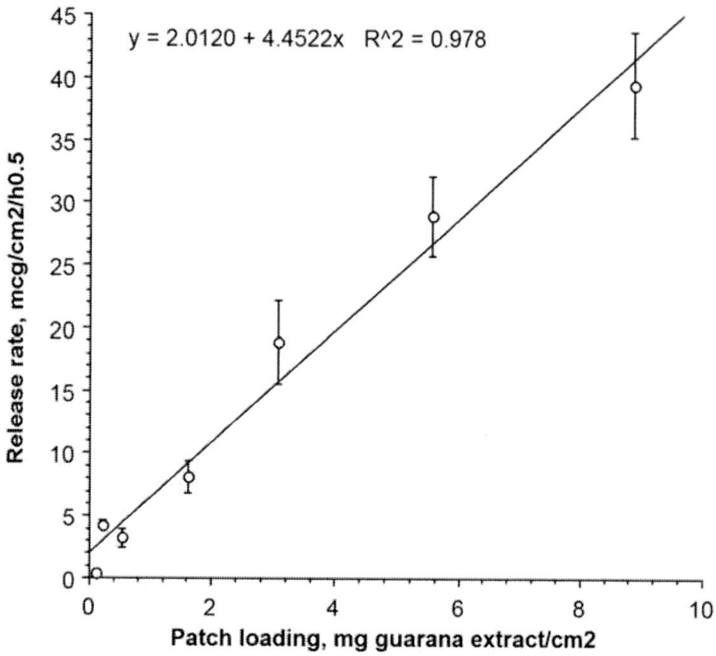

Figure 4. Correlation between guarana loading in model drug-in-adhesive patch and caffeine release rate of (n = 4, ± SD).

Caffeine as a non-ionic drug, crystal violet (CV) as a cationic drug solute, and phenol red as an anionic drug solute were chosen as model drugs to perform the drug release experiment. Results show that the release ratio of caffeine in the hydrogels is not affected by the ionicity of hydrogels. The CV strongly interacted with the anionic hydrogel; thus, the CV release ratio is very low. CV is only adsorbed on the skin layer of the cationic hydrogel due to charge repulsion and is released rapidly. The result of phenol red (anionic solute) release in the hydrogels is contrary to CV. In addition, the partition coefficients and the drug delivery behaviour of the present gels were also investigated.

In formulating a drug-in-adhesive patch for guarana, linear relationships between the amount of caffeine liberated from the model patches per unit time were observed up to 8.8 mg cm^{-2}, indicating 0-order release kinetics and no dump effect, despite the loadings being visibly in excess of the solubility (Heard et al 2006) (Figure 4).

5.6. Chemical Enhancement

For many drugs development of effective transdermal systems is unobtainable due to low rates of delivery. Caffeine exhibits relatively high rates of transdermal delivery. However, as it is very much a standard model permeant there are numerous papers in the literature that investigate the enhancement of penetration. Methods of enhancing the rate of delivery across skin are generally classed as either Physical/Biophysical (Section 5.7) of Chemical, where molecules are formulated with the drug or applied as a pre-treatment with the aim causing either a (reversible) modulation of the barrier function or as recent research suggests, by co-permeation or pull effect (Heard et al, 2006)

Bonina et al (1993) investigated the effects of Labrasol (LBS) (glycolysed ethoxylated C8/C10 glycerides), Labrafil (LBF) (glycolysed ethoxylated glycerides), Transcutol (TSC) (diethylene glycol monoethyl ether) and DPPG (propylene glycol dipelargonate) on the flux across excised human skin of the lipophilic testosterone (TST) and the hydrophilic caffeine (CAF) and on the affinity of the human stratum corneum for these drugs are compared taking propylene glycol (PG) and liquid petrolatum (LP) as reference vehicles. DPPG and LBF enhance CAF flux relative to PG while LBS and TSC increase the stratum corneum affinity for TST relative to LP. However, the materials tested enhance neither the flux of nor the stratum corneum affinity for both drugs with respect to either reference. On the other hand, a saturated solution of DPPG in PG enhances both properties for both drugs relative to PG. Such effects are ascribed to the ability of DPPG to interact with the lipid bilayers and to that of PG to promote DPPG penetration into stratum corneum and to create interaction sites in such a tissue.

Thakur et al (2007) examined the in vitro permeation of caffeine, theophylline, and theobromine across human skin with the aid of six chemical enhancers. It was found that oleic acid was the most potent enhancer for all three methylxanthines. Further optimization studies with different solvents showed that caffeine transport could be enhanced to give flux values up to 585 $\mu g\ cm^{-2}\ h^{-1}$. An additional study involving a buccal tissue equivalent showed that this membrane was more permeable than skin for all model actives tested and would offer an alternate way of delivery.

Touitou et al (1994b) reported high flux of caffeine through the skin was obtained from an aqueous solution containing an enhancing mixture of 20% Transcutol and 10% oleic acid. The presence of the enhancers resulted in caffeine flux 40 times greater than in their absence. The high flux of caffeine through the skin in vitro which was obtained using the enhancing composition was shown to be parallel to increased serum concentrations of drug in rats in vivo. Application of caffeine in aqueous solution containing enhancing mixture resulted in high serum concentrations of 50-60 $\mu g\ mL^{-1}$ after 1 h, which remained high for at least 12 h following. The use of phosphatidylcholine as a skin permeation enhancer was probed by Kim et al (2002) using caffeine as a model active. Lipid vesicles were prepared by the micro-the fluidization process and the encapsulation efficiency of caffeine was found to be very low due to the instability of the liposome structure and the water solubility of caffeine. However, the amount of absorbed caffeine was nearly independent of the encapsulation efficiency and the vesicle size, but increased with the increase of phosphatidylcholine concentration. These results indicated that phosphatidylcholine could act as a penetration enhancer, irrespective of its presence in vesicular form or solubilized form.

The enhancing activity of pre-treatment solutions consisting of monounsaturated (oleic acid) and palmitoleic and poly-unsaturated (linoleic) fatty acids in benzyl alcohol (BA) was determined on the permeation of caffeine, methyl paraben and butyl paraben by Nanayakkara et al (2005). At 5% (w/w) fatty acids in BA, only pre-treatment solutions containing palmitoleic acid (PA) increased the permeation of MP when compared to pre-treatment with

BA alone, whereas at higher concentrations (10 and 20% w/w), all pre-treatment solutions except 10% OA produced a significant increase in MP flux ($P < 0.05$). The general order of fatty acid effectiveness at any concentration was PA > LA > OA. At 20% (w/w) fatty acids in BA, all pre-treatment solutions significantly enhanced the permeation of all three penetrants ($P<0.05$) and an inverse relationship between penetrant lipophilicity and enhancement effect was observed. The permeation of BP was enhanced to a similar extent by all three fatty acids, whereas PA caused a significantly greater enhancement in the flux of both MP and CF when compared to CIA, LA and controls ($P<0.05$). It was proposed that the synergetic enhancement mechanisms of fatty acids and BA in pre-treatment solutions were augmenting the polar route by way of interactions with both polar and non-polar regions of stratum corneum lipids. The dermal absorption of caffeine and testosterone through SLS-treated human skin in vitro was studied by Wakefield et al (2006).

Southwell and Barry (1984) compared the permeation of model drugs, aspirin and caffeine, under the influence of penetration enhancers 2-pyrrolidone (2-P) and dimethylformamide (DMF), with their penetration through normal and fully hydrated cadaver skin. The in vitro finite dose technique was used to mimic physiological conditions and the drugs were applied in acetone. The penetration rate versus time profile for a finite dose reached a maximum rate J_{max} at time T_{max}. For caffeine 2-P significantly increased J_{max} and the % dose penetrated in 48 h ($P = 0.031$). DMF significantly increased J_{max}, decreased T_{max} and increased the % dose penetrated in 48 h ($P = 0.031$).

A number of natural products have been found to possess skin penetration enhancing properties, in particular, terpenes. A combination of terpenes in PG provided significant enhancement of the permeation of caffeine through hairless mouse skin. The most active compounds (+)-neomenthol and geraniol increased permeation by between 13-fold and 16-fold (Godwin and Michniak, 1999). In a study by Cole and Heard (2007) the potential of Aloe Vera juice as a skin permeation enhancer was probed. For caffeine and mefenamic acid no significant enhancements occurred between Aloe Vera and water a vehicles ($p > 0.05$) although for other permeants enhancements were observed, with enhancement potential dependent upon the molecular weight of the drug in formulation. A new mechanistic rationale is proposed whereby larger drug solutes inhibit the permeation of Aloe Vera components, but also are then able to interact more effectively with the enhancing factor and be subject to the pull effect.

5.7. Physical/Biophysical Enhancement

Physical/biophysical enhancements occur by disruption caused by physical contact or the application of an external energy source that is disruptive to the skin barrier function. One of the simplest methods is the process of occlusion, or the application of an air or fluid-tight seal over the area of application. A study by Treffel et al (1993) compared the in vitro permeation profiles of two molecules with different physicochemical properties under *occlusion* versus unoccluded conditions. Human abdominal skin samples were mounted on Dianorm(R) Teflon(R) macro 1 cells and Franz diffusion cells which represented occluded or unoccluded conditions, respectively. Our data show that occlusion increased the permeation of citropten (lipophilic compound) 1.6 times whereas that of caffeine (amphiphilic compound) remained unchanged. This lack of penetration enhancement under occluded conditions has also been observed by other authors, especially concerning hydrophilic and slightly lipophilic molecules. Our results support the view that occlusion does not necessarily increase the percutaneous absorption of a chemical.

The effect of increased *pressure* was investigated on the percutaneous absorption of caffeine in vitro on Franz diffusion cells, using excised human skin (Treffel et al 1992). 50 μΛ of either a 320 μg mL^{-1} or a 15 μg mL^{-1} acetone solution of caffeine were pipetted onto the surface of each skin sample, which represented caffeine skin deposits of 5 mug/cm2 and 240 μg cm^{-2} respectively. During each experiment, a pressure device delivering 0.25 bar over the atmospheric pressure was applied for the first 30 min on half of the cells. At 2, 4, 6, 8, 12 and 24 h the aqueous dermal bathing solution, containing 14 g L^{-1} albumin, was removed and assayed. With the applied dose of 5 μg cm^{-2} no statistical difference was found between the cumulated absorbed amount under atmospheric pressure and increased pressure. On the other hand, with the applied dose of 240 μg cm^{-2}, the permeation of caffeine was 1.8 times higher under increased pressure than the permeation under atmospheric pressure ($p < 0.05$). This enhancing effect of increased pressure was probably connected to either an improved transappendageal route during the percutaneous absorption process or a higher stratum corneum filling-up.

The effect of *heat* on the transdermal delivery of model penetrants of differing lipophilicity in vitro was investigated by Akomeah et al (2004). Saturated suspensions of the model penetrants; methyl paraben (MP), butyl paraben (BP) and caffeine (CF) in deionised water (vehicle) were used to attain maximal thermodynamic activity. Franz cell experiments were performed at temperatures ranging from 23 to 45 °C using the infinite dose method. Artificial membrane studies showed the penetrant diffusivity (diffusion coefficient) in the vehicle to be totally dependent on temperature and not changes in donor solubility. Epidermal flux and retention of all penetrants was found to be affected by temperature. The amount of penetrant retained in the epidermis was found to be in the order BP > CF > MP whilst the transdermal fluxes increased in the order MP > BP > CF with increasing receptor temperature. Estimated epidermal diffusivity of MP was found to be significantly affected by temperature ($P \leq 0.05$) compared to BP and CF. Using Arrhenius plots, a lower activation energy was recorded for CF and may suggest a difference in permeation kinetics compared to the other penetrants.

The effect of *solar irradiation* on ex vivo dermatomed hairless rat skin samples maintained in culture on flow-through diffusion cells for at least 24 h was evaluated by 3-(4,5-dimethylthiazol-2-yl)-2,5-diphenyl tetrazolium bromide assay and by histological observations (Gelis et al., 2002). Transepidermal water loss (TEWL) measurements and kinetic analysis of the permeation of both tritiated water and ^{14}C caffeine through the skin were performed after full-spectrum solar exposure involving the use of a xenon arc solar simulator. After a UV exposure of less than 420 mJ cm^2, skin integrity and permeation of both water and caffeine did not change significantly. In contrast, after a 420 mJ cm^{-2} UV exposure, the epidermis appeared more contracted, associated with an increase of 55% of TEWL and 220% of the skin permeation of tritiated water after 6 h. The data suggested a dramatic alteration of the skin barrier integrity. Moreover, the flux of ^{14}C caffeine increased rapidly by 338% of the absorption of water 12 h after irradiation. These results reveal the presence of a threshold UV exposure that would not modify skin penetration.

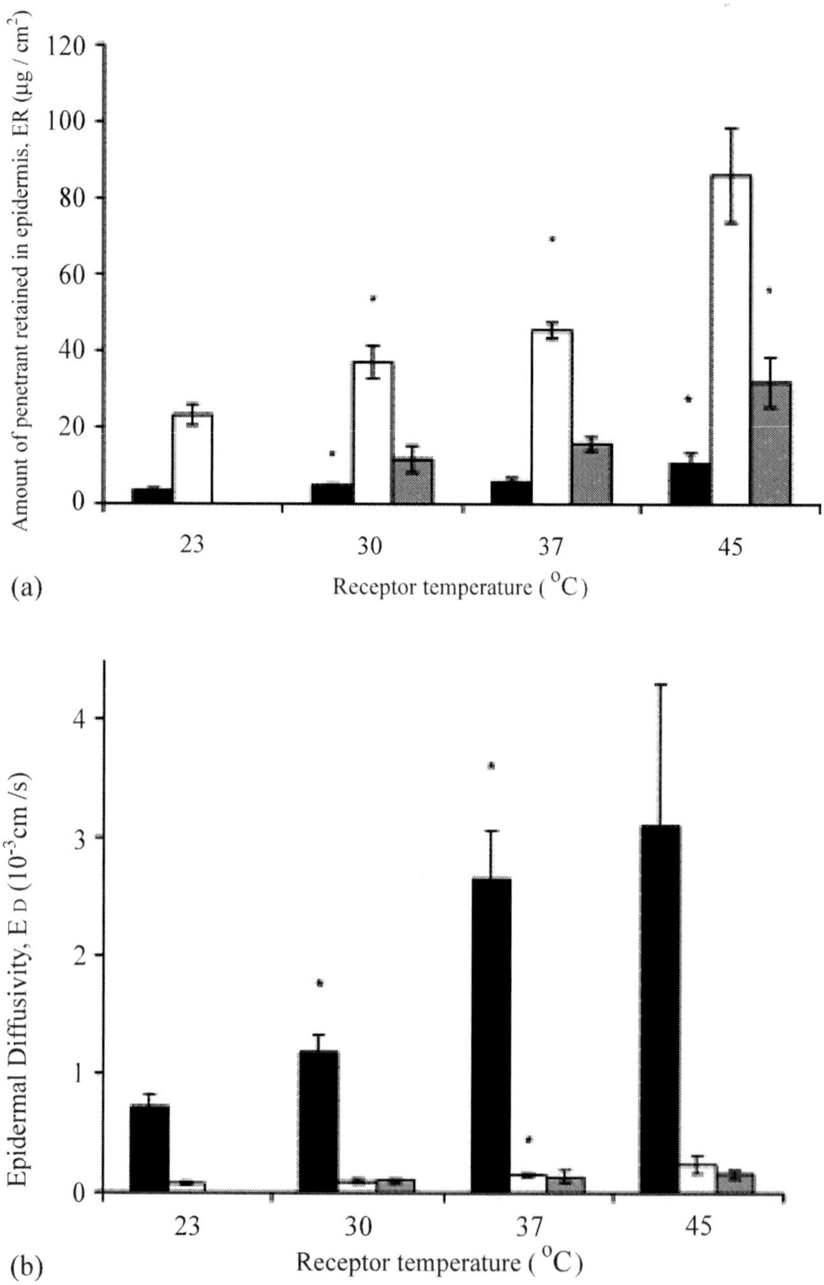

*Significantly different from the amount of penetrant retained/diffusivity at the lower preceding receptor temperature for same penetrant ($p \leq 0.05$) (Akomeah et al 2004).

Figure 5. Effect of temperature on (a) epidermal retention (b) epidermal diffusivity of methyl paraben, butyl parabens and caffeine at different temperatures (mean ± SD, ≥3).

The roles played by various ultrasound-related phenomena, including cavitation, thermal effects, generation of convective velocities, and mechanical effects, in the enhancement of transdermal drug delivery by *sonophoresis* (Mitragotri et al., 1995). Our experimental findings suggest that among all the ultrasound-related phenomena evaluated, cavitation plays the dominant role in sonophoresis using therapeutic ultrasound (frequency range, 1-3 MHz; intensity range, 0-2 W cm^{-2}). Furthermore, confocal microscopy results indicate that cavitation occurs in the keratinocytes of the stratum corneum upon ultrasound exposure. It is hypothesized that oscillations of the cavitation bubbles induce disorder in the stratum corneum lipid bilayers, thereby enhancing transdermal transport. Evidence supporting this hypothesis is presented using skin electrical resistance measurements. Finally, a theoretical model is developed to predict the effect of ultrasound on the transdermal transport of drugs. The model predicts that sonophoretic enhancement depends most directly on the passive permeant diffusion coefficient, rather than on the permeability coefficient through the skin. Specifically, permeants passively diffusing through the skin at a relatively slow rate are expected to be preferentially enhanced by ultrasound. The experimentally measured sonophoretic transdermal transport enhancement for seven permeants, including estradiol, testosterone, progesterone, corticosterone, benzene, butanol, and caffeine, agree quantitatively with the model predictions. These experimental and theoretical findings provided quantitative guidelines for estimating the efficacy of sonophoresis in enhancing transdermal drug delivery.

The effect of low-frequency *sonophoresis* on fentanyl and caffeine permeation through human and hairless rat skin was studied in vitro was studied by Boucard et al. (2001). Experiments were performed using 20 kHz ultrasound applied at either continuous or discontinuous mode and with an average intensity of 2.5 W cm^{-2}. The results showed that low-frequency ultrasound enhanced the transdermal transport of both fentanyl and caffeine across human and hairless rat skin. This was explained by both increasing flux during sonication and shortening the lag time. Discontinuous mode was found to be more effective in increasing transdermal penetration of fentanyl while transdermal transport of caffeine was enhanced by both continuous and pulsed mode. Histological and electron microscopy studies showed that human and hairless rat skin was unaffected by ultrasound exposure. Further studies will be necessary to determine the relative contribution of ultrasound parameters in low-frequency ultrasound-induced percutaneous enhancement of drug transport.

Sonophoresis were directly compared against chemical enhancers for their effects on the transdermal permeation of caffeine and morphine through hairless mouse skin in vitro (Monti et al., 2001). The three chemical enhancers, tested in combination with propylene glycol, were benzalkonium chloride oleyl alcohol and oc-terpineol. Low-frequency (40 KHz) low-power (< 0.5 W cm^{-2}) and high-frequency ultrasound (1.5-3.0 MHz) ultrasound was examined. The high-frequency ultrasound of caffeine did not result in statistically significant enhancement of caffeine, while low frequency produced a small but significant increase of the enhancement factor. However, the effect of ultrasound on caffeine permeation was lower than that produced by chemical enhancers, in particular oleic acid. The conclusion was that sonophoretic delivery of caffeine is inferior to the use of oleic acid.

5.8. Caffeine as a Test Substance Comparing Different Membrane Types

The validity of in vitro methodologies for modelling in vivo skin permeation is of clear importance in the development of topical drug delivery systems. Over the years membranes from many different sources have been proposed and, as illustrated below, caffeine has featured as a benchmark model permeant. However, even the use of human skin membranes is far from straightforward or unified. Full thickness, heat separated epidermis, dermatomed skin have all been used. The intrinsic variation of permeability within human skin complicates the picture even further.

Alhough widely used as a model permeant, caffeine (by virtue of its polarity) does not behave typically and abnormal distribution in k_p data has been reported (Khan et al., 2005). From another angle, Akomeah et al. (2007) probed the *intrinsic variability in human skin* permeability associated with model penetrants of differing lipophilicity, caffeine, methyl paraben, and butyl paraben was examined in a standardized intra-laboratory study (Franz cell experiments) using epidermal tissue from various human donors. The high variability in CF permeation compared to the parabens suggested the in vitro skin permeation of solutes becomes more sensitive to intra- and/or inter-subject variation in skin lipid content, appendageal density, and imperfections (pores, cracks) as the hydrophilic nature of the solute increases. Such variability in skin permeability suggests a difference in caffeine permeation kinetics relative to the parabens (Figure 5).

The effect of *skin thickness* on the percutaneous penetration and distribution of test compounds with varying physicochemical properties using in vitro systems was also investigated recently (Wilkinson et al., 2006). Percutaneous penetration of caffeine testosterone and propoxur was determined through skin of varying thicknesses under occluded conditions was measured using flow through cells for 8-24 h. The maximum flux of caffeine was increased with decreasing skin thickness, although these differences were found to be non-significant. The presence of caffeine in the skin membrane was not altered by skin thickness. A complex relationship exists between skin thickness, lipophilicity and percutaneous penetration and distribution.

Racial differences in the in vivo percutaneous absorption of caffeine were probed by Lotte et al. (1993]. Black, Caucasian and Asian subjects were treated with a 30 min topical application on the upper outer arm of 1 μmol cm^{-2} ^{14}C-labeled permeant, and the percutaneous absorption was determined by both urinary excretion and stripping technique. Amounts of caffeine absorbed were 1.06 +/- 0.17% (A), 1.01 +/- 0.19% (B) and 0.96 +/- 0.12% (C). No statistical difference ($P > 0.05$) was found in percutaneous absorption of benzoic acid, caffeine or acetylsalicylic acid between the various groups.

Southwell and Barry (1984) compared the permeation of model drugs, aspirin and caffeine, under the influence of penetration enhancers 2-pyrrolidone (2-P) and dimethylformamide (DMF), with their penetration through normal and fully *hydrated* cadaver skin. Hydration significantly increased ($P = 0.031$) J_{max} and % dose penetrated in 48 h for caffeine. Aspirin data followed this same trend. The apparent diffusion coefficient of aspirin and caffeine through human skin increased with hydration. As hydration appears to act on skin lipids, these drugs probably penetrate, at least in part, through a lipid route in the stratum corneum.

In vivo, the situation if further complicated by clearance due to cutaneous blood flow. Auclair et al. (1991) used a bipediculated dorsal flap was created in the *hairless rat*. Results showed that a hydrophilic compound poorly absorbed (urea) was insensitive to cutaneous blood flow modifications whereas compounds readily absorbed (caffeine, amphiphilic; urea on stripped skin) or slightly absorbed (progesterone, lipophilic) exhibited local concentration phenomena in relation to cutaneous blood flow lowering. Hairless rat was also used in vivo (Rougier et al. 1990) to determine that for a given thickness of stratum corneum and a given anatomical site, the penetration flux value of a substance depends only on its stratum corneum/vehicle partition coefficient. A combination of terpenes in propylene glycol provided significant enhancement of the permeation of caffeine through *hairless mouse* skin. The most active compounds (+)-neomenthol and geraniol increased permeation by between 13-fold and 16-fold (Godwin and Michniak, 1999).

Porcine skin has become a common model for human skin in drug delivery experiments and used in the determination of transdermal delivery of caffeine from green tea (Batchelder et al. 2004), Guarana (Heard et al., 2006) and as a model permeant using Aloe vera as a potential penetration enhancer (Cole and Heard, 2007). The *isolated perfused porcine skin flap* (IPPSF) was proposed as an alternative in vitro tool for examining the pharmacokinetics and mechanisms of percutaneous absorption (Carver et al., 1989).

Netzlaff et al. (2006) studied the suitability of *bovine udder skin* as a possible replacement material for use in in vitro permeability tests. We investigated the barrier strength of bovine udder skin against four different substances, and its histology and lipid profile, in comparison with pig skin and heat-separated human epidermis. Pig and human skin were found to be equally permeable, whilst bovine udder skin seemed to exhibit a weaker, but less variable, barrier against caffeine, benzoic acid, testosterone, and flufenamic acid.

Cultured skin has received much recent attention. Gay et al. (1992) used caffeine and 3 other model permeants to propose that an organotypic skin culture (living skin equivalent) can be used as model systems for studying certain aspects of chemically induced dermal irritation. In all cases the LSE was more permeable than human skin with k_p values ranging from $0.56 \pm 0.10 \times 10^{-3}$ cm h^{-1} for hydrocortisone to $29 \pm 5 \times 10^{-3}$ cm h^{-1} for water penetration.

Lotte et al. (2002) examined the reproducibility of various industrial reconstructed human skin models. The reproducibility of 3 industrial models - EpiDerm, Episkin and SkinEthic - was tested regarding the permeation and skin absorption of caffeine (as well as lauric acid and mannitol. For all the models, the intra-batch reproducibility was greater than the inter-batch reproducibility. According to the batches tested, the larger difference in terms of reproducibility between the 3 models was observed in the case of mannitol, a very poor permeant. In this case, the best reproducibility was observed with EpiDerm and Episkin. Moreover, the rank order of the 3 compounds applied, in terms of permeation and skin absorption, was the same as that expected from ex vivo human skin. Such results revealed human skin models as a promising means to test in vitro permeation and percutaneous absorption of topical products.

EpiDerm® and Episkin® were also the subject of an examination Dreher et al. (2002), involving the influence on caffeine's and a-tocopherol's cutaneous bioavailability of cosmetic vehicles such as a water-in-oil emulsion, an oil-in-water emulsion, a liposome dispersion and a hydrogel applied at finite dose using the reconstructed human skin models. It was demonstrated that the rank order of solute permeability could be correctly predicted when the preparation was applied at a finite dose in human skin models, at least when solutes with far different physicochemical properties such as caffeine and alpha-tocopherol were used.

Exposure to chemicals absorbed by the skin can threaten human health. Schaefer-Korting measured the permeation of the OECD standard compounds, caffeine and testosterone, through commercially available *reconstructed human epidermis* (RHE) RHE models was compared to that of human epidermis and animal skin (Schafer-Korting et al., 2006). In comparison to human epidermis, the permeation of the chemicals was overestimated when using RHE. The following ranking of the permeation coefficients for testosterone was obtained: SkinEthic® > EpiDerm®, Episkin® > human epidermis, bovine udder skin, pig skin. The ranking for caffeine was: SkinEthic, EPISKIN > bovine udder skin, EpiDerm, pig skin, human epidermis. The inter-laboratory and intra-laboratory reproducibility was good. Long and variable lag times, which are a matter of concern when using human and pig skin, did not occur with RHE.

Sometimes workers use *synthetic membranes* as a model for skin delivery, in the belief that a simple polymeric matrix can be a suitable model for the more heterogenous and complex skin. The work of Dias et al. (1999) showed that the diffusion of caffeine in a saturated solution through epidermal tissue was significantly slower than through the synthetic membranes. The steady state flux for epidermal tissue and silicone values were 6.65±0.16 and 57.55±1.13 μg cm^{-2} h^{-1} respectively. Using the solubility of 25.8 mg mL^{-1}, these values can be converted to permeability coefficients of, respectively: 2.58 x 10^{-4} and 2.23 x 10^{-3} cm h^{-1}. A comparison between the epidermal permeation and silicone permeation showed no correlation. The conclusion was that a synthetic membrane cannot be used predictively to estimate the efficiency of formulations on skin.

5.9. Reverse Transcutaneous

The outward migration of molecules through the skin has been recognised for a number of years as potentially the basis of a biomedical monitoring system. Conner et al. (1991) proposed a Bandaid-like transcutaneous chemical collection device to study the phenomenon of outward transcutaneous chemical migration, allowing collection and quantitation of chemicals that diffuse directly through the skin from within the body. Devices were placed on the skin of normal male volunteers. Twenty-four hours later subjects took caffeine by mouth. Blood samples were collected and TCD were removed at various times after drug intake and analyzed by HPLC for caffeine. Studies of the sweating effect were carried out in a similar manner, except that one arm of each subject was maintained at 40-degrees-C to induce local sweating, the other arm acted as a non-sweating control. The amount of caffeine collected was linearly related to the AUC. Sweating seemed to have a large (40%) contribution to transdermal collection in the early period (5.5 h) of the study, but this difference was much less (14%) at longer collection times (10 h).

Conclusion

There is clearly much interest in the study of the delivery of caffeine into and across the skin. We have seen that caffeine offers some important pharmacologic activities in the context of numerous dermatological disorders. Stimulant, weight loss and anti-cellulite products comprise the main commercial products containing caffeine. Much of the published articles relate to caffeine as a model permeant in the investigation of other variables and techniques in topical drug delivery investigations, this practice is expected to continue even though the route through the skin taken by this drug may be dissimilar to other test compounds.

References

Ademola JI, Wester RC, Maibach HI. Cutaneous metabolism of theophylline by the human skin. *Journal Of Investigative Dermatology* 1992, 98, 310-314.

Akomeah FK, Nazir T, Martin GP, Brown MB Effect of heat on the percutaneous absorption and skin retention of three model penetrants. *European Journal Of Pharmaceutical Sciences* 2004, 21, 337-345.

Akomeah, FK, Martin, GP, Brown, MB. Variability in human skin permeability in vitro: Comparing penetrants with different physicochemical properties. *Journal Of Pharmaceutical Sciences* 2007, 96, 824-834.

Amato, M, Isenschmid, M, Huppi, P. Percutaneous CAFFEINE application in the treatment of neonatal apnea. *European Journal Of Pediatrics* 1991, 150, 592-594.

Amato M, Huppi P, Isenschmid M, Schneider H. Developmental aspects of percutaneous caffeine absorption in premature-infants. *American Journal of Perinatology* 1992, 9, 431-434.

Andersen, T, Fogh, J. Weight loss and delayed gastric emptying following a South American herbal preparation in overweight patients. *J. Hum. Nutr. Diet.* 2001, 14, 243-50.

Auclair F, Besnard M, Dupont C, Wepierre J. Importance of blood-flow to the local-distribution of drugs after percutaneous-absorption in the bipediculated dorsal flap of the hairless rat. *Skin Pharmacology* 1991, 4, 1-8 1991.

Barrett, D, Rutter, N. Transdermal delivery and the premature neonate. *Critical Reviews In Therapeutic Drug Carrier Systems* 1994, 11, 1-30.

Batchelder RJ, Calder RJ, Thomas CP, Heard CM In vitro transdermal delivery of the major catechins and caffeine from extract of Camellia sinensis. *International Journal Of Pharmaceutics* 2004, 283, 45-51.

Bertin, C, Zunino, H, Pittet, JC, Beau, P, Pineau, P, Massonneau, M, Robert, C, Hopkins, J. A double-blind evaluation of the activity of an anti-cellulite product containing retinol, caffeine, and ruscogenine by a combination of several non-invasive methods. *Journal Of Cosmetic Science* 2001, 52, 199-210.

Bonina FP, Carelli V, Dicolo G, Montenegro L, Nannipieri E. Vehicle effects on in-vitro skin permeation of and stratum-corneum affinity for model-drugs caffeine and testosterone. *International Journal Of Pharmaceutics* 1993, 100, 41-47.

Boucaud, A, Machet, L, Arbeille, B, Machet, MC, Sournac, M, Mavon, A, Patat, F, Vaillant, L. In vitro study of low-frequency ultrasound-enhanced transdermal transport of fentanyl and caffeine across human and hairless rat skin. *International Journal Of Pharmaceutics* 2001, 228, 69-77.

Carver MP, Williams PL, Riviere JE. The isolated perfused porcine skin flap .3. percutaneous-absorption pharmacokinetics of organophosphates, steroids, benzoic-acid, and *caffeine Toxicology And Applied Pharmacology* 1989, 97, 324-337.

Chambinremoussenard, O, Treffel, P, Bechtel, Y, Agache, P. Surface recovery and stripping methods to quantify percutaneous-absorption of caffeine in humans. *Journal Of Pharmaceutical Sciences* 1993, 82, 1099-1101.

Cole, L, Heard, C. Skin permeation enhancement potential of Aloe Vera and a proposed mechanism of action based upon size exclusion and pull effect. *International Journal Of Pharmaceutics* 2007, 333, 10-16.

Conner DP, Millora E, Zamani K, Nix D, Almirez RG, Rhynekirsch P, Peck CC. Transcutaneous chemical collection of caffeine in normal subjects - relationship to area under the plasma concentration-time curve and sweat production. *Journal Of Investigative Dermatology* 1991, 96, 186-190.

Deplanque, G, Vincent, F, Mah-Becherel, MCM, Cazenave, JP, Bergerat, JP, Klein-Soyer, C. caffeine does not cause override of the G2/M block induced by UVc or gamma radiation in normal human skin fibroblasts. *British Journal Of Cancer* 2000, 83, 346-353.

Dias, M, Farinha, A, Faustino, E, Hadgraft, J, Pais, J, Toscano, C. Topical delivery of caffeine from some commercial formulations. *International Journal Of Pharmaceutics* 1999, 182, 41-47.

Dreher, F, Fouchard, F, Patouillet, C, Andrian, M, Simonnet, JT, Benech-Kieffer, F. Comparison of cutaneous bioavailability of cosmetic preparations containing caffeine or alpha-tocopherol applied on human skin models or human skin ex vivo at finite doses. *Skin Pharmacology And Applied Skin Physiology* 2002, 15, 40-58.

Feldman, RJ, Maibach, HI. Absorption of some organic compounds through the skin in man. *J. Invest. Dermatol.* 54, 399-404, 1970.

Frantz SW, Dittenber DA, Eisenbrandt DL, Watanabe PG. Evaluation of a flow-through in vitro skin penetration chamber method using acetone-deposited organic-solids. *Journal Of Toxicology-Cutaneous And Ocular Toxicology* 1990, 9, 277-299.

Fujiki H, Suganuma M, Okabe S, Sueoka E, Suga K, Imai K, Nakachi K, Kimura S. Mechanistic findings of green tea as cancer preventive for humans. *Proceedings of the society for experimental biology and medicine* 1999, 220, 225-228.

Gay R, Swiderek M, Nelson D, Ernesti A. The living skin equivalent as a model invitro for ranking the toxic potential of dermal irritants. *Toxicology in vitro* 1992, 6, 303-315.

Gee, GC, Method for treatment of sores and lesions of the skin. International Application No. PCT/US2004/019892 *Priority Date* 23.06.2003

Gelis, C, Mavon, A, Delverdier, M, Paillous, N, Vicendo, P. Modifications of in vitro skin penetration under solar irradiation: Evaluation on flow-through diffusion cells. *Photochemistry And Photobiology* 2002, 75, 598-604.

Godwin, DA, Michniak, BB. Influence of drug lipophilicity on terpenes as transdermal penetration enhancers. *Drug Development And Industrial Pharmacy* 1999, 25, 905-915.

Heard, CM, Johnson, S, Moss, G, Thomas, CP. In vitro transdermal delivery of caffeine, theobromine, theophylline and catechin from extract of Guarana, *Paullinia Cupana*. *International Journal Of Pharmaceutics* 2006, 317, 26-31.

Heard, CM, Kung, D, Thomas, CP. Skin penetration enhancement of mefenamic acid by ethanol and 1,8-cineole can be explained by the pull effect, *International Journal of Pharmaceutics*. 2006, 321, 167-170.

Hikima, T, Tojo, K, Maibach HI. Skin metabolism in transdermal therapeutic systems. *Skin Pharmacology And Physiology* 2005, 18, 153-159.

Hoshino, H, Tanooka, H. Caffeine enhances skin tumor-induction in mice. *Toxicology Letters* 1979, 4, 83-85 1979.

Huang, MT, Xie, JG, Wang, ZY, Ho, CT, Leu, YR, Wang, CX, Hard, GC, Conney, AH. Effects of tea, decaffeinated tea, and caffeine on UVB light-induced complete carcinogenesis in SKH-1 mice: Demonstration of caffeine as a biologically important constituent of tea. *Cancer Research* 1997, 57, 2623-2629.

Illel B, Schaefer, H. Wepierre J, Doucet O. Follicles play an important role in percutaneous-absorption. *Journal Of Pharmaceutical Sciences* 1991, 80, 424-427.

Itoh, T, Linn, S, Kamide, R, Tokushige, H, Katori, N, Hosaka, Y, Yamaizumi, M. Xeroderma pigmentosum variant heterozygotes show reduced levels of recovery of replicative DNA synthesis in the presence of caffeine after ultraviolet irradiation. *Journal Of Investigative Dermatology* 2000, 115, 981-985.

Khan, GM, Frum, Y, Sarheed, O, Eccleston, GM, Meidan, VM. Assessment of drug permeability distributions in two different model skins. *International Journal Of Pharmaceutics* 2005, 303, 81-87.

Kim C, Shim J, Han S, Chang I. The skin-permeation-enhancing effect of phosphatidylcholine: caffeine as a model active ingredient. *Journal Of Cosmetic Science* 2002, 53, 363-374.

Koo, S-W, Hirakawa, S, Fujii, S, Kawasumi M, Nghiem P. Protection from photodamage by topical application of caffeine after ultraviolet irradiation. *Photobiology*, 2007, 156, 957-964.

Koot, P, Deurenberg, P. Comparison of changes in energy-expenditure and body temperatures after caffeine consumption. *Annals of Nutrition and Metabolism* 1995, 39, 135-142.

Kramata, P, Lu, YP, Lou, YR, Cohen, JL, Olcha, M, Liu, S, Conney, AH. Effect of administration of caffeine or green tea on the mutation profile in the p53 gene in early mutant p53-positive patches of epidermal cells induced by chronic UVB-irradiation of hairless SKH-1 mice. *Carcinogenesis* 2005, 26, 1965-1974.

Lee, WF, Chiu, RJ. Thermoreversible hydrogel. XVII. Investigation of the drug release behavior for [N-isopropylacrylamide-co-trimethyl acrylamidopropyl ammonium iodide-co-3-dimethyl (methacryloyloxyethyl) ammonium propane sulfortate] copolymeric hydrogels. *Journal Of Applied Polymer Science* 2002a, 86, 1592-1598.

Lee WF, Chiu RJ. Investigation of charge effects on drug release behavior for ionic thermosensitive hydrogels. *Materials Science and Engineering C-Biomimetic And Supramolecular Systems* 2002b, 20, 161-166.

Lehmann AR, Kirkbell S, Effects of caffeine and theophylline on DNA-synthesis in unirradiated and UV-irradiated mammalian-cells. *Mutation Research* 26 (2): 73-82 1974

Levischaffer, F, Touitou, E. Xanthines inhibit 3t3 fibroblast proliferation. *Skin Pharmacology* 1991, 4, 286-290.

Lotte C, Wester RC, Rougier A, Maibach HI. Racial-differences in the in vivo percutaneous-absorption of some organic-compounds - a comparison between black, caucasian and asian subjects. *Archives Of Dermatological Research* 1993, 284, 456-459.

Lotte C, Patouillet C, Zanini M, Messager A, Roguet R Permeation and skin absorption: Reproducibility of various industrial reconstructed human skin models. *Skin Pharmacology and Applied Skin Physiology* 2002, 15, 18-30.

Lou, YR, Lu, YP, Xie, JG, Huang, MT, Conney, AH. Effects of oral administration of tea, decaffeinated tea, and caffeine on the formation and growth of tumours in high-risk SKH-1 mice previously treated with ultraviolet B light. *Nutrition And Cancer-An International Journal* 1999, 33, 146-153.

Lu, YP, Lou, YR, Li, XH, Xie, JG, Brash, D, Huang, MT, Conney, AH. Stimulatory effect of oral administration of green tea or CAFFEINE on ultraviolet light-induced increases in epidermal wild-type p53, p21(WAF1/CIP1), and apoptotic sunburn cells in SKH-1 mice. *Cancer Research* 2000, 60, 4785-4791.

Lu, YP, Lou, YR, Li, XH, Xie, JG, Lin, Y, Shih, WJ, Conney, AH. Stimulatory effect of topical application of caffeine on UVB-induced apoptosis in mouse skin. *Oncology* Research 2001, 13, 61-70.

Lu, YP, Lou, YR, Xie, JG, Peng, QY, Liao, I, Yang, CS, Huang, MT, Conney, AH. Topical applications of caffeine or (-)-epigallocatechin gallate (EGCG) inhibit carcinogenesis and selectively increase apoptosis in UVB-induced skin tumors in mice. *Proceedings Of The National Academy Of Sciences Of The United States Of America* 2002, 99, 12455-12460.

Lu, YP, Lou, YR, Peng, QY, Xie, JG, Conney, AH. Stimulatory effect of topical application of caffeine on UVB-induced apoptosis in the epidermis of p53 and Bax knockout mice. *Cancer Research*, 2004, 64, 5020-5027.

Lu, YP, Lou, YR, Liao, J, Xie, JG, Peng, QY, Yang, CS, Conney, AH. Administration of green tea or caffeine enhances the disappearance of UVB-induced patches of mutant p53 positive epidermal cells in SKH-1 mice. *Carcinogenesis* 2005, 26, 1465-1472.

Lu, YP, Lou, YR, Xie, JG, Peng, QY, Zhou, S, Lin, Y, Shih, WJ, Conney, AH. Caffeine and caffeine sodium benzoate have a sunscreen effect, enhance UVB-induced apoptosis, and inhibit UVB-induced skin carcinogenesis in SKH-1 mice. *Carcinogenesis,* 2007a, 28, 199-206.

Lu, YP, Nolan, B, Lou, YR, Peng, QY, Wagner, GC, Conney, AH. Voluntary markedly exercise together with oral caffeine stimulates UVB light-induced apoptosis and decreases tissue fat in SKH-1 mice. *Proceedings Of The National Academy Of Sciences Of The United States Of America* 2007b, 104, 12936-12941.

Mitani, H, Ryu, A, Suzuki, T, Yamashita, M, Arakane, K, Koide, C. Topical application of plant extracts containing xanthine derivatives can prevent UV-induced wrinkle formation in hairless mice. *Photodermatology Photoimmunology and Photomedicine*, 2007, 23, 86-94.

Mitragotri, S, Edwards, DA, Blankschtein, D, Langer, R. Mechanistic study of ultrasonically-enhanced transdermal drug-delivery. *Journal of Pharmaceutical Sciences* 1995, 84, 697-706.

Monti, D, Giannelli, R, Chetoni, P, Burgalassi, S. Comparison of the effect of ultrasound and of chemical enhancers on transdermal permeation of caffeine and morphine through hairless mouse skin in vitro. *International Journal Of Pharmaceutics* 2001, 229, 131-137.

Mourgues A, Charmette C, Sanchez J, Marti-Mestres G, Gramain P. EO/EP copolymer membranes as reservoir in a transdermal therapeutic system for caffeine delivery - Modeling and simulation. *Journal Of Membrane Science* 2004, 241, 297-304.

Nanayakkara, GR, Bartlett, A, Forbes, B, Marriott, C, Whitfield, PJ, Brown, MB. The effect of unsaturated fatty acids in benzyl alcohol on the percutaneous permeation of three model penetrants. *International Journal Of Pharmaceutics* 2005, 301, 129-139.

Nangia, A, Camel, E, Berner, B, Maibach, H. Influence of skin irritants on percutaneous-absorption. *Pharmaceutical Research* 1993, 10, 1756-1759.

Narayanan, PK, Rudnick, JM, Walthers, EA, Crissman, HA. Modulation in cell cycle and cyclin B1 expression in irradiated HeLa cells and normal human skin fibroblasts treated with staurosporine and caffeine. *Experimental Cell Research* 1997, 233, 118-127.

Netzlaff, F, Schaefer, UF, Lehr, CM, Meiers, P, Stahl, J, Kietzmann, M, Niedorf, F. Comparison of bovine udder skin with human and porcine skin in percutaneous permeation experiments. *Alternatives To Laboratory Animals* 2006, 34, 499-513.

Nicoli S, Amoretti V, Colombo P, Santi P Bioadhesive transdermal film containing caffeine. *Skin Pharmacology and Physiology* 2004, 17, 119-123.

PharmGkb. The Pharmacogenetics and Pharmacogenomics Knowledge Base (http://www.pharmgkb.org). Accessed 7 December 2007.

Potts, M. Use of caffeine in the treatment of herpes simplex virus infections (WO/1991/007969).

Potts, RO, Guy RH. Predicting skin permeability. *Pharmaceutical Research* 1992, 9, 663-669.

Rahman, MS, Gallo, MA, Umbreit, TH, Zatz, JL. Investigation of the invitro interaction of various vehicles with hairless mouse skin. *Journal Of The Society Of Cosmetic Chemists* 1992, 43, 251-258.

Rothwell, K. Dose-related inhibition of chemical carcinogenesis in mouse skin by caffeine. Nature 1974, 252, 69-70.

Rougier A, Rallis M, Krien P, Lotte C. In vivo percutaneous-absorption - a key role for stratum-corneum vehicle partitioning. *Archives Of Dermatological Research* 1990, 282, 498-505.

Sahl, WJ, Glore, S, Garrison, P, Oakleaf, K, Johnson, SD. Basal-cell carcinoma and life-style characteristics. *International Journal Of Dermatology* 1995, 34, 398-402.

Sainio, EL, Rantanen, T, Kanerva, L. Ingredients and safety of cellulite creams. *European Journal Of Dermatology* 2000,10, 596-603.

Schafer-Korting M, Bock U, Gamer A, Haberland A, Haltner-Ukomadu E, Kaca M, Kamp H, Kietzmann M, Korting HC, Krachter HU, Lehr CM, Liebsch M, Mehling A, Netzlaff F, Niedorf F, Rubbelke MK, Schafer U, Schmidt E, Schreiber S, Schroder KR, Spielmann

H, Vuia A. Reconstructed human epidermis for skin absorption testing: Results of the German pre-validation study. *ATLA-Alternatives To Laboratory Animals* 2006, 34, 283-294.

Sekkat, N, Naik, A, Kalia, YN, Glikfeld, P, Guy, RH. Reverse iontophoretic monitoring in premature neonates: feasibility and potential. *Journal Of Controlled Release* 2002, 81, 83-89.

Sekkat N, Kalia YN, Guy RH. Porcine ear skin as a model for the assessment of transdermal drug delivery to premature neonates. *Pharmaceutical Research* 2004, 21, 1390-1397.

Shiraki, K, Rapp F. Effects of caffeine on herpes simplex virus. *Intervirology*. 1988, 29, 235-40.

Shiraki K, Ando T, Imakita, M, Kurokawa, M, Kuraishi Y, Niimura, M, Kageyama, S. Caffeine inhibits paresthesia induced by herpes simplex virus through action on primary sensory neurons in rats. *Neuroscience Research*, 1998, 31, 235-240.

Southwell, D, Barry, BW. Penetration enhancers for human-skin - mode of action of 2-pyrrolidone and dimethylformamide on partition and diffusion of model compounds water, normal-alcohols, and caffeine, Journal OF Investigative Dermatology 1983, 80, 507-514.

Stüttgen, G, Neumann, D. Inhibition of dermographism in human skin after topical application of caffeine. *Archiv. Fur. Dermatologische. Forschung.* 1972 242, 229-232.

Swanson, DL, Barnes, SA, Koon, SJM, El-Azhary, RA. Caffeine consumption and methotrexate dosing requirement in psoriasis and psoriatic arthritis. *International Journal Of Dermatology* 2007, 46, 157-159.

Tagliabue, A, Terracina, D, Cena, H, Turconi, G, Lanzola, E, Montomoli, C. Coffee induced thermogenesis and skin temperature. *International Journal Of Obesity* 1994, 18, 537-541.

Teichmann, A, Richter, H, Knorr, F, Antoniou, C, Sterry, W, Lademann, J. Investigation of the penetration and storage of a shampoo formulation containing caffeine into the hair follicles by in vivo laser scanning microscopy. *Laser Physics Letters*, 2007, 4, 464-468.

Touitou E, Junginger HE, Weiner ND, Nagai T, Mezei M. Liposomes as carriers for topical and transdermal delivery. *Journal Of Pharmaceutical Sciences* 1994a, 83, 1189-1203.

Touitou E, Levischaffer F, Dayan N, Alhaique F, Riccieri F. Modulation of caffeine skin delivery by carrier design - liposomes versus permeation enhancers. *International Journal Of Pharmaceutics* 1994b, 103, 131-136.

Thakur, RA, Michniak, BB, Meidan, VM. Transdermal and buccal delivery of methylxanthines through human tissue in vitro. *Drug Development And Industrial Pharmacy* 2007, 33, 513-521.

Treffel, P, Muret, P, Muretdaniello, P, Coumesmarquet, S, Agache, P. Effect of occlusion on in vitro percutaneous-absorption of 2 compounds with different physicochemical properties. *Skin Pharmacology* 1992, 5, 108-113.

Treffel, P, Panisset, F, Humbert, P, Remoussenard, O, Bechtel, Y, Agache, P. Effect of pressure on in-vitro percutaneous-absorption of caffeine. *Acta Dermato-Venereologica* 1993, 73, 200-202.

Valcic, S, Timmermann, BN, Alberts, DS, Wachter, GA, Krutzsch, M, Wymer, J, Guillen, JM. Inhibitory effect of six green tea catechins and caffeine on the growth of four selected human tumor cell lines. *Anti-Cancer Drugs* 1996, 7, 461-468.

van de Sandt JJM, van Burgsteden JA, Cage S, Carmichael PL, Dick I, Kenyon S, Korinth G, Larese F, Limasset JC, Maas WJM, Montomoli L, Nielsen JB, Payan JP, Robinson E, Sartorelli P, Schaller KH, Wilkinson SC, Williams FM. In vitro predictions of skin absorption of caffeine, testosterone, and benzoic acid: a multi-centre comparison study. *Regulatory Toxicology And Pharmacology* 2004, 39, 271-281.

Vonka V, Petrovska P, Borecky L, Roth Z. Increased effects of topically applied interferon on herpes-simplex virus-induced lesions by caffeine. *Acta. Virologica* 1995, 39, 125-130.

Wakefield, JC, Pendlington, RU, Lockley, DJ, Williams, FM. Dermal absorption of caffeine and testosterone through SLS-treated human skin in vitro. *Drug Metabolism Reviews* 2006, 38, 149-150.

Wilkinson, SC, Maas, WJM, Nielsen, JB, Greaves, LC, van de Sandt, JJM, Williams, FM. Interactions of skin thickness and physicochemical properties of test compounds in percutaneous penetration studies. *International Archives Of Occupational And Environmental Health* 2006, 79, 405-413.

Williams, AC. Topical and transdermal drug delivery. *Pharmaceutical Press*, London, 2003.

Yamada, K, Takezawa, J, Ezaki, O. Translesion replication in cisplatin-treated xeroderma pigmentosum variant cells is also caffeine-sensitive: features of the error-prone DNA polymerase(s) involved in UV-mutagenesis. *DNA Repair* 2003, 2, 909-924.

Yoshida, Y, Yamamura, J, Sato, H, et al. Efficacy of Cafon gel on cutaneous infection with herpes simplex virus (HSV)-2 and acyclovir-resistant HSV in mice. *J. Dermatol. Sci.* 1996, 13, 237-241.

Yamamura, J, Koyasu, M, Sato, H, Kurokawa, M, Yoshida, Y, Amahabu, Y, Shiraki, K. Topical treatment of cutaneous herpes simplex virus-1 infection in mice with a specially formulated caffeine gel (Cafon). *Journal of Dermatological Science* 1996, 12, 50-55.

Zajdela, F, Latarjet, R. Inhibiting effect of caffeine on induction of skin cancers by ultraviolet rays in mice. *Comptes Rendus Hebdomadaires Des Seances De L Academie Des Sciences Serie* D 1973, 277, 1073-1076.

Zesch, A, Schaefer, H, Stuttgen, G. Quantitative distribution of percutaneously applied caffeine in the human-skin. *Archives Of Dermatological Research* 1979, 266, 277-283.

In: Caffeine and Health Research
Editor: Kenneth P. Chambers

ISBN 978-1-60456-437-2

Chapter III

Coffee Lipid Class Variation during Storage

***Gulab N. Jham*[1], *Vidigal Muller*[1] *and Paulo Cecon*[2]**
Universidade Federal de Viçosa, [1]Labarótorio de Pesquisas de Produtos Naturais (LPPN), [2]Departamentos de Química and Informática, Viçosa, MG 36.570-000, Brazil.

Abstract

Despite little literature on coffee lipids, it has been hypothesized that they lower coffee quality through hydrolysis of the triacylglycerols during storage releasing free fatty acids, which are in turn oxidized to produce compounds producing off-flavour. Coffee is stored for extended periods by small producers in Brazil to fetch better market prices. As a part of our coffee-breeding program aiming to improve the quality of Brazilian coffee, we plan to evaluate the role of lipids during storage, developing initially methods (TLC-thin layer chromatography, HLPC-LSD-high performance liquid chromatography with light sensitive detection and HPLC with refractive index detection) for their determination. In this study experiments were carried out to evaluate the variation of lipid classes (free fatty acids, fatty acids after oil hydrolysis, triacylglycerols-TAG and terpene esters-TE) during coffee storage. Three types of coffee beans (immature, random mixture and cherry) picked in Viçosa, MG, Brazil (a region traditionally considered to be a producer of low quality coffee), were dried by two widely used procedures (dryer and open air cement patio) and stored on wood shelves in a house without neither temperature nor humidity control for 19 months. We tried to reproduce storage conditions used by small farmers in Brazil. At 4, 7, 10, 13, 16 and 19 months of storage, a part of samples was withdrawn and lipid classes were analyzed using the methods developed in our laboratory. The experiment consisted of thirty-six treatments in a randomised block design with three repetitions. The following treatments (T) were used: immature coffee beans dried in a dryer (T_1) and on a patio (T_2); a random mixture of coffee beans dried in a dryer (T_3) and on a patio (T_4) and cherry coffee beans dried in a dryer (T_5) and on a patio (T_6). In these treatments, samples were stored for four months followed by analysis of lipid classes. The procedure was repeated for immature, random and cherry coffee beans after 7, 10, 13, 16 and 19 months of storage corresponding to treatments T_7-T_{12},

T_{13}-T_{18}, T_{19}-T_{24}, T_{25}-T_{30} and T_{31}-T_{36}, respectively. Lipid class data were statistically analyzed through variance and regression. The qualitative factors (type of coffee and type of drying) and the averages were compared by the Tukey test at 5% probability. The quantitative factor (months of storage) and the averages were chosen based on the significance of regression coefficients using the t test at 5% probability and determination coefficients (r^2). While apparently random variation was observed in a few cases, no effects of storage time, storage type and coffee type were found on the lipid classes. These results contradict literature studies where a small number of samples were studied utilizing short storage times.

1. Introduction

Most Brazilian coffee produced for internal consumption is considered to be of low quality. A number of factors such as poor post-harvesting practices (Informe Agropecuário, 1997), fungal contamination (Zambolin et al., 1996) and the presence of undesired compounds (Spadone et al., 1990) have been reported as possible causes. Despite little literature on coffee lipids, it has been hypothesized that they lower coffee quality through hydrolysis of the triacylglycerols during storage releasing free fatty acids, which are in turn oxidized to produce compounds producing off-flavour. Degradation of free amino acids, sugars and oxidation of lipids in coffee stored for one year has been reported with coffee quality loss (Multon et al., 1973). Increased free fatty acids content has been associated to long storage in subtropical conditions and may be due to enzymatic activity. The latter is assumed also to be a cause of flavour deterioration (Wajda & Walczky, 1978). In a simulated study, linoleic acid (L), which is susceptible to oxidation, was reported to be reduced in rancid beans with respect to fresh beans; while palmitic acid (P) remained unaltered (Fourney et al., 1982). Higher concentrations of free fatty acids in *robusta* than in *arabica* coffee beans were linked to rough processing or storage conditions (Speer et al., 1993).

In Brazil, coffee is often stored over extended periods of times by small producers to obtain better prices. However, the long-term storage effects on coffee quality and chemical composition have been little studied (Multon et al., 1973; Wajda & Walczky, 1978; Speer et al., 1993). No such studies have been carried out under Brazilian conditions. Such studies are very important since it is known that small variations in storage temperature and humidity may have profound influence on coffee quality (Illy & Viani, 1995).

Our coffee breeding program aims to study the role of lipids in coffee quality and initially methods were developed for their determination. We reported lipid classes and the TAG molecular species by TLC (thin layer chromatography) (Nikolova-Damyanova et al., 1998). HPLC-LSD (high performance liquid chromatography-light sensitive detector) (Jham et al., 2003) and HPLC-RID (high performance liquid chromatography-refractive index detector) (Jham et al., 2005) methods were reported for the identification and determination of relative % of individual TAG molecular species in eight coffee types. More recently, liquid chromatography-mass spectrometry (LC-MS) (Segall et al., 2005) for determination of coffee TAGs has also been reported. In addition, effects of coffee type and drying procedures on lipid classes and TAG molecular species by TLC were reported on a few coffee samples (Jham et al., 2001). We now report the variation of coffee lipid classes (free fatty acids, fatty acids after oil hydrolysis, triacylglycerols-TAGs and terpene esters-TE) of three type of coffee beans (immature, random mixture and cherry) dried by two widely used procedures (dryer and open air cement patio) stored for nineteen months in Viçosa in the State of Minas Gerais, Brazil.

2. Methods and Materials

2.1. Coffee Samples

The details have been described before (Nikanva-Dayanova et al., 1998) and hence will be briefly described. About 10 kg of coffee (Catuaí Vermelho, *Coffea arabica* L) were harvested in Viçosa, MG by the "derriça" method (coffee beans were hand-removed from the tree and allowed to drop on the floor covered with cloth). From this sample, a random mixture was obtained by separating 5 kg and the rest was used to obtain immature and cherry beans by placing the coffee sample in a tank containing 50 L of water. The dry beans floated immediately and were separated while the immature and cherry beans remained at the bottom of the tank. After draining the water tank, the immature and the cherry beans were hand-separated and allowed to air-dry for 20 h. The three types of coffee beans (immature, random mixture and cherry) were divided in roughly six equal parts and dried by two methods (dryer and patio). A dryer prototype developed by the Agricultural Engineering Dept. of Universidade Federal de Viçosa was used for drying with the air temperature at 45°C for several hours until humidity was 11% (Jham et al., 2003, 2005). For patio drying, coffee samples were spread on a cement floor and dried for several days until a humidity of 14% was attained. All samples were stored in jute bags on wooden racks in a house without control of neither temperature nor humidity. After 4, 7, 10, 13 and 19 months of storage, about 1 kg of each of the coffee samples was withdrawn, lipids extracted and analysed (oil, acidity, TAGs and fatty acids after hydrolysis). Treatments used in this study are described in Table 1.

2.2. Chemical Analysis

2.2.1. Oil Extraction

The oil was extracted from the coffee beans in a Soxhlet extractor for 6 h using hexane as the solvent. The solvent was evaporated at 40^0C in a rotatory evaporator, dried over anhydrous sodium sulphate, filtered, re-evaporated, weighed, stored at –10°C. The samples were thawed to room temperature for chemical analysis (acidity, free fatty acids and fatty acids after hydrolysis and main lipid classes-TE and triacylglycerols).

Table 1. Description of the treatments (T) used in the study

T	Description
T_1	Immature coffee beans dried in a dryer and analyzed after four months of storage
T_2	Immature coffee beans dried on a patio and analyzed after four months of storage
T_3	Random mixture of coffee beans dried in a dryer and analyzed after four months of storage
T_4	Random mixture of coffee beans dried on a patio and analyzed after four months of storage
T_5	Cherry coffee beans dried in a dryer and analyzed after four months of storage
T_6	Cherry coffee beans dried on a patio and analyzed after four months of storage
T_7	Immature coffee beans dried in a dryer and analyzed after seven months of storage
T_8	Immature coffee beans dried on a patio and analyzed after seven months of storage
T_9	Random mixture of coffee beans dried in a dryer and analyzed after seven months of storage
T_{10}	Random mixture of coffee beans dried on a patio and analyzed after seven months of storage
T_{11}	Cherry coffee beans dried in a dryer and analyzed after seven months of storage
T_{12}	Cherry coffee beans on a patio and analyzed after seven months of storage
T_{13}	Immature coffee beans dried in a dryer and analyzed after ten months of storage
T_{14}	Immature coffee beans obtained dried on a patio and analyzed after ten months of storage
T_{15}	Random mixture of coffee beans dried in a dryer and analyzed after ten months of storage
T_{16}	Random mixture of coffee beans dried on a patio and analyzed after ten months of storage
T_{17}	Cherry coffee beans obtained dried in a dryer and analyzed after ten months of storage
T_{18}	Cherry coffee beans dried on a patio and analyzed after ten months of storage
T_{19}	Immature coffee beans dried in a dryer and analyzed after thirteen months of storage
T_{20}	Immature coffee beans dried on a patio and analyzed after thirteen months of storage
T_{21}	Random mixture of coffee beans dried in a dryer and analyzed after thirteen months of storage
T_{22}	Random mixture of coffee beans dried on a patio and analyzed after thirteen months of storage
T_{23}	Cherry coffee beans dried in a dryer and analyzed after thirteen months of storage
T_{24}	Cherry coffee beans dried on a patio and analyzed after thirteen months of storage
T_{25}	Immature coffee beans obtained dried in a dryer and analyzed after sixteen months of storage
T_{26}	Immature coffee beans on a patio and analyzed after sixteen months of storage
T_{27}	Random mixture of coffee beans dried in a dryer and analyzed after sixteen months of storage
T_{28}	Random mixture of coffee beans dried on a patio and analyzed after 16 months of storage
T_{29}	Cherry coffee beans dried in a dryer and analyzed after sixteen months of storage
T_{30}	Cherry coffee beans obtained dried on a patio and analyzed after sixteen months of storage
T_{31}	Immature coffee beans dried in a dryer and analyzed after nineteen months of storage
T_{32}	Immature coffee beans dried on a patio and analyzed after nineteen months of storage
T_{33}	Random mixture of coffee beans dried in a dryer and analyzed after nineteen months of storage
T_{34}	Random mixture of coffee beans dried on a patio and analyzed after nineteen months of storage
T_{35}	Cherry coffee beans dried in a dryer and analyzed after nineteen months of storage
T_{36}	Cherry coffee beans dried on a patio and analyzed after nineteen months of storage

2.2.2. *Coffee Oil Acidity*

Titrable acidity was determined by Association of Official Analytical Chemists method (1984) expressing it as oleic acid using 0.5g of sample and using 0.01 mol/L for titration.

2.2.3. *Identification of the Main Lipid Classes by Analytical Silica Gel TLC*

Reference mixture of lipid classes was prepared by mixing equal aliquots of 10% solutions of docosane, cholesteryl_oleate, methyl oleate, oleyl alcohol, cholesterol, 1,3-

diolein, 1-monoolein-rac-glycerol, L-α dioleylphosphatidyl choline (all purchased form Sigma-Aldrich Chemie GmbH, Germany), triacylglycerol fraction from sunflower oil in dichloromethane. A reference TAG mixture was prepared by mixing equal quantities of TAGs from lard and sunflower oils. To this mixture 100 g kg^{-1} of tristearin was added to increase the proportion of the trisaturated TAG (SSS; S, saturated acyl residue). This mixture was used to identify the TAGs from SSS to DDD (D, dienoic acyl residues). Pure TAG fractions with known composition from tangerine and linseed oils (Tarandjiiska et al., 1996) were used to identify the TAGs.

The lipid class composition was determined by analytical silica gel TLC. An aliquot of the 1% lipid solution in dichloromethane was applied on 4 cm x 19 cm glass plates (ca 0.200 mm thick layer). The lipid classes were identified by comparison with a reference lipid mixture (20 μL of 1% solution in dichloromethane), which was applied alongside each plate. The plates were developed with ca. 4 ml petroleum ether-acetone, 100:8 (by volume). The lipid zones were detected by spraying with 50% ethanolic sulphuric acid and heating at 200°C on a metal plate with temperature control.

2.2.4. Isolation, Purification and Quantification of Lipid Classes by Preparative Silica Gel TLC

An aliquot of the 10% stock solution was applied on 20 cm x 20 cm plates (ca. 1 mm thick layer) and developed with petroleum ether-acetone 100:8 (by volume). The separated zones were detected by spraying the edge of each plate with 2,7-dichlorofluorescein. Partial acylglycerols, free fatty acids and polar lipids, which migrated below the sterols in this system, were collected jointly, and the components were isolated on a second preparative silica TLC plate with mobile phase light petroleum-acetone-acetic acid (70:30:1, by volume). All zones form the two plates were scrapped, transferred to small glass columns and eluted with ethyl ether. The solvent was evaporated under stream of nitrogen and the residue was weighed in small glass containers (of known weight) to a constant weight.

2.2.5. Quantitative (%) Fatty Acid Composition of Oil by Gas Chromatography (GC)

Hydrolysis of the oil and methylation were carried out as described (Jham et al., 1982). The fatty acid methyl esters were identified by standards. A Shimadzu gas chromatograph, model 17-A fitted with FID, auto sampler and an integration system was used. Fused silica capillary columns (30 m x 0.25 mm; film thickness of 0.25 μm) coated with the Carbowax stationary phase were purchased from Supelco. The GC oven temperature was increased from 60^0C to 240^0C at a rate of 6^0C/min.

2.3. TAG Determination

The detailed procedures for the identification of individual coffee TAG by HPLC-LSD (Jham et al., 2003) and HPLC-RID were described (Jham et al., 2005). A LC-MS procedure to determine the TAG composition has also been described (Segall et al., 2005). In these procedures, crude oil was injected into the HPLC and the individual TAG identified with standards and literature procedures (Christy, 1987, Nikolova-Damyanova et al., 1990). With the LSD, a linear gradient of acetonitrile (solvent A) and dichloromethane-dichloroethane (8:2, v/v) (solvent B) was generated from 55% A to 65% B over 40 minutes. The flow rate was 0.5 mL/min. The mobile phase with RID was acetonitrile/acetone (1:1, v/v) at a flow rate of 2 mL/min. A Techsphere ODS column (5 μm, 250 x 4.6 mm id, HPLC Technology, Herts, England) equipped with a Techsphere ODS guard-column (5 μm, 10 x 4.6 mm, HPLC Technology, Herts, England) was used in both cases.

2.4. Statistical Analysis

The experiment was arranged in subdivided parcels, with the parcels in a 3x2 factorial scheme [(three types of coffee beans-immature, random mixture and cherry coffee beans) and two types of drying procedures-dryer and patio)] and the sub parcels being storage time (4, 7, 10, 13, 16 and 19 months) in a completely randomised design with 3 repetitions. Data on lipid classes (acidity, fatty acid after hydrolysis, TE and TAG) were statistically analysed through variance and regression. The qualitative factors (type of coffees and types of drying) the averages were compared by the Tukey test at 5% probability. The quantitative factor (months of storage) and the models were chosen based on the significance of regression coefficients using the t test at 5% probability and determination coefficient (r^2) and the biological phenomenon.

3. Results and Discussion

The storage conditions used in this study attempted to simulate the conditions used by small coffee producers. Hence, a simple house with wooden racks without control of the temperature nor humidity was utilized.

3.1. Coffee Oil Acidity

No effect of storage time on acidity the coffee types or type of drying was noted, i.e., as the storage time increased the coffee acidity did not change (Table 2). However, a significant effect of coffee type was noted on acidity, with higher values being obtained for cherry coffee beans as compared to immature coffee beans (Table 3). A higher coffee acidity was verified for patio drying than for conventional drying (Table 4). Unfortunately, comparisons of our results with the literature values will be difficult since no such studies have been conducted. However, it is generally empirically accepted that cherry coffee beans are considered to have lower acidity than the immature coffee beans.

Table 2. Adjusted regression equations for coffee acidity as a function of storage time for three types of coffee and two types of drying

Type of coffee beans	Adjusted equation
Immature	$\hat{Y} = 3.99$
Random mixture	$\hat{Y} = 4.53$
Cherry beans	$\hat{Y} = 5.22$
Type of drying	
Conventional	$\hat{Y} = 3.65$
Patio	$\hat{Y} = 5.51$

Table 3. Average acidity* for the three types of coffees as a function of storage time

Storage time (months)	Immature coffee beans	Random mixture of coffee beans	Cherry coffee beans
4	3.57 c	4.02 b	4.60 b
7	3.80 b	4.02 b	4.93 a
10	4.41 c	4.97 b	5.52 a
13	4.50 c	510 b	5.78 a
16	3.70 c	4.52 b	5.15 a
19	3.92 c	4.57 b	5.37 a

*Averages followed by same small letter in a column do not differ by the Tukey test at 5% probability.

Table 4. Average acidity* for combinations of storage time and drying

Storage time (months)	Type of drying	
	Dryer	Patio
4	3.17 b	4.98 a
7	3.39 b	5.10 a
10	3.95 b	5.98 a
13	4.24 b	6.05 a
16	3.54 b	5.37 a
19	3.64 b	5.60 a

*Averages followed by same small letter in a column do not differ by the Tukey test at 5% probability.

3.2. Oil

The % oil obtained in this study is in agreement with the literature value (8.7-12.2%) reported for crude coffee beans (Belitz & Grosh, 1988) and our study (Nikalova-Damyanova et al., 1998).

No effect of storage time was noted for any of the coffee types or drying types with the average % oil being $\hat{Y}$ =10.82. However, the quantity of oil behaved differently with respect to coffee type and drying type. For all the coffee types studied, a higher oil value was found for conventional drying as compared to patio drying. In relation to type of drying, a higher % of oil was obtained for immature coffee beans than for cherry beans (Table 5).

Table 5. Average oil* (%) as a function of coffee bean type and storage type

Type of coffee beans	Type of drying	
	Dryer	Patio
Immature	12.02 aA	10.50 bA
Random mixture	11.27 aB	10.46 bA
Cherry	10,70 aC	9.95 bB

*Averages followed by same small letter in a column do not differ by the Tukey test at 5% probability.

Table 6. Adjusted regression equations for the % of palmitic acid (P) and linoleic acid (L) as a function of storage time, coffee type and drying

Type of coffee beans	Type of drying	Variable	Adjusted equations
Immature	Dryer	P	$\hat{Y} = 38.23$
Immature	Patio	P	$\hat{Y} = 40.19$
Random mixture	Dryer	P	$\hat{Y} = 39.87$
Random mixture	Patio	P	$\hat{Y} = 37.87$
Cherry	Dryer	P	$\hat{Y} = 40.86$
Cherry	Patio	P	$\hat{Y}$ 41.91
Immature	Dryer	L	$\hat{Y} = 40.05$
Immature	Patio	L	$\hat{Y} = 39.68$
Random mixture	Dryer	L	$\hat{Y} = 37.77$
Random mixture	Patio	L	$\hat{Y} = 36.73$
Cherry	Dryer	L	$\hat{Y} = 37.38$
Cherry	Patio	L	$\hat{Y} = 39.40$

3.3. Fatty Acid (FA) Composition of Coffee Oil after Lipid Hydrolysis

The fatty acids identified in all oils after hydrolysis were miristic (14:0), palmitic (16:0), palmitoleic (16:1), stearic (18:0), oleic (cis 9-18:1), linoleic acid (cis 9,12-18:2), linolenic (cis 9,12, 15-18:32) , arahidic (20:0) and bechenic (22:0) acids The major acids were the P and L acids (~40% each) corresponding to about 80% of the total FA. These results are in agreement with the literature studies (Kaufmann & Hamsagar, 1963; Speer et al., 1993) and with our study (Nikalova-Damyanova et al., 1998).

No effect of storage time in any of the coffee types and storage types was observed on the relative % of both P and L, i.e., as the storage time increased the % of the acids did not change (Table 6). After seven months of storage, for immature coffee beans there was no effect of type of drying for P and L acids (Tables 7 and 8). However, cherry coffee beans presented higher % of P for all storage times and types of drying. In general, immature coffee beans presented the highest % for all storage and drying types. This result was not in agreement with that of Fourney et al., 1982 who reported through simulated experiments that the % of L, susceptible to oxidation was reduced in rancid beans with respect to fresh beans while that of P remained practically unaltered.

Table 7. Average palmitic acid (%)* as a function of storage time, type of coffee and drying

Type of coffee beans	Storage time (months) 4		7		10	
	Type of drying					
	Dryer	Patio	Dryer	Patio	Dryer	Patio
Immature	38.43 bB	42.80aA	35.96bB	42.40abA	40.76aA	38.83aA
Random mixture	41.46 aA	35.80bB	43.00aA	39.80bB	39.00aA	36.80aA
Cherry	40.36abB	43.23aA	43.30aA	44.30aA	40.29aA	38.50aA

Type of coffee beans	Storage time (months) 13		16		19	
	Type of drying					
	Dryer	Patio	Dryer	Patio	Dryer	Patio
Immature	37.16bA	38.41bA	41.60aA	41.91aA	35.46A	36.80bA
Random mixture	41.16aA	36.60bB	33.70bB	40.66aA	38.10abA	37.57bA
Cherry	40.70aA	41.50aA	39.83aB	42.70aA	40.66aA	41.23

*Averages followed by same small letter in a column do not differ by the Tukey test at 5% probability.

Table 8. Average linoleic acid* (%) as a function of storage time, type of coffee and drying

Type of coffee	Storage time (months) 4		7		10	
	Type of drying					
	Dryer	Patio	Dryer	Patio	Dryer	Patio
Immature	40.83 aA	40.86 aA	43.16 aA	38.80 bB	39.13 aA	40.00 aA
Random mixture	38.00 bA	35.63 bB	37.16 bA	36.36 cA	38.63 aA	38.30 aA
Cherry	37.50 bB	41.50 aA	36. 19 bB	41.74 aA	37.31 aB	39.89 aA

Type of coffee beans	Storage time (months) 13		16		19	
	Type of drying					
	Dryer	Patio	Dryer	Patio	Dryer	Patio
Immature	39.83 aA	40.80 aA	38.5 0abA	37.36 aA	38.83 aA	40.27 aA
Random mixture	36.60 bA	36.78 bA	39.56 aA	35.86 abB	36.70 aA	37.44 bA
Cherry	37.70 abB	41.63 aA	37.00 bA	33.9 4bB	38.60 aA	38.21 abA

*Averages followed by same small letter in a column do not differ by the Tukey test at 5% probability.

3.4. Triacylglycerols (TAGs) and Terpene Esters (TE)

The methodology used for lipid class analysis is presented is presented in Figure 1 (Jham et al., 2004). The most abundant class was the TAGs (~75%) followed by substantial amounts of terpene esters (~14%) (Table 9). In addition, all samples contained small amounts of sterol esters, partial acylglycerols, polar lipids, free fatty acids and unidentified material. These results were in agreement with our previous studies (Nikalova-Damyanova et al., 1998) and literature study (Kaufmann & Hamsagar, 1962). Small amounts (0.5%-2.5%) of free fatty acids have been reported in coffee (Speer et al., 1993), although their origin was not discussed.

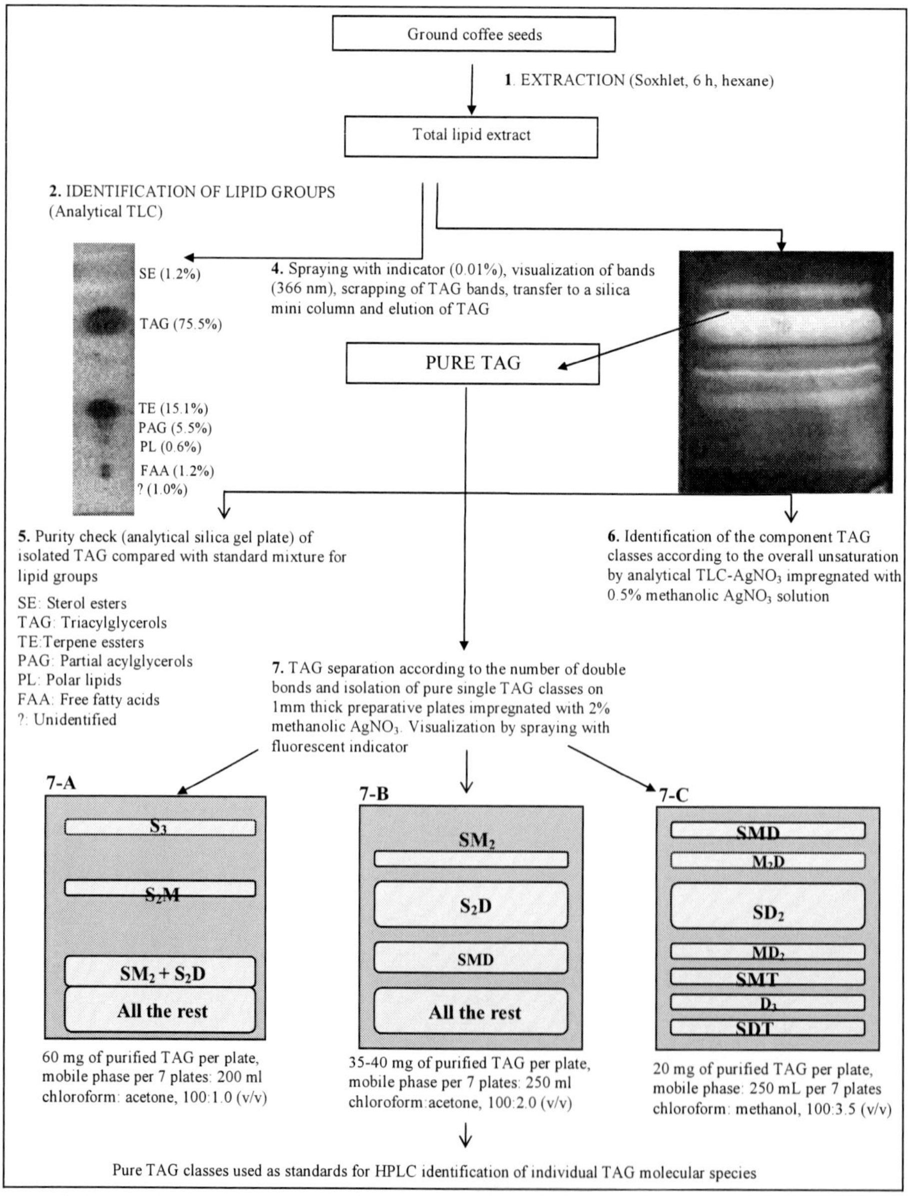

Figure 1. Fluxogram for the separation of coffee triacylglycerols.

Table 9. Average TAG (%) for the three types of coffee

Type of coffee beans	TAG
Immature	73.18 a
Random mixture	72.91 a
Cherry beans	72.95 a

*Averages followed by the same letter in a column indicate no significant difference at 5% probability by the Scot-Knott test.

No effects of bean type, drying type nor storage time was noted on the TAGs composition, although some apparently random variation was observed. This result was in agreement with our previous study (Jham et al., 2001) where a small number of samples were evaluated. It has been hypothesized in the literature that the TAGs are degraded during storage releasing free fatty acids, which are in turn oxidized to produce compounds responsible for off-flavour. Degradation of free amino acids, sugars and oxidation of lipids in coffee stored for one year has been reported along with loss of the coffee quality (Multon et al., 1973, Wajda & Walczky, 1978).

No effects of bean type, drying type and storage time were noted on the TE (Table 10) composition. The chemical structure of the TE has not been yet determined.

Table 10. Average terpene esters *(%) as a function of storage time, type of coffee and drying

Type of coffee beans	Storage time (months)					
	4		7		10	
	Type of drying					
	Dryer	Patio	Dryer	Patio	Dryer	Patio
Immature	14.13 a	15.10 a	13.43aa	14.83 a	14.10 a	14.43 a
Random mixture	15.10 a	15.26 a	14.30 a	14.63 a	14.60 a	14.96 a
Cherry	14.87 a	15.20 a	14.73 a	14.83 a	13.50 a	14.50 a

Type of coffee beans	Storage time (months)					
	13		16		19	
	Type of drying					
	Dryer	Patio	Dryer	Patio	Dryer	Patio
Immature	13.17 a	14.53 a	14.60 a	14.67 a	14.91 a	15.00 a
Random mixture	15.44 a	13.46 a	13.90 a	14.70 a	15.65 a	15.10 a
Cherry	14.34 a	14.60 a	14.67 a	14.86 a	14.71 a	15.00 a

*Averages followed by same small letter in a column do not differ by the Tukey test at 5% probability.

3.5. TAG Molecular Species of Crude Coffee Oils

The average TAG composition (%) of six coffee samples obtained with a crude hexane extract using LSD is presented in Table 11. Twelve TAG molecular species were identified in all the samples with a representative % composition being LLL (5.88%), StLLn (1.88%), OLL (4.93%), PLL (26.92%), OOL (1.05%), StLL (5.15%), POL (11.38%), PPL (25.98%), POO+ALL (1.43%), PStL (9.67%), PPO (2.38%) and PStO (3.64%) (in order of elution, Ln-linolenic, L-linoleic, O-oleic, P-palmitic and St-stearic acid residues). A solvent gradient was utilized to separate the TAG molecular species (Figure 2). As reported, the TAG molecular species did not vary with coffee type and drying type (Jham et al., 2003).

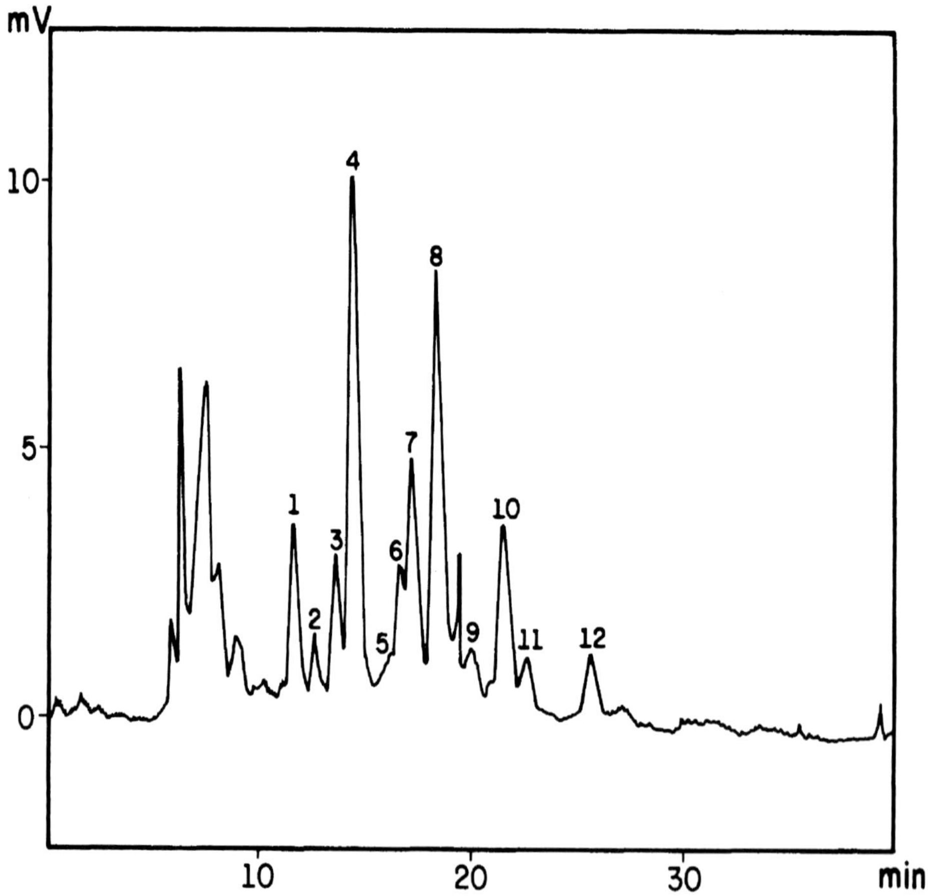

Figure 2. Typical chromatogram obtained on analysis of a crude hexane extract using a light sensitive detector Peaks 1 to 12 are LLL, SLLn, OLL, PLL, OOL, StLL, POL, PPL, POO + ALL, PStL, PPO and PStO (Ln-linolenic, L-linoleic, O-oleic, P-palmitic and St- stearic acid residues). The five peaks eluting before peak 1 corresponded to the more polar compounds (free acids, monacylglycerols and diacylglycerols) found in the crude coffee extract (Nikolova-Damyanova, B., Velikova, & Jham, 1998).

Table 11. Average TAG* composition (%) of six coffee samples obtained with a crude hexane extract using a light sensitive detector LSD**

T	LLL	StLLn	OLL	PLL	OOL	StLL	POL	PPL	POO+ALL	PStL	PPO	PStO
T_1	5.88 a	1.83 a	4.93 a	26.92 a	1.05 a	5.15 a	11.38 a	25.98 a	1.43 a	9.67 a	2.38 a	3.64 a
T_3	5.69 a	1.90 a	5.23 a	26.74 a	1.42 a	5.41 a	11.41 a	25.15 a	1.35 a	9.71 a	2.35 a	3.58 a
T_5	6.41 a	1.71 a	5.30 a	26.89 a	0.98 a	5.28 a	11.16 a	25.18 a	1.63 a	9.58 a	2.05 a	3.64 a
T_2	6.45 a	1.75 a	5.60 a	27.18 a	0.81 a	5.79 a	11.25 a	23.90 a	1.31 a	9.88 a	2.88 a	3.75 a
T_3	5.92 a	1.84 a	5.65 a	27.54 a	1.66 a	5.28 a	11.88 a	24.80 a	1.63 a	9.84 a	2.87 a	3.02 a
T_6	5.68 a	1.92 a	5.52 a	26.88 a	1.53 a	4.94 a	11.91 a	25.33 a	1.56 a	9.71 a	2.33 a	3.62 a

*Averages followed by same small letter in a column do not differ by the Tukey test at 5% probability;

**Jham et al. 2003;

T: See Table 1 for the treatment description;

Ln-linolenic, L-linoleic, O-oleic, P-palmitic and St- stearic acid residues

Preparative silver ion thin-layer chromatography (Ag-TLC) was also utilized for the preparative isolation of TAG classes according to the degree of unsaturation (Jham et al., 2005, Figure 2). These were used as standards to identify TAGs species from eight coffee samples evaluate effects of bean type, drying procedures and geographic origin on the TAG composition by means of RP-HPLC using a refractive index detector (RID).

Acetonitrile/acetone (1:1, v/v) was used as elution solvent. The following nine TAGs species were identified in all the coffee samples: LLL (5.78%), SLLn (2.06%), OLL (5.15%), PLL (29.72%), StLL + POL (14.80%), PPL + OOL (22.94%), ALL, PStL + POO (9.65%) and PStO (3.78%). In agreement with our previous studies, no effects of bean type, drying procedures and geographic origin on the TAG composition were found. It has been demonstrated that although resolution with RP-HPLC/RID was poorer as compared to the previously described RP-HPLC-light scattering detector (RP-HPLC/LSD) approach, in general the results were in good agreement. Thus, despite the limitation of the RP-HPLC/RID, the method is suitable for monitoring the TAG composition of coffee stored over prolonged period of time or to determine relative percentage of the resolved TAGs.

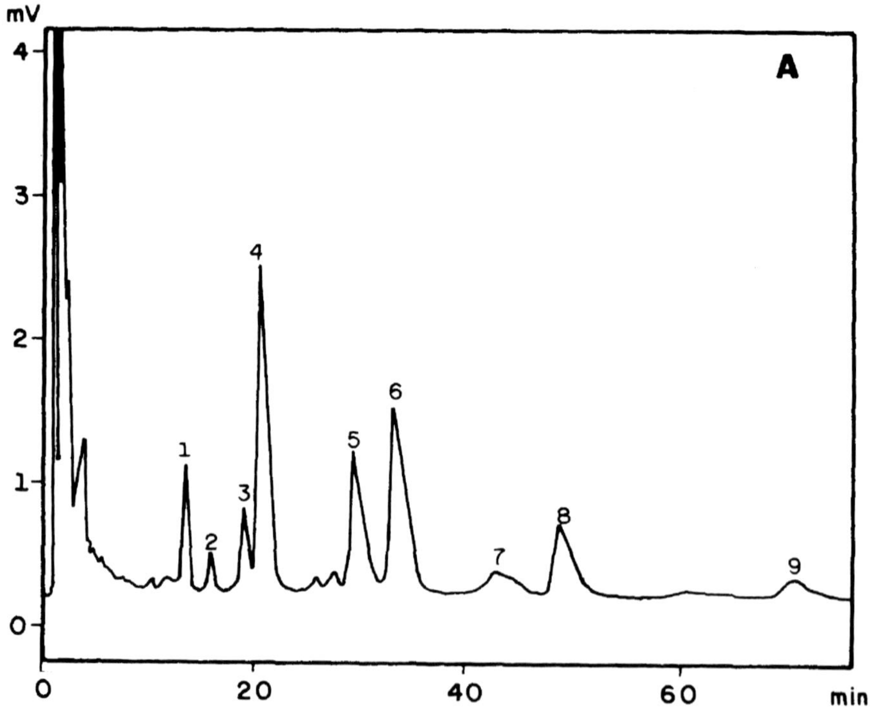

Figure 3. Typical chromatogram obtained on analysis of a crude hexane extract using a refractive index detector. Peaks 1-9 correspond to LLL, StLLn, OLL, PLL, StLL + POL, PPL + OOL, ALL, PStL + POO and PStO (Ln-linolenic, L-linoleic, O-oleic, P-palmitic and St-stearic acid residues).

Table 12. Comparison of average TAG composition* (%) of six coffee samples obtained with a crude hexane extract using a refractive index detector (RID) and a light sensitive detector (LSD)**

T***	% TAG composition in crude hexane										
	LLL		StLLn		OLL		PLL		StLL+POL		
	RID	LSD	RID	LSD	RID	LSD	RID	LSD	RID	LSD****	
										StLL	POL
T_1	5.78 abA	5.85 bA	2.06	1.83	5.15	5.69	29.72	27.89	14.80	5.00	10.93
	(1, 2)	(1, 3)	(2, 2)	(2, 3)	(3, 2)	(3, 3)	(4, 2)	(4, 3)	(5, 2)	(6, 3)	(7, 3)
T_3	6.05 aA	5.69 bB	1.82	1.86	5.05	5.50	29.32	27.92	15.76	5.21	11.01
T_5	5.88 abB	6.41 aA	2.26	1.78	5.00	5.48	29.44	28.16	15.53	5.08	10.76
T_2	5.77 bB	5.65 aA	1.90	1.79	4.92	5.69	30.18	27.06	15.13	5.44	11.00
T_3	5.75 abcB	5.68 bA	1.97	1.87	5.28	5.88	29.14	27.14	15.4.8	4.94	11.61
T_6	5.74 abA	5.92 bA	2.04	1.81	5.21	5.65	29.77	26.93	15.16	5.08	11.48
GA*****	-	-	1.95	1.86	5.19B	5.62A	29.46A	27.45B	15.37B	16.35A	
VC(%)	2.54		10.43		4.83		4.28		5.43		

T***	% TAG composition in crude hexane							
	PPL+OOL			PStL+POO			PStO	
	RID	LSD****		RID	LSD****		RID	LSD
		PPL	OOL		PStL	POO		
T_1	22.94	23.08	0.95	9.65	9.65	1.10	3.78 abA	3.62 abA
	(6, 2)	(8, 3)	(5, 3)	(8, 2)	(10, 3)	(9, 3)	(9, 2)	(12, 3)
T_3	23.72	25.15	1.32	10.90	9.71	1.35	2.99 aB	3.56 abA
T_5	22.54	22.18	0.98	11.96	9.58	1.63	3.38 abA	3.62 abA
T_2	23.16	20.90	0.81	11.23	9.88	1.31	2.85 abB	3.77 aA
T_3	22.34	22.53	1.33	11.79	9.71	1.56	3.34 abA	3.55 abA
T_6	22.63	21.46	1.00	10.82	9.84	1.63	3.62 abA	3.01 abB
GA*****	22.75B	23.35A		11.21A	11.17A		-	-
VC(%)	4.20			5.32			9.37	

*Averages followed by at least one lower case letter in the column or upper case letter in the row do not differ by the Tukey test (5% probability);

** Jham et al. 2004;

*** See Table 1 for description of treatments;

****For comparison of statistical data, the sum of TAG molecular species obtained with the LSD was compared to the RID results;

*****No interaction between treatments and detector but differences in two detectors were obtained;

T: treatment; GA: general average; VC: variation coefficient;

Ln=linolenic, L=linoleic, O=oleic, P=palmitic and St= stearic acid residues;

% TAG in the first row followed by two numbers in parentheses represents the peak number in Fig. 2;

PPO (~5%) detected by LSD not considered;

ALL (~5%) detected by RID not considered

4. Conclusion

Although variation in lipid class was noted in some treatments, it appeared to be random. Hence, it appears that the lipid classes do not vary during storage using the methodology in this study. However, a more detailed study, using HPLC should be conducted to determine the variation of individual TAGs during storage. In order to draw definite conclusions, these studies should be conducted simultaneously with cup quality tests. The role of volatile compounds in coffee quality should also be investigated.

References

Association of Official Analytical Chemists. *Official Methods of Analysis*. (1984). 4th ed., 1-1141.

Belitz, H. D. & Grosh, W. (1988). *Food Chemistry*. Berlin, Springer Verlag.

Christie, W. W. (1987). *High Performance liquid Chromatography and Lipids*. Oxford, Pergamon.

Fourney, G. E., Cros, E. & Vicent, J. C. (1982). Estudo preliminaire de l'oxydation de l'huile de café. In: *Proc. 10th ASIC Coll.*, 235-246.

Illy, A. & Viani, R. (1995). *Expresso coffee: The Chemistry of Quality*, London, Academic.

González, A. G., Pablos, F., Martín, M. J., León-Camacho, C. & Valdenebro, M. S. (2001). HPLC analysis of tocopherols and triglycerides in coffee and their use as authentication parameters. *Food Chemistry*, *73*, 93-101.

Informe Agropecuário (1997). Qualidade do Café. 18, 1-76.

Jham, G. N., Teles, F. F. F. & Campos, L. 1982. Use of aqueous HCl/MeOH as esterification reagent for analysis of fatty acids derived from soybean lipids. *Journal of American Oil Chemists Society*, *59*, 132-133.

Jham, G. N., Velikova, R. Muller H., Nikolova-Damyanova, B. & Cecon, P. R. (2001). Lipid classes and triacylglycerols in coffee samples from Brazil: effects of coffee type and drying procedures. *Food Research International*, *34*, 111-115.

Jham, G. N., Nikolova-Damyavova, B., Viera, M., Natalino, R. & Rodrigues, A. C. (2003). Determination of triacylglycerol composition of eight coffee samples by RP-HPLC. *Phytochemical Analysis*, *13*, 99-104.

Jham, G. N., Velikova, R., Nikolova-Damyavova, B., Rabelo. S. C., Silva, J. C. T., Souza, P. K., Moreira, M.V. & Cecon, P. R. (2005). Preparative silver ion TLC/RP-HPLC determination of coffee triacylglycerol molecular species. *Food Research International*, *38*: 121-126.

Kaufmann, H. P. & Hamsagar, R. S. (1962). Zur Kentnis der Lipoide der Kaffeebohne. I: Ueber Fettsaure des Cafestols. *Fette Seifen Anstrichmiffel*, *64*, 206-213.

Multon, J. L., Poisson, B. & Cachaginer, M. (1973). Evolution de plusieurs caratéristiquers d'un café Arabica au cours d'un stockage expérimental effectuéà 5 humidités relatives et 4 températures différentes. In: *Proc. 6th ASIC Coll.*, 268-277.

Nikolova-Damyanova, B., Velikova, R. & Jham, G. N. (1998). Lipid classes, fatty acid composition and triacylglycerol molecular species in crude coffee beans harvested in Brazil. *Food Research International*, *31*, 479-486.

Nikolova-Damyanova B, Christie W. W, Herslof, B. (1990). The structure of the triglycerides of meadowfoam oil. *Journal of the American Oil Chemists Society*, *67*, 503-507.

Segall, S. D., Artz, W. E., Raslan, D. S., Jham, G. N. & Takahashi, J. A. (2005). TAG Composition of Coffee Beans (*Coffea canephora* L.) by Reversed-Phase High Performance Liquid Chromatography and Tandem Mass Spectroscopy. In preparation.

Spadone, J. C., Takeoke, G. & Liardon, R. (1990). Analytical investigation of Rio off-flavor in green coffee. *Journal of Agriciculture and Food Chemistry, 38*, 226-233.

Speer, K., Sehat, N. & Montang A. (1993). Fatty acids in coffee. In: *Proc. 15th ASIC Coll.*, 583-592.

Wajda, P. & Walczyk, D. (1978). Relationship between acid values of extracted fatty matter and age of green coffee bean. *Journal of Science Food Agriculture*, *29*, 237-245.

Tarandjiiska, R., Marekov, I., Nikolova-Damyanova, B. & Amidzhin, B. (1996). Determination of molecular species of triacylglycerols classes and molecular species in seed oils with high content of linolenic fatty acids. *Journal of Science and Food Agriculture*, *72*, 403-410.

Zambolim, L., Sondahl, M. & Fernandes, N. T. (1996). *Microorganismos associados à qualidade de bebida de café. Relatório Anual sobre a Qualidade da Bebida.* Universidade Federal de Viçosa, Viçosa – MG. 1-55.

In: Caffeine and Health Research
Editor: Kenneth P. Chambers
ISBN 978-1-60456-437-2

Chapter IV

Caffeine and HIV

Johanna A. Smith and René Daniel
Division of Infectious Diseases - Center for Human Virology,
Kimmel Cancer Center, Thomas Jefferson University,
Philadelphia, PA, USA

Abstract

Caffeine's psychostimulatory effects are well known. These are mediated by the blockage of adenosine A2A receptors on the surface of nerve cells. However, caffeine can also enter the cells and affect a number of intracellular proteins. Some of these proteins are involved in the replication of the human immunodeficiency virus type 1 (HIV-1). As a consequence, caffeine may affect the HIV-1 life-cycle at at least three steps (integration, expression and Vpr-mediated growth arrest). Several caffeine-related compounds have been shown to have similar effects. Some of these compounds are used for the treatment of diseases other than HIV-1 infection. In this article, we summarize the current evidence for each of the described effects of caffeine and caffeine-related compounds, as published by us and others, as well as future directions of the field. In addition, we include new results addressing and explaining the underlying reasons behind some of the controversies in the field. Finally, we discuss the molecular mechanism underlying the described effects of caffeine and caffeine-related compounds on HIV-1 replication and potential consequences for the treatment of HIV-1 infection.

Introduction: Caffeine Effects

Caffeine is likely the most popularly consumed pharmacologically active substance throughout the globe. This trimethylxanthine is named so for the three methyl groups on carbons 1, 3, and 7 of xanthine (a purine base, depicted in figure 1). When ingested, caffeine is rapidly absorbed in the stomach and small intestines, and peak levels are detected in the plasma within two hours [1].

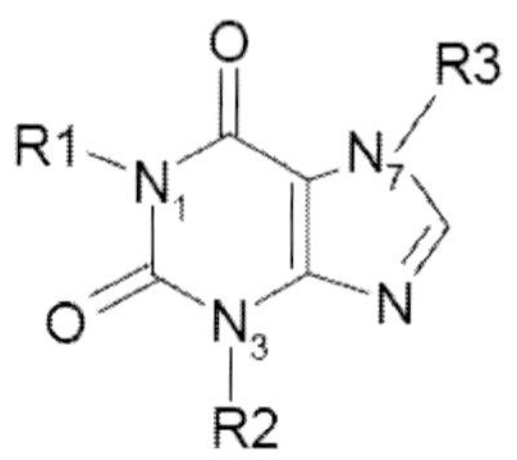

Caffeine	R1 = R2 = R3 = CH3
Theobromine	R1 = H, R2 = R3 = CH3
Theophylline	R1 = R2 = CH3, R3 = H
Paraxanthine	R1 = R3 = CH3, R2 = H

Figure 1. Molecular formula of the trimethylxanthine, caffeine, and its three primary metabolites: theobromine, theophylline, and paraxanthine.

Caffeine diffuses rapidly throughout the body, however there is no long term accumulation of the compound in the body. In the liver caffeine is broken down into three primary metabolites: paraxanthine, theobromine, and theophylline (depicted in figure 1, theobromine and theophylline are also found naturally in a variety of plants along with caffeine). The half-life of caffeine is approximately 3-4 hours in humans, although this can increase in the presence of oral contraceptives [2], pregnancy [3, 4], or liver disease. Caffeine is known to affect diverse systems of the body including the cardiovascular, nervous, respiratory, and renal systems [5]. Worldwide, people use caffeine as a stimulant and to ward off somnolence.

Caffeine is therapeutically administered for the treatment of bronchial asthma, preterm infant apnea, headaches, and postprandial hypotension and obesity [1, 5, 8]. The caffeine metabolite theophylline is clinically used as an effective central stimulant as well in the treatment of bronchial asthma, pulmonary edema, preterm infant apnea, myocardial stimulant to increase coronary flow, and as a diuretic [5]. Theobromine has also been used as a diuretic, to treat asthma, and as a cardiac stimulant, although it is the least active stimulant of the naturally occurring methylxanthines [5].

Caffeine's psychoactive stimulant effects are presumably due to the blockage of A2A adenosine receptors on the surface of nerve cells [6, 7]. The presence of caffeine prevents the neurotransmitter, adenosine, from activating inhibitory neurons, thereby increasing motor activity. This occurs at caffeine plasma levels reached following the ingestion of caffeine containing beverages, which is generally up to 10 to 50 μM. At higher caffeine concentrations, such as those between 0.1 and 1 mM [it should be noted that plasma concentrations above 0.25 mM are generally lethal [1]], phosphodiesterase (PDE) activity is repressed [8]. PDEs cleave the cyclic nucleotide phosphodiester bond between the phosphorus and oxygen atoms at the 3'-position with inversion of configuration at the phosphorus atom [9, 10]. Some PDEs are highly specific for hydrolysis of cAMP (PDE4, PDE7, PDE8), some are highly cGMP-specific (PDE5, PDE6, PDE9), and some have mixed specificity (PDE1, PDE2, PDE3, PDE10). Precise modulation of PDE function in cells is critical for maintaining cyclic nucleotide levels within a narrow rate-limiting range of concentrations. Early evidence showed that caffeine is a non-selective inhibitor of PDEs and elevates cyclic AMP levels in cells [11, 12].

When caffeine is administered to cells at levels higher than necessary to inhibit PDE activity (over 100 μM), there are also profound effects on cellular responses to DNA damage. Caffeine has been shown to sensitize cells to ionizing radiation, which induces DNA double strand breaks. The drug is thus referred to as a radiosensitizing agent and inhibitor of the DNA damage response. Caffeine modifies cellular responses to DNA damage through the inhibition of two related protein kinases (called ATM and ATR, discussed below) which are crucial for the execution of appropriate repair of diverse forms of DNA lesions. These kinases are susceptible to caffeine inhibition both *in vitro* and *in vivo* [13-16]. The IC_{50} for both of these proteins falls within the 1-2 mM range *in vitro* [15]. This property has rendered caffeine a fundamental research tool used to investigate the DNA damage response.

The DNA Damage Response

The DNA damage response is regulated by two related kinases, ATM (ataxia telangiectasia mutated) and ATR (ataxia-telangiectasia and Rad3-related), which belong to the PI-3K-related group of kinases. This group of large proteins includes yeast and mammalian kinases that bear a signature (kinase) domain at their carboxyl termini. Three members of this family, DNA-PK, ATM and ATR, have been implicated in mammalian DNA repair. ATM and ATR are caffeine targets *in vitro*, and possibly *in vivo* [14, 15]. ATM and ATR phosphorylate a common motif, S/TQ [17]. Despite this shared motif, gene knock-out studies in mice suggest little redundancy among the functions of these kinases [18]. DNA-PK and ATM act primarily in response to DNA double strand breaks, while ATR has been traditionally regarded as a responder to replication stress [17]. However, recently ATR has also been implicated in the response to double strand breaks [19-21]. DNA-PK also is fundamental to V(D)J recombination, and the induction of apoptosis [22].

The ATM gene is mutated in the human ataxia telangiectasia syndrome (A-T), a radiosensitivity and genome stability disorder, characterized by progressive cerebellar degeneration and increased cancer incidence. Cells derived from A-T patients and from atm -/- mice display sensitivity to ionizing radiation, chromosomal instability, and defects in cell cycle checkpoints. The regulation of checkpoints by ATM has been studied extensively and a number of ATM substrates have been identified. ATM mediates growth arrest in response to DNA damage by phosphorylation of these substrates [17, 18]. Checkpoint regulation thus seems to be a major ATM function. However, ATM also appears to play a direct role in DNA repair at the sites of DNA damage. Its kinase activity is activated by free DNA ends *in vitro* [23]. Moreover, a significant fraction of ATM co-sediments with damaged DNA in cell-free systems [24]. Finally, ATM was shown to phosphorylate the BRCA1 protein in response to ionizing radiation [25, 26]. BRCA1 is a tumor suppressor gene mutated in 50% of familial breast and ovarian cancers. BRCA1-deficient cells display spontaneous chromosomal abnormalities and DNA repair deficiencies [27, 28]. The exact role of BRCA1 in DNA repair is unclear; however, BRCA1 seems to control homologous double-strand break DNA repair and physically associates with proteins implicated in this DNA repair system, including Rad51 [27, 29].

In addition to BRCA1 phosphorylation, double-strand DNA breaks induce extensive phosphorylation of a member of the H2A family, H2AX, at the sites of DNA damage in chromatin [30, 31]. This histone modification (termed γH2AX) appears to have a critical role in signaling DNA damage and/or the subsequent repair of these breaks [32, 33]. Phosphorylation occurs at a consensus site for PI-3K-related kinases, in the C-terminal tail of this histone. ATM seems to be a principal kinase responsible for H2AX phosphorylation at sites of double strand breaks [34], and/or the retention of the phosphorylated state of the histone. ATM is recruited to double strand break sites by the Mre11/Rad50/Nbs1 sensor complex which enables the damage signal to be transmitted to the proper effectors [35-40].

Finally, two members of the RecQ family of helicases, the BLM and WRN proteins, were shown to be ATM substrates. The BLM protein is mutated in Bloom's syndrome, which is characterized by genomic instability and elevated rates of most types of cancer [BS, [41]]. At a cellular level, BLM is involved in maintaining genome integrity and its absence leads to accumulation of DNA breaks [42]. At molecular level, BLM is required for correct localization of the Mre11/Rad50/Nbs1 DNA repair complex at sites of DNA damage, such as stalled replication forks [43]. *In vitro*, BLM promotes branch migration of Holliday junctions and is thus involved in homologous DNA repair [44]. The WRN protein is mutated in Werner's syndrome, which is typically characterized by premature aging, again including increased incidence of cancer [WS, [45]]. At the cellular level, WS cells also exhibit genomic instability and hypersensitivity to agents causing DNA damage and in particular interfering with the replication process [46-48]. The role of WRN in DNA repair is not yet understood, however, similar to BRCA1 and BLM, WRN localizes to sites of DNA damage [48]. Taken together, these data indicate a dual function for ATM in both DNA repair and cell cycle checkpoint control.

Until recently no disease had been associated with an ATR deficiency. However, ATR-Seckel syndrome is now recognized as a disease due to inadequacies of ATR expression. It is an autosomal recessive disorder caused by mutations in said protein. The disease is characterized by developmental delay, microcephaly, characteristic facial features, growth and mental retardation, and DNA repair deficiencies. In mice, the ATR knock-out is embryonic lethal indicating that this protein is indispensable to organismal survival [49, 50]. Nevertheless, studies with an inducible transdominant-negative ATR mutant have implied that ATR also functions in cell cycle checkpoint control [51]. ATR and ATM seem to be operating in similar pathways. Both ATM and ATR phosphorylate p53. However, ionizing radiation induces p53 phosphorylation primarily by ATM, whereas UV radiation induces phosphorylation by ATR. Nevertheless, ATM and ATR may also respond to the same type of DNA damage and some data suggest that phosphorylation is sequential [18]. Although ATR was not originally thought to respond to double strand breaks, it has been recently shown to do so by localizing to break sites subsequent to ATM and the MRN complex [19-21]. In any case, the ATM and ATR pathways overlap to a certain degree. In addition, it has been observed that ionizing radiation induces ATR foci that presumably accumulate at sites of DNA damage [52]. These foci also contain BRCA1 [53, 54]. ATR phosphorylates BRCA1 in response to ionizing radiation, and, unlike ATM, also in response to UV light and stalled DNA replication forks [54]. Likewise, ATR phosphorylates H2AX, WRN and the BLM proteins in response to these genotoxic insults [48, 55].

It has been established that caffeine disrupts DNA damage-activated cell cycle checkpoints through the responses elicited through ATM and ATR. For example, it has been shown that caffeine eliminates p53 activation and G1 arrest, G2/M arrest and S phase delay in response to DNA damage [56-67]. Nevertheless, it seems that not all caffeine effects are due to disruption of DNA damage checkpoints. It has been shown that caffeine-mediated checkpoint abrogation does not correlate with the level of caffeine-induced radiosensitization [68]. It is thus likely that caffeine acts on both cell cycle checkpoints and directly on DNA repair.

Caffeine and HIV: The HIV Life-Cycle

The human immunodeficiency virus (HIV) is an enveloped RNA retrovirus. Infection of a susceptible cell is initiated upon binding of exposed viral components to certain receptors on the target cell's surface (figure 2, #1). Subsequently, the virion and cell membranes fuse, and the viral core is deposited into the cytoplasm (figure 2, #1).

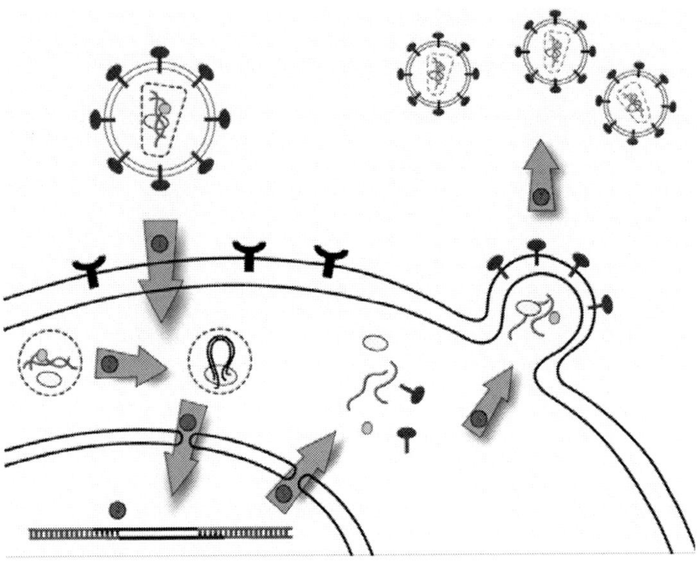

Figure 2. The life-cycle of HIV-1. Entry of an HIV particle into a cell is initiated upon binding of viral surface proteins to receptors on the target cell. The viral envelope fuses with the cell's lipid bilayer and the viral core is deposited into the cytoplasm (1). The viral enzyme reverse transcriptase converts the RNA to DNA (2), and the preintegration complex enters the nucleus (3). Viral DNA is then inserted into the host's genome (4, for details see figure 3) in the process of integration which depends on the viral enzyme integrase, as well as host cellular co-factors. The viral genome is then transcribed to produce RNA copies of the full-length genome, as well as transcripts which will be converted to polypeptids. These components exit the nucleus (5) and assemble at the plasma membrane. Particles bud from the plasma membrane (6) and are released from the cell (7).

The retroviral enzyme reverse transcriptase catalyzes reverse transcription, which converts the viral genetic material from RNA to DNA (figure 2, #2), which subsequently enters the nucleus in a complex with the viral enzyme integrase (figure 2, #3). The viral double stranded DNA product can then be incorporated into the genome of the host cell in a process called integration [figure 2, #4, [69-71]].

This stage of the HIV life-cycle can not be completed without the involvement of certain host cell DNA repair co-factors (see below). Once the viral genetic material has been successfully inserted into host cell DNA, the virus is capable of replication. Transcription of the stably transduced viral genome (now called a provirus) proceeds in order to produce viral proteins, as well as two RNA copies of the viral genome. These components accumulate at the plasma membrane to assemble viral particles which then release from the infected cell [figure 2, #5 – 7, [69, 71].

Caffeine and HIV: Integration and Postintegration Repair

Integration is an essential stage in the HIV life-cycle. The first two steps are catalyzed by the viral enzyme integrase, and are denoted processing and joining (Figure 3B) [72, 73]. First integrase removes two nucleotides from the 3' ends of the viral DNA (processing), to create "sticky", nucleophilic ends which can then attack host DNA, creating a double stranded break while inserting it's own genetic material between the DNA ends (Figure 3B). Now the 3' viral ends are joined to the host 5' DNA ends, but there is a 5 base pair gap left between the viral 5' ends and host 3' ends [74]. To complete integration, the viral 5' nucleotide overhangs are cleaved (Figure 3C), the gap repaired (Figure 3D), and ends ligated (Figure 3E) in the process of postintegration repair [75, 76].

Postintegration repair has been shown to be mediated by host cellular DNA repair mechanisms by multiple laboratories. Because host cellular co-factors have the potential of being attractive targets of anti-HIV-1 therapies (thereby circumventing the viral mutation rate problem), the elucidation of postintegration repair mechanisms is being actively sought by multiple groups.

In order to study early stages of the retroviral life-cycle – which include entry, reverse transcription, nuclear import of viral DNA and requisite proteins, and integration – retroviral based vectors are commonly employed. A vector can be thought of as a vehicle used to stably introduce exogenous DNA into the genome of a cell. Retrovirus-based vectors consist of recombinant viruses with only select genes present in the viral particle [71]. Also packaged in the particle are viral proteins which are necessary for all of the early steps in retroviral replication. However, the genes which encode these proteins are not included within the recombinant viral genome. This means that once integration occurs, the viral life-cycle is terminated. Vectors made for most applications are therefore replication-defective because the viral DNA which integrates lacks the necessary genes to produce new virions. In addition to delivering a therapeutic gene into a cell of interest, these genetically altered viruses are useful tools to study the process of integration. Such vectors are constructed to contain a "reporter gene" which enables one the ability to quantify infected cells.

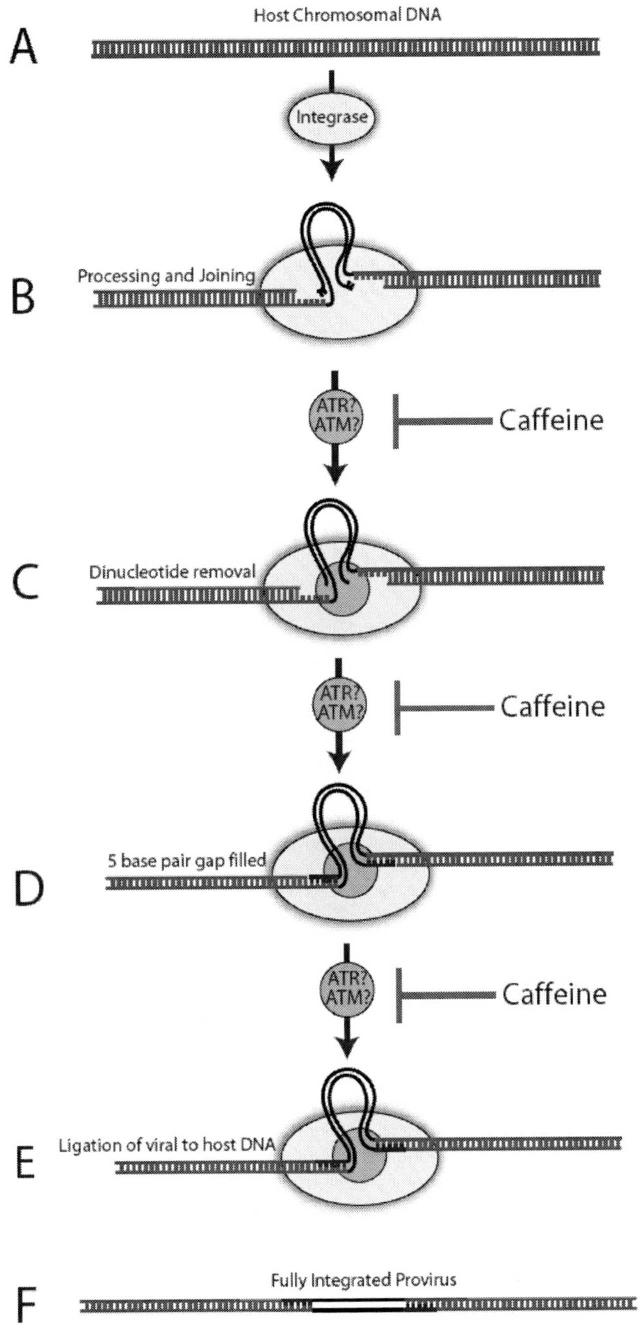

Figure 3. Integration and postintegration repair. Integration is a process of the incorporation of viral DNA into the host cell genome. The first two steps (called processing and joining) are catalyzed by integrase (B). Integrase cleaves a dinucleotide from 3' viral ends, which are then joined to host cell DNA, producing a double stranded break. The final step, postintegration repair (C – E), is facilitated by host cellular DNA damage response proteins. To complete postintegration repair, two nucleotides from 5' viral ends are excised (C), the five base pair gap is filled (D), and viral ends are ligated to host DNA ends (E), to create a fully integrated provirus (F). Host cell co-factors (ATM/ATR) play a role in one or more of the steps of postintegration repair.

Common reporter genes include the *lacZ*, EGFP (enhanced green fluorescent protein), and luciferase genes. Once integration is complete, the cell is referred to as "stably transduced" because it's genome now contains the viral vector, which will then be passed on to all daughter cells. It is because of this attribute that much effort is being made to advance the field of gene therapy using retroviral vectors.

Caffeine and HIV: Host Co-factors Involved in Postintegration Repair

The first host cellular DNA repair co-factors observed to play a role in HIV integration were those of the nonhomologous end joining (NHEJ) double strand break repair pathway. It was first found that cells deficient in DNA-PK (DNA-dependent protein kinase) were induced to undergo apoptosis in response to infection with retrovirus-based vectors [77]. As well as increased cell death, the number of stably transduced cells has been shown to be 5-10-fold lower in cells deficient of elements of the NHEJ pathway. These results were dependent on the presence of the active integrase enzyme. We therefore suggested that DNA repair proteins may be required for the completion of efficient retroviral integration (in the postintegration repair step).

DNA-PK belongs to the same PI-3K-related protein kinase family as the previously mentioned ATM and ATR. Residual integration occurring in DNA-PK-deficient cells was shown to be facilitated by the ATM protein kinase [77]. To investigate the role of ATM and the closely related ATR protein, caffeine was utilized as an inhibitor of these two proteins (but not DNA-PK), and was shown to dramatically decrease integration in a dose-dependent manner [78]. Experiments conducted on the human cervical cancer HeLa cell line infected in the absence or presence of caffeine at varying amounts (1-4 mM, all utilized concentrations are non-toxic to cells and do not inhibit HeLa cell growth) showed that caffeine inhibited stable transduction of both HIV-1 and ASV (avian sarcoma virus)-based vectors. Cells exposed to 4 mM of caffeine were only infected roughly at 10% when normalized to cells infected in the absence of the drug. This reduction was not due to viral DNA synthesis, nor its nuclear import.

Caffeine could have an effect on the joining reaction of viral to host DNA. Alternatively, the stability of the junctions could be influenced by the presence of caffeine. Therefore an important technique was employed to detect the junctions present in cell DNA following infection [78]. Alu-PCR is a nested PCR technique [78] which takes advantage of the fact that primate DNA contains short repetitive Alu units throughout the genome, over one million copies [79, 80]. During the first round of PCR, one primer anneals to a portion of the Alu sequence, while the other primer's target is in the LTR of the virus. A portion of the first round product is then used in a second PCR reaction (alternatively, real time PCR may be used for the second round as a more sensitive method) which utilizes two LTR primers, both within the sequence that was expanded in the first round, therefore it is a "nested" PCR technique. Then the final products may be run on an agarose gel, and then using a radioactive probe, subjected to southern hybridization to quantitate. This method was used to detect host to virus junctions 24 hours after infections with the ASV vector. Infection in the presence of caffeine reduced the junctions detectable in a dose dependent manner, with an 88% decrease in samples infected with 4 mM caffeine. This difference could be explained by inhibition of integrase mediated processing or joining, or the instability of the virus-host DNA intermediate in the presence of the drug. However, Daniel *et al.* showed *in vitro* that the catalytic activity of integrase was unaffected by caffeine up to 10 mM [78]. Therefore another hypothesis was suggested, which was that the unrepaired integration intermediate promotes cell death, thereby removing those cells from the population.

To more directly investigate the role of ATR in HIV integration, transduction efficiency was examined in cells capable of induced expression of a transdominant-negative ATR mutant. Knocking out the ATR gene is lethal in mice, and cells in culture die quickly once the ATR gene is removed [19, 49, 50]. In order to study ATR function the GM847/ATRkd fibroblast cell line was constructed to inducibly express a kinase dead form of the ATR protein denoted as ATRkd [ATR kinase dead, [51]] in the presence of doxycycline, because ATRkd is under the control of a doxycycline dependent promoter. Such ATRkd expressing cells are viable, and show DNA repair defects which are different from those of ATM-deficient cells.

Because caffeine is a non specific inhibitor of ATM and ATR, the effect of caffeine on ATM-deficient cells (AT22IJE-T, a cell line derived from primary A-T fibroblasts) was investigated alongside ATM-proficient cells (AT22IJE-T, cells complemented with a vector encoding wild-type ATM). In this study, stable transduction was shown to be independent of ATM, as caffeine inhibited both ATM-deficient and proficient cells at comparable rates. Besides ATR and ATM, the related kinase mTOR is also sensitive to caffeine, so HeLa cells were treated with rapamycin, an inhibitor specific to mTOR, and infected. However, this drug had no observable effect on transduction. This together with the data on transduction of ATM-deficient cells therefore implicated ATR as the caffeine target involved in postintegration repair [78].

In the work discussed above, experiments were conducted solely on normally cycling cells. ATM and ATR play multiple roles in the DNA damage response including the induction of cell cycle checkpoints, as well as physical repair of DNA. At concentrations that stimulate radiosensitization *in vivo*, caffeine also inhibits ATM and ATR catalytic activity *in vitro* [14, 15]. If cell cycle checkpoint induction is required to complete efficient integration, it is possible that the caffeine effect could be resulting from the abrogation of ATR/ATM dependent cell cycle checkpoints. It was therefore important to further investigate the caffeine effect on non-mitosing cells because if the caffeine effect on HIV replication was through the mechanism of inhibiting ATR controlled cell cycle checkpoints, the caffeine effect would not be seen if the cells were already nondividing prior to infection [81]. Nocodazole is an agent used to arrest cell growth at M phase as it disrupts mitotic spindle function by binding to β-tubulin. The human kidney cell line 293T was growth arrested using nocodazole, and infected with an HIV-1-based vector alongside exponentially dividing cultures in the presence of varying amounts of caffeine. Interestingly, the effect of caffeine on transduction efficiencies of both growth arrested cells and dividing cells were sensitive to caffeine, responding in a dose-dependent manner [81]. In cells infected in the presence of 1 mM caffeine, transduction was reduced by approximately 25% when compared to cells infected in the absence of caffeine. Two mM of caffeine reduced transduction by over 50%, and 4 mM reduced transduction by about 80%, in both dividing and nondividing cells.

To investigate the caffeine effect on cells growth arrested using another mechanism, mouse embryonic fibroblasts (MEFs) were arrested in G1 by contact inhibition. Although arrested MEFs were transduced at significantly lower rates than dividing MEFs (at least 6-fold lower), transduction of both sets were very sensitive to caffeine, with a dose dependent response similar to that of infected 293T cells. The caffeine effect on infected, terminally differentiated human neurons and macrophages was also studied, and in both cases, caffeine significantly decreased transduction of the HIV-1 based vector. At just 1 mM, caffeine had a profound impact on transduction of terminally differentiated macrophages, decreasing transduction by almost 6-fold. All caffeine concentrations used were non-toxic to cells. Taken together, the data suggest that the caffeine effect is due at least in part by the inhibition of ATR, and this inhibition is not due to the inhibition of cell cycle checkpoint induction.

It has been suggested that the inhibition of HIV transduction by caffeine was due to inhibition of CMV-driven expression of the integrated reporter gene [82]. Another group also found caffeine to have no effect on HIV-1 transduction [83]. This led Nunnari *et al.* to investigate the effect of caffeine and other methylxanthines on the replication of infectious HIV-1 strains. First, human peripheral blood mononuclear cells (PBMCs) from uninfected individuals were infected with HIV-1 NL4-3 (a T-cell-line tropic replication competent strain), in the presence of caffeine, theophylline, theobromine, paraxanthine, or NL4-3 alone [84]. Infections were measured using a p24 antigen assay which measures the quantity of the p24 protein, a component of the viral core of HIV, in order to quantitate viral infectivity. Cells were assayed 3, 7, and 21 days post infection (dpi). At three days post infection, HIV-1 p24 values of theobromine and paraxanthine treated samples were only 50% of that of samples infected in the absence of methylxanthines. A more striking inhibitory effect was seen in caffeine and theophylline treated samples. At 2 dpi a 9-fold reduction was observed. This difference decreased over time, which was gathered to be due to the removal of the drugs from the cultures. Additionally, the macrophage-tropic HIV-1 replication competent ADA strain was used in this work, and interestingly the results of methylxanthine inhibition were even more profound. In fact, the IC_{50} of theophylline inhibition was found to be 60 μM which is well within the range of current pharmacologically utilized concentrations found in plasma of theophylline treated patients [28-110 μM, [85]]. In the presence of the highest utilized concentration of theophylline (4 mM) the p24 antigen readout was approximately 15-fold lower in cultures infected in the presence of either theophylline or caffeine than that of cells infected in the absence of methylxanthines. The IC_{50} of caffeine inhibition was also lower in ADA infected cells (verses infection with the NL4-3 strain) and found to be 100 μM. From here it was concluded that caffeine and structurally similar methylxanthines suppress replication of wild-type infectious HIV-1 strains.

It had been shown formerly that caffeine suppression of retrovirus-based vectors was due to the integration step of the retroviral life cycle, because the other early steps of infection remained unaffected by caffeine [78]. In this study [84], the early steps in the HIV-1 life-cycle were investigated to determine if it was also the case in fully infectious HIV-1 which contained the wild-type HIV-1 envelope, as opposed to the pseudotyped envelopes used in preceding works. HIV-1 DNA synthesis, HIV-1 nuclear import, and HIV-1 DNA integration were measured and compared in samples infected with and without caffeine, in order to determine which step was responsible for the caffeine effect. PBMCs were infected with the NL4-3 strain of replication competent virus, and infected with one or none of the methylxanthines (caffeine, theophylline, theobromine, or paraxanthine). Caffeine and other methylxanthines did not have a noteworthy effect on HIV-1 DNA synthesis, nor the formation of 2-LTR circle DNA junctions, which suggest that the methylxanthines do not affect entry, or the nuclear import of the HIV-1 pre-integration complex. However, when levels of integrated viral DNA were determined 24 hpi, a 4- to 50-fold reduction was found in methylxanthine treated samples using the Alu-PCR method. Then we sought out to determine the levels of unspliced RNA in samples, because integration begins to take place around 4-8 hpi, so at 24 hours, the HIV RNA expressed is derived from integrated proviral DNA. As expected, HIV-1-specific RNA levels were down in caffeine-treated samples, correlating with decreased integration events, supporting the hypothesis that caffeine suppresses HIV infection at the integration phase [84].

However, the affect of methylxanthines on the late steps of the HIV-1 life-cycle were also pursued. Using the ACH-2 cell line, which produces HIV-1 virions upon stimulation with phorbol myristate acetate (PMA), we observed that neither virion production nor p24 antigen expression were affected with the presence of methylxanthines. Experiments were conducted on both stimulated and unstimulated ACH-2 cells. This suggests that the methylxanthines tested do not reduce HIV-1 replication *via* the post-integrative steps. Furthermore, in PBMC infected cells, caffeine was shown to suppress the phosphorylation of ATR and ATM targets, including BRCA1 (Ser 1423) and p53 (Ser 15), which are shown to be expressed at increased levels in response to infection with HIV-1. In other words, the wild-type HIV-1 strain, NL4-3, triggers the ATR and ATM-dependent DNA damage response. This response is suppressed by certain methylxanthines. Our hypothesis remains that HIV-1 and certain other retroviruses trigger host cellular DNA repair mechanisms to be activated in order to facilitate postintegration repair. It would also seem likely that proteins of the DNA damage response may play a role in the reconstitution of chromatin structure following viral to host DNA joining. Although the highest levels of methylxanthines used would be toxic to humans, it is noteworthy that theophylline had a considerable effect on the inhibition of HIV-1 replication at concentrations that are currently observable in plasma samples of those who consume the drug to treat unrelated diseases. However, more effective inhibitors will be needed before pursuing the possibility of inhibiting DNA repair kinases to ward off HIV infection. Additionally, side effects of therapeutic inhibitors will need to be meticulously investigated.

So why has the effect of caffeine on integration not been universally observed? Lau *et al.* pointed out that with the use of siRNA (targeting proteins involved in the DNA damage response or control, non specific sequences) results are not convincing, because even the control siRNA alters transduction readouts, which may at least partially explain the discrepancies [86]. Another rationale likely involves complications resulting from utilized markers. Colony assays appear to be more conclusive when detecting the role of DNA repair proteins in postintegration repair as opposed to other reporters that are routinely assayed shortly after infection [86]. In addition, some markers (for instance EGFP) have been shown to be expressed from unintegrated DNA for as long as one week after infection [87]. We have also noticed a significant amount of EGFP expressed from unintegrated DNA (albeit at a lower intensity), and this expression may be included in the portion of the cell population that is scored positive for EGFP (and therefore considered to contain integrated proviral DNA). This is demonstrated in figure 4. HeLa cells were infected with an HIV-1 based vector containing the EGFP (enhanced green fluorescent protein) reporter gene, either in the presence of an integrase inhibitor (figure 4C), caffeine (figure 4D), or pentoxifylline (figure 4E, structurally similar to caffeine, discussed below), or in the absence of any drug. Two days post infection, EGFP was measured by FACS (fluorescence activated cell scanner) analysis.

The expression from unintegrated DNA can be quantified when careful attention is paid to the gating of the individual cell populations. This can be done by examining the histogram of the HeLa cells exposed to the inhibitor specific to the integrase enzyme (L-731,988), which blocks the joining step of integration, without affecting steps prior to joining [88]. Compared to cells infected in the absence of any compound, HeLa cells exposed to L-731,988 lack the peak on the far right of the histogram seen in cells infected without any drugs.

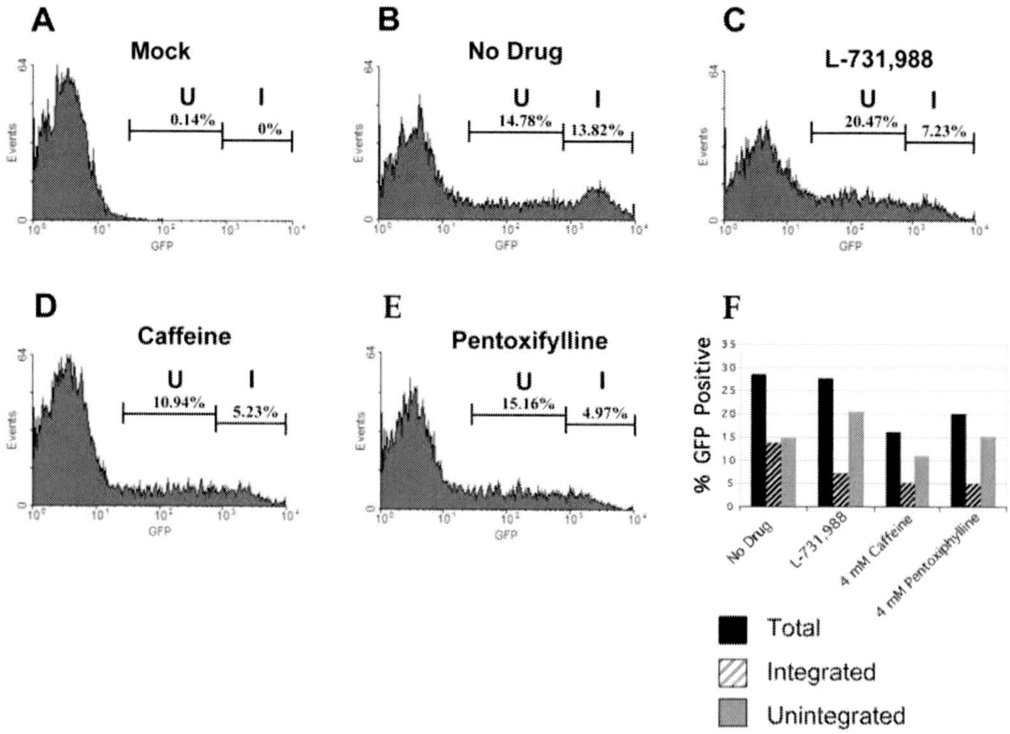

Figure 4. Effect of pentoxifylline on HIV-1 transduction of an EGFP marker. Exponentially dividing HeLa cells were infected with the HIV-1-based vector and exposed to L-731,988, caffeine, pentoxifylline, or in the absence of any drug. Two days post-infection, cells were analyzed by flow cytometry. (A) Uninfected cells. (B) Cells infected in the absence of a drug. (C) Cells infected in the presence of 10 μM concentration of the integrase inhibitor, L731,988. (D) Cells infected in the presence of 4 mM caffeine. (E) Cells infected in the presence of 4 mM pentoxifylline. (F) Comparison of fractions of cells expressing EGFP from unintegrated and integrated DNA in each sample. "I" – cells expressing EGFP from integrated DNA, "U" – cells expressing EGFP from unintegrated DNA.

However, between the main cell population on the left and the highly expressing EGFP population on the right, is a significant fraction of cells that are considered "EGFP positive" because in the uninfected cells (figure 4A) there is no such population. Because L-731,988 inhibits joining of viral to host DNA, this expression must derive from unintegrated DNA. Thus, we scored this portion of the population as "U" for unintegrated, and the peak containing the cell population expressing the highest levels of EGFP as "I" for integrated. As shown in figure 4B, the EGFP reporter was expressed in approximately 28% of infected cells. Comparison with cells that were treated with the integrase inhibitor demonstrated that the reporter was expressed from integrated vector DNA in only a fraction of cells (labeled "I"), 13.82% in these experiments (figure 4B, see also F). Consistent with our previously published data, caffeine treatment also resulted in the reduction of the percentage of cells in fraction I, likely due to failure of postintegration repair, which is required for completion of the integration process (figure 4D, F). In contrast, caffeine treatment resulted in only a minor reduction of the fraction U, from 14.78% (figure 4B, no drug) to 10.94%, which is again consistent with published results (Figure 3D, F) [89]. Treatment with a caffeine-related compound, pentoxifylline, also caused reduction in the fraction I from 13.82 to 4.97% (figure 4E, F), but did not have any significant effect on the U fraction.

All of the methylxanthines discussed so far are products of caffeine metabolism. Another methylxanthine, pentoxyfylline (briefly mentioned above), is a chemically modified methylxanthine (structure see figure 5) currently used for the treatment of vaso-oclusive diseases, leg ulcers [90], and sickle cell disease [91]. Intriguingly, this compound has shown a certain potential in early clinical trials to treat patients with AIDS [92]. The mechanism of HIV replication inhibition at that time was presumed to be due to the fact that pentoxifylline suppresses tumor necrosis factor alpha (TNFα) production and nuclear factor-kappa B (NF-κB) [92-96]. TNFα is a cytokine which has many functions. In the context of HIV, it plays a role in T cell activation [97] and inducing HIV-1 expression in infected cells [98]. The latter is conducted by upregulating the transcription factor NF-κB [99, 100] which is a major activator of HIV LTR. Caffeine, however, does not seem to have this inhibitory effect on LTR expression. In fact, it has been revealed that caffeine is an inducer of LTR expression [101].

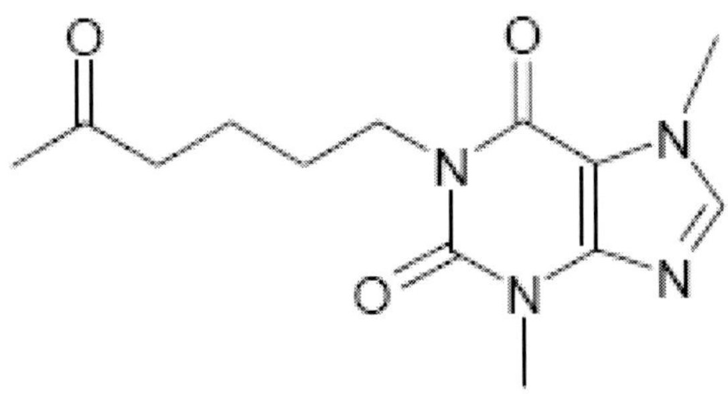

Figure 5. Pentoxifylline. Molecular formula of pentoxifylline, a chemically modified xanthine.

Although exogenous TNFα addition in pentoxifylline treated HIV-1-infected T cells restored NF-κB activation, it did not affect the suppression of p24, likely suggesting that pentoxifylline suppresses HIV through a method distinct from NF-κB or TNFα suppression

[102]. Therefore it seems that the pentoxifylline effect is multifaceted, likely involving more than just the inhibition of TNFα and NF-κB, which limit HIV expression due to LTR suppresssion. To study this effect, we conducted experiments using HIV-1 based vectors with reporter genes under the control of the cytomegalovirus (CMV) promoter (as opposed to replication competent virus used in other pentoxifylline studies which is under control of LTR driven expression).

We found that pentoxifylline inhibits transduction by an HIV-1-based vector containing the *lac*Z reporter gene [103]. The first step in determining whether or not pentoxifylline affects other portions of the HIV-1 life-cycle besides repressing LTR promoter function, we infected the human kidney fibroblast 293T cell line in the presence of pentoxifylline, caffeine (as a control, because it impedes postintegration repair), or no methylxanthine with the vector. Pentoxifylline reduced stable transduction more dramatically than caffeine, with an IC_{50} of 100 μM, while that of caffeine was 1 mM. Pentoxyfilline was non-toxic at all utilized concentrations.

In these experiments cells were assayed two days post infection with a β-galactosidase assay. The *lac*Z reporter gene present in this vector encodes for the bacterial β-galactosidase enzyme, which turns the transduced cells blue, and can be visualized under the microscope. Alternatively, cell lysates can be stained and measured for absorbance using a spectrophotometer. Two days is sufficient for the *lac*Z gene to be abundantly expressed from the provirus in most cell lines.

To investigate the possibility that the pentoxifylline effect could be due to suppression of the CMV promoter, 293T cells were stably transduced in the absence of the drug. Forty-eight hours later pentoxifylline or caffeine was added to cultures, and exposed for 24 hours. Twenty-four hours after removal of the drug, a β-galactosidase assay was conducted and blue cells counted. Neither methylxanthine suppressed expression of the *lac*Z reporter. However, at the highest concentrations used of both pentoxifylline and caffeine, there were slightly higher numbers of *lac*Z positive cells. The effect of these drugs on transient expression of plasmid *lac*Z DNA was also examined. The day following transfection, the drugs were added to *lac*Z transfected 293T cells. A β-galactosidase assay was done twenty four hours following removal of the drugs. As expected, there was no significant effect on *lac*Z transient expression from transfected cells. Taken together these data show that pentoxifylline suppresses transduction of HIV-1-based vectors without any effect on promoter function. Similar to the previously described studies, in order to verify which stage of the HIV-1 life-cycle was susceptible to pentoxifylline, levels of viral DNA synthesis, nuclear import, and integrated DNA had to be addressed. As seen before with other methylxanthines, late products of reverse transcription and 2-LTR circle formation was roughly equivalent in all samples. On the other hand, levels of integrated DNA differed significantly in a dose dependent manner according to pentoxifylline concentration. In fact, using densitometry analysis of the Alu-PCR final product, at 4 mM of pentoxifylline, the level of integrated DNA was measured to be more than 10-fold less than that measured from cells infected without the drug.

We have shown previously that ATR function is necessary for efficient HIV-1 transduction. Since ATR was reported to be a pentoxifylline target [15] effects of pentoxifylline on ATR-deficient cells was examined using the GM847/ATRkd cell line, which can be induced with doxycycline to express ATRkd. As seen before, cells expressing functional ATR were transduced approximately 5-fold higher than cells expressing the dominant negative mutant form of the kinase. Interestingly, the effect of pentoxifylline in cells expressing ATRkd was reduced. At the highest concentration of pentoxifylline, cells infected with doxycycline, were only reduced about 3-fold, compared to cells infected with doxycycline, but without pentoxifylline. On the other hand, in the absence of doxycycline, pentoxifylline decreased the efficiency of stable transduction by about 10-fold when compared to samples infected without the methylxanthine.

Taken together this data suggests that there is another mechanism involved in the pentoxifylline inhibition of HIV-1 replication, besides the TNFa/NF-κB effect, and this newly uncovered mechanism involves the suppression of the ATR kinase. Postintegration repair consists of trimming 5' viral ends, filling in the five base pair gap that exists between viral ends and host DNA. Then the ends must be ligated, and chromatin structure reconstituted in the vicinity where the virus was inserted. ATR could play a role in one or more of these steps. Alternatively, since part of ATR's major function is cell cycle checkpoint control, ATR could trigger checkpoints to halt the cell cycle long enough for postintegration repair to take place. However, we have shown that caffeine and other methylxanthines suppress transduction of HIV-1 based vectors, and infection of replication competent virus in non-dividing cells where the cell cycle is already arrested or terminated. Therefore, the methylxanthine effect is not due to the inhibition of cell cycle checkpoints, but rather through a direct effect on DNA repair.

Vpr Induced Cell Cycle Arrest

In addition to an effect on postintegration repair and LTR-driven expression, caffeine and it's target ATR have been implicated in the induction of cell cycle arrest by the HIV-1 viral protein R (Vpr). The HIV-1 protein Vpr has been shown to induce G2 phase arrest [104-109] and apoptosis [110-115]. This growth arrest is believed to be due to the inactivation of the cyclin-dependent kinase Cdc2 (a protein downstream of ATM and ATR) which must be activated to induce the cell cycle from G2 to M [104-106]. Notably, this Vpr-induced arrest has been shown to be overcome by methylxanthines [116, 117]. Together, these data suggest that Vpr stimulates cell cycle arrest by means of a DNA damage-responsive pathway [116]. Therefore, it would be conceivable that the effect of caffeine on HIV replication may at least in part be mediated by the Vpr-mediated cell cycle arrest. However, our data showed that caffeine represses even transduction of HIV-1-based vectors that lack Vpr [81]. Thus, the caffeine effect on Vpr function is unrelated to caffeine's effect on postintegration repair.

Vpr-induced G2 checkpoint induction is independent of ATM [118]. Therefore, Roshal *et al.* examined the possibility of ATR as the kinase accountable for Vpr-induced arrest [119]. To do so, this group used a pharmacological inhibitor of ATR (LY294002) as well as the less specific inhibitor caffeine, to treat HeLa cells and then infected them with an HIV-1-based vector encoding either Vpr and GFP or GFP alone. G2 arrest depended on the presence of Vpr in the HIV vector. Also, samples treated with either LY294002 or caffeine were much less sensitive to the growth arrest. Two different ATRkd inducible cell lines were used to investigate the role of this possible Vpr mediated G2 arrest. Cells expressing the mutant form of the kinase were largely alleviated of the cell cycle checkpoint induction. Knockdown experiments were also conducted with siRNA targeting ATR. Similarly, it was concluded that the knockdown of ATR minimized the occurrence of Vpr-induced G2 arrest.

Together, the data propose that ATR function is required for G2 arrest mediated by the viral protein Vpr. It is not clear whether Vpr directly causes damage to DNA or whether it causes a signal that imitates damage by activating a sensor in the DNA damage response cascade. Interestingly it has been revealed that Vpr-mediated G2 arrest provokes BRCA1 and γH2AX nuclear foci formation through a mechanism which requires Rad17 and Hus1 [120] indicative of host cellular responses to replication stress [121, 122]. It has also been suggested that Vpr directly induces the formation of double strand breaks [123]. This Vpr mediated response may assist in the elucidation of the mechanisms of cytopathic effects resulting from HIV-1 infection. Taken together, Vpr induces ATR-dependent growth arrest, which is reversible by caffeine. However, it is not clear if this Vpr effect has any role in HIV-1 replication or pathogenesis.

Role for ATM in Integration

As noted above, we were first to report that ATM is involved in postintegration repair [124]. However, we found only residual integration events to depend on ATM in cells that lack functional DNA-PK. In contrast, a very intriguing and thorough study was completed by the O'Connor group suggesting that the ATM kinase is in fact crucial for efficient HIV-1 replication [86]. This group did so by using both genetic and pharmacological systems to study the role of ATM in retroviral replication. This study provides proof of concept that use of a specific inhibitor to a DNA repair protein may be a feasible, novel approach to targeting HIV-1 while avoiding drug resistance. Such an approach may be feasible for caffeine related compounds as well, especially since pentoxifylline has already been used in clinical trials for the treatment of AIDS.

In this study, ATM knockout mouse embryonic stem cells and human fibroblasts from A-T patients were used to test transduction efficiencies, when compared to respective cells containing functional ATM using two different HIV-1-based vectors. ATM-deficient cells were transduced at rates between 10-20% when normalized to that of ATM proficient cells. Furthermore, using A-T fibroblast cells complemented with the wild-type form of ATM, the deficiency was rescued in the presence of functional ATM. Next it was shown that HIV-1 infection activates the DNA damage response controlled primarily by ATM, and there was enhanced cell death in ATM-deficient cells.

Using a new, small molecule inhibitor specific to ATM (KU-55933), the drug was found to profoundly inhibit HIV-1 vector transduction of Jurkat lymphoblast cells with an IC50 value of only 1 μM. In the presence of 10 μM of KU-55933 transduction was reduced to approximately 10% of that in the absence of the drug. Interestingly, the drug also did not have much effect on the residual transduction that was observed in A-T fibroblast cells, while the infectivity of the ATM-proficient fibroblast cells was significantly supressed in the presence of KU-55933. Again, the decrease of infection was due to the postintegration repair step based on late RT products, 2-LTR junctions, and integrated DNA PCR data. Notably, the ability of KU-55933 to inhibit HIV-1 transduction was extended to both wild-type strains of HIV-1, as well as drug resistant strains, which illustrates the potential significance of targeting cellular enzymes in HIV-1 patients with diverse strains of the virus.

This study convincingly illustrates the critical role that ATM plays in postintegration repair, even though initial studies demonstrated that this kinase played only a secondary role, in the absence of NHEJ [124]. What is the reason for this inconsistency? Lau *et al.* suggests the discrepancy is due to the different cell lines utilized to study the role of DNA damage response proteins in integration [86]. It is also possible that because the DNA damage response pathways are overlapping and complex, it is hard to differentiate between the major protein kinases involved, especially as in the case of ATM/ATR because these two proteins are sometimes found to be implicated in the same interconnected pathway. Our new, yet unpublished data, which utilize primary cells, indicate that differences among cell lines are the likely explanation of these disparities. ATM thus may play a more significant role in postintegration repair than previously envisaged.

Conclusion

In summary, caffeine and related compounds inhibit HIV-1 replication and vector transduction. Interestingly, caffeine has been shown to increase transcriptional activation of the viral LTR. The mechanism of the caffeine inhibitory effect on HIV is through inhibition of important host DNA repair proteins which the virus exploits to facilitate postintegration repair. Caffeine was also shown to inhibit the Vpr-induced growth arrest of HIV-1-infected cells. However, it is not yet clear if this effect of caffeine has any significance in HIV-1 replication and pathogenesis. Caffeine-related compounds also inhibit HIV-1 replication. These data suggest that caffeine-based compounds could be eventually developed into antivirals for the treatment of HIV-1 infection.

References

[1] Garattini, S., ed. Caffeine, Coffee, and Health. *Metabolism of Caffeine and Other Components of Coffee*, ed. M.J. Arnaud. 1993, Raven Press: New York.

[2] Meyer, F.P., et al., Zeitverlauf der Hemmung der Coffeinelimination unter dem Einfluss des oralen Depotkontrazeptivum Deposiston. Hormonale Kontrazeptiva und Coffeinelimination. *Zentralblatt fur Gynakologie*, 1991. 113(6): p. 297-302.

[3] McKim, E.M., Caffeine and its effects on pregnancy and the neonate. *Journal of Nurse-Midwifery*, 1991. 36(4): p. 226-31.

[4] Ortweiler, W., et al., Bestimmung der Elimination von Koffein und Metamizol in der Schwangerschaft und im Wochenbett als in vivo-Methode zur Charakterisierung verschiedener Zytochrom P-450-abhangiger Biotransformationsreaktionen. *Biomedica Biochimica Acta*, 1985. 44(7-8): p. 1189-99.

[5] Garattini, S., ed. Caffeine, Coffee, and Health. Mechanism of Action of Caffeine, ed. J.W. Daly. 1993, *Raven Press*: New York.

[6] Mandel, H.G., Update on caffeine consumption, disposition and action. *Food and Chemical Toxicology*, 2002. 40(9): p. 1231-4.

[7] Vaugeois, J.M., Signal transduction: positive feedback from coffee.[comment]. *Nature*, 2002. 418(6899): p. 734-6.

[8] Sawynok, J. and T.L. Yaksh, Caffeine as an analgesic adjuvant: a review of pharmacology and mechanisms of action. *Pharmacological Reviews*, 1993. 45(1): p. 43-85.

[9] Burgers, P.M., et al., Stereochemistry of hydrolysis of adenosine 3':5'-cyclic phosphorothioate by the cyclic phosphodiesterase from beef heart. *Journal of Biological Chemistry,* 1979. 254(20): p. 9959-61.

[10] Goldberg, N.D., et al., 18O-Labeling of guanosine monophosphate upon hydrolysis of cyclic guanosine 3':5'-monophosphate by phosphodiesterase. *Journal of Biological Chemistry*, 1980. 255(21): p. 10344-7.

[11] Corbin, J.D. and S.H. Francis, Cyclic GMP phosphodiesterase-5: target of sildenafil. *Journal of Biological Chemistry*, 1999. 274(20): p. 13729-32.

[12] Rall, T.W. and E.W. Sutherland, Formation of a cyclic adenine ribonucleotide by tissue particles. *Journal of Biological Chemistry*, 1958. 232(2): p. 1065-76.

[13] Blasina, A., et al., Caffeine inhibits the checkpoint kinase ATM. *Current Biology*, 1999. 9(19): p. 1135-8.

[14] Hall-Jackson, C.A., et al., ATR is a caffeine-sensitive, DNA-activated protein kinase with a substrate specificity distinct from DNA-PK. *Oncogene*, 1999. 18(48): p. 6707-13.

[15] Sarkaria, J.N., et al., Inhibition of ATM and ATR kinase activities by the radiosensitizing agent, caffeine. *Cancer Research*, 1999. 59(17): p. 4375-82.

[16] Zhou, B.B., et al., Caffeine abolishes the mammalian G(2)/M DNA damage checkpoint by inhibiting ataxia-telangiectasia-mutated kinase activity. *Journal of Biological Chemistry*, 2000. 275(14): p. 10342-8.

[17] Shiloh, Y., ATM and ATR: networking cellular responses to DNA damage. *Current Opinion in Genetics and Development*, 2001. 11(1): p. 71-7.

[18] Durocher, D. and S.P. Jackson, DNA-PK, ATM and ATR as sensors of DNA damage: variations on a theme? *Current Opinion in Cell Biology*, 2001. 13(2): p. 225-31.

[19] Cortez, D., et al., ATR and ATRIP: partners in checkpoint signaling. *Science*, 2001. 294(5547): p. 1713-6.

[20] Jazayeri, A., et al., ATM- and cell cycle-dependent regulation of ATR in response to DNA double-strand breaks. *Nature Cell Biology*, 2006. 8(1): p. 37-45.

[21] Zou, L. and S.J. Elledge, Sensing DNA damage through ATRIP recognition of RPA-ssDNA complexes.[see comment]. *Science*, 2003. 300(5625): p. 1542-8.

[22] Burma, S. and D.J. Chen, Role of DNA-PK in the cellular response to DNA double-strand breaks. *DNA Repair*, 2004. 3(8-9): p. 909-18.

[23] Gately, D.P., et al., Characterization of ATM expression, localization, and associated DNA-dependent protein kinase activity. Molecular Biology of the Cell, 1998. 9(9): p. 2361-74.

[24] Costanzo, V., et al., Reconstitution of an ATM-dependent checkpoint that inhibits chromosomal DNA replication following DNA damage. *Molecular Cell*, 2000. 6(3): p. 649-59.

[25] Cortez, D., et al., Requirement of ATM-dependent phosphorylation of brca1 in the DNA damage response to double-strand breaks. [see comment]. *Science*, 1999. 286(5442): p. 1162-6.

[26] Gatei, M., et al., Role for ATM in DNA damage-induced phosphorylation of BRCA1. *Cancer Research*, 2000. 60(12): p. 3299-304.

[27] Moynahan, M.E., et al., Brca1 controls homology-directed DNA repair. *Molecular Cell*, 1999. 4(4): p. 511-8.

[28] Xu, X., et al., Centrosome amplification and a defective G2-M cell cycle checkpoint induce genetic instability in BRCA1 exon 11 isoform-deficient cells. *Molecular Cell*, 1999. 3(3): p. 389-95.

[29] Scully, R., et al., Association of BRCA1 with Rad51 in mitotic and meiotic cells. *Cell*, 1997. 88(2): p. 265-75.

[30] Rogakou, E.P., et al., Megabase chromatin domains involved in DNA double-strand breaks in vivo. *Journal of Cell Biology*, 1999. 146(5): p. 905-16.

[31] Rogakou, E.P., et al., DNA double-stranded breaks induce histone H2AX phosphorylation on serine 139. *Journal of Biological Chemistry*, 1998. 273(10): p. 5858-68.

[32] Celeste, A., et al., Genomic instability in mice lacking histone H2AX. *Science*, 2002. 296(5569): p. 922-7.

[33] Downs, J.A., N.F. Lowndes, and S.P. Jackson, A role for Saccharomyces cerevisiae histone H2A in DNA repair. *Nature*, 2000. 408(6815): p. 1001-4.

[34] Burma, S., et al., ATM phosphorylates histone H2AX in response to DNA double-strand breaks. *Journal of Biological Chemistry*, 2001. 276(45): p. 42462-7.

[35] Bartek, J., J. Falck, and J. Lukas, CHK2 kinase--a busy messenger. *Nature Reviews Molecular Cell Biology*, 2001. 2(12): p. 877-86.

[36] Carson, C.T., et al., The Mre11 complex is required for ATM activation and the G2/M checkpoint. *EMBO Journal*, 2003. 22(24): p. 6610-20.

[37] Kitagawa, R., et al., Phosphorylation of SMC1 is a critical downstream event in the ATM-NBS1-BRCA1 pathway. *Genes and Development*, 2004. 18(12): p. 1423-38.

[38] Lee, J.H. and T.T. Paull, Direct activation of the ATM protein kinase by the Mre11/Rad50/Nbs1 complex. *Science*, 2004. 304(5667): p. 93-6.

[39] Lee, J.H. and T.T. Paull, ATM activation by DNA double-strand breaks through the Mre11-Rad50-Nbs1 complex.[see comment][erratum appears in Science. 2005 Jun 24;308(5730):1870]. *Science*, 2005. 308(5721): p. 551-4.

[40] Uziel, T., et al., Requirement of the MRN complex for ATM activation by DNA damage. *EMBO Journal*, 2003. 22(20): p. 5612-21.

[41] German, J., Bloom's syndrome. *Dermatologic Clinics*, 1995. 13(1): p. 7-18.

[42] Li, W., et al., Absence of BLM leads to accumulation of chromosomal DNA breaks during both unperturbed and disrupted S phases. *Journal of Cell Biology*, 2004. 165(6): p. 801-12.

[43] Franchitto, A. and P. Pichierri, Bloom's syndrome protein is required for correct relocalization of RAD50/MRE11/NBS1 complex after replication fork arrest. *Journal of Cell Biology*, 2002. 157(1): p. 19-30.
[44] Karow, J.K., et al., Oligomeric ring structure of the Bloom's syndrome helicase. *Current Biology*, 1999. 9(11): p. 597-600.
[45] Mohaghegh, P. and I.D. Hickson, DNA helicase deficiencies associated with cancer predisposition and premature ageing disorders. *Human Molecular Genetics*, 2001. 10(7): p. 741-6.
[46] Franchitto, A., et al., Catalytic inhibition of topoisomerase II in Werner's syndrome cell lines enhances chromosomal damage induced by X-rays in the G2 phase of the cell cycle. *International Journal of Radiation Biology*, 2000. 76(7): p. 913-22.
[47] Pichierri, P., et al., Werner's syndrome lymphoblastoid cells are hypersensitive to topoisomerase II inhibitors in the G2 phase of the cell cycle. *Mutation Research*, 2000. 459(2): p. 123-33.
[48] Pichierri, P., F. Rosselli, and A. Franchitto, Werner's syndrome protein is phosphorylated in an ATR/ATM-dependent manner following replication arrest and DNA damage induced during the S phase of the cell cycle. *Oncogene*, 2003. 22(10): p. 1491-500.
[49] Brown, E.J. and D. Baltimore, ATR disruption leads to chromosomal fragmentation and early embryonic lethality. *Genes and Development*, 2000. 14(4): p. 397-402.
[50] De Klein, A., et al., Targeted disruption of the cell-cycle checkpoint gene ATR leads to early embryonic lethality in mice. *Current Biology*, 2000. 10(8): p. 479-82.
[51] Cliby, W.A., et al., Overexpression of a kinase-inactive ATR protein causes sensitivity to DNA-damaging agents and defects in cell cycle checkpoints. *EMBO Journal*, 1998. 17(1): p. 159-69.
[52] Tibbetts, R.S., et al., A role for ATR in the DNA damage-induced phosphorylation of p53. *Genes and Development*, 1999. 13(2): p. 152-7.
[53] Scully, R., et al., Dynamic changes of BRCA1 subnuclear location and phosphorylation state are initiated by DNA damage. *Cell*, 1997. 90(3): p. 425-35.
[54] Tibbetts, R.S., et al., Functional interactions between BRCA1 and the checkpoint kinase ATR during genotoxic stress. *Genes and Development*, 2000. 14(23): p. 2989-3002.
[55] Osborn, A.J., S.J. Elledge, and L. Zou, Checking on the fork: the DNA-replication stress-response pathway. *Trends in Cell Biology*, 2002. 12(11): p. 509-16.
[56] Griffiths, T.D., J.G. Carpenter, and D.B. Dahle, DNA synthesis and cell survival after X-irradiation of mammalian cells treated with caffeine or adenine. International Journal of Radiation Biology and Related Studies in Physics, *Chemistry and Medicine*, 1978. 33(5): p. 493-505.
[57] Jung, T. and C. Streffer, Effects of caffeine on protein phosphorylation and cell cycle progression in X-irradiated two-cell mouse embryos. *International Journal of Radiation Biology*, 1992. 62(2): p. 161-8.
[58] Kastan, M.B., et al., Participation of p53 protein in the cellular response to DNA damage. *Cancer Research*, 1991. 51(23 Pt 1): p. 6304-11.

[59] Kimler, B.F., et al., Modification of radiation-induced division delay by caffeine analogues and dibutyryl cyclic AMP. International Journal of Radiation Biology and Related Studies in Physics, *Chemistry and Medicine*, 1982. 41(1): p. 47-58.

[60] Lau, C.C. and A.B. Pardee, Mechanism by which caffeine potentiates lethality of nitrogen mustard. *Proceedings of the National Academy of Sciences of the United States of America*, 1982. 79(9): p. 2942-6.

[61] Lucke-Huhle, C., Alpha-irradiation-induced G2 delay: a period of cell recovery. *Radiation Research*, 1982. 89(2): p. 298-308.

[62] Murnane, J.P., et al., Effects of methylated xanthines on mammalian cells treated with bifunctional alkylating agents. *Nature*, 1980. 285(5763): p. 326-9.

[63] Painter, R.B., Effect of caffeine on DNA synthesis in irradiated and unirradiated mammalian cells. *Journal of Molecular Biology*, 1980. 143(3): p. 289-301.

[64] Rowley, R., Reduction of radiation-induced G2 arrest by caffeine. *Radiation Research*, 1992. 129(2): p. 224-7.

[65] Tolmach, L.J., R.W. Jones, and P.M. Busse, The action of caffeine on X-irradiated HeLa cells. I. Delayed inhibition of DNA synthesis. *Radiation Research*, 1977. 71(3): p. 653-65.

[66] Tomasovic, S.P. and W.C. Dewey, Comparative studies of the effects of drugs on X-ray-induced G2 delay. *Radiation Research*, 1978. 74(1): p. 112-28.

[67] Valenzuela, M.T., et al., Variation in sensitizing effect of caffeine in human tumour cell lines after gamma-irradiation. *Radiotherapy and Oncology*, 2000. 54(3): p. 261-71.

[68] Ribeiro, J.C., et al., Caffeine-increased radiosensitivity is not dependent on a loss of G2/M arrest or apoptosis in bladder cancer cell lines. *International Journal of Radiation Biology*, 1999. 75(4): p. 481-92.

[69] Coffin, J.M., S.H. Hughes, and H.E. Varmus, Retroviruses. 1997, Plainview, NY: Cold Spring Harbor Laboratory Press.

[70] Craigie, R., HIV integrase, a brief overview from chemistry to therapeutics. *Journal of Biological Chemistry*, 2001. 276(26): p. 23213-6.

[71] Flint, S.J., et al., Principles of Virology. *Molecular Biology, Pathogenesis, and Control*. 2000, Washington, DC: ASM Press.

[72] Craigie, R., T. Fujiwara, and F. Bushman, The IN protein of Moloney murine leukemia virus processes the viral DNA ends and accomplishes their integration in vitro. *Cell*, 1990. 62(4): p. 829-37.

[73] Katz, R.A., et al., The avian retroviral IN protein is both necessary and sufficient for integrative recombination in vitro. *Cell*, 1990. 63(1): p. 87-95.

[74] Vincent, K.A., et al., Host sequences flanking the HIV provirus. *Nucleic. Acids. Res.*, 1990. 18(20): p. 6045-7.

[75] Skalka, A.M. and R.A. Katz, Retroviral DNA integration and the DNA damage response. *Cell Death and Differentiation*, 2005. 12 Suppl 1: p. 971-8.

[76] Smith, J.A. and R. Daniel, Following the path of the virus: the exploitation of host DNA repair mechanisms by retroviruses. *ACS Chemical Biology* [Electronic Resource], 2006. 1(4): p. 217-26.

[77] Daniel, R., R.A. Katz, and A.M. Skalka, A role for DNA-PK in retroviral DNA integration. *Science*, 1999. 284(5414): p. 644-7.

[78] Daniel, R., et al., Evidence that the retroviral DNA integration process triggers an ATR-dependent DNA damage response. *Proceedings of the National Academy of Sciences of the United States of America*, 2003. 100(8): p. 4778-83.
[79] Batzer, M.A. and P.L. Deininger, Alu repeats and human genomic diversity. *Nature* Reviews Genetics, 2002. 3(5): p. 370-9.
[80] Lander, E.S., et al., Initial sequencing and analysis of the human genome.[see comment][erratum appears in Nature 2001 Aug 2;412(6846):565 Note: Szustakowki, J [corrected to Szustakowski, J]]. *Nature*, 2001. 409(6822): p. 860-921.
[81] Daniel, R., et al., Caffeine inhibits human immunodeficiency virus type 1 transduction of nondividing cells. Journal of Virology, 2005. 79(4): p. 2058-65.
[82] Dehart, J.L., et al., The ataxia telangiectasia-mutated and Rad3-related protein is dispensable for retroviral integration. *J. Virol*, 2005. 79(3): p. 1389-96.
[83] Ariumi, Y., et al., DNA damage sensors ATM, ATR, DNA-PKcs, and PARP-1 are dispensable for human immunodeficiency virus type 1 integration. *J. Virol*, 2005. 79(5): p. 2973-8.
[84] Nunnari, G., et al., Inhibition of HIV-1 replication by caffeine and caffeine-related methylxanthines. *Virology*, 2005. 335(2): p. 177-84.
[85] Ohnishi, A., et al., Differential pharmacokinetics of theophylline in elderly patients. *Drugs and Aging*, 2003. 20(1): p. 71-84.
[86] Lau, A., et al., Suppression of HIV-1 infection by a small molecule inhibitor of the ATM kinase. *Nat. Cell Biol.*, 2005. 7(5): p. 493-500.
[87] Daniel, R., et al., Evidence that stable retroviral transduction and cell survival following DNA integration depend on components of the nonhomologous end joining repair pathway. *J. Virol*, 2004. 78(16): p. 8573-81.
[88] Hazuda, D.J., et al., Inhibitors of strand transfer that prevent integration and inhibit HIV-1 replication in cells. *Science*, 2000. 287(5453): p. 646-50.
[89] Daniel, R., et al., Evidence that the retroviral DNA integration process triggers an ATR-dependent DNA damage response. Proc Natl Acad Sci U S A, 2003. 100(8): p. 4778-83.
[90] Jull, A., et al., Pentoxifylline for treating venous leg ulcers.[update of Cochrane Database Syst Rev. 2002;(1):CD001733; PMID: 11869606]. *Cochrane Database of Systematic Reviews*, 2007(3): p. CD001733.
[91] Sherer, J.T. and P.H. Glover, Pentoxifylline for sickle-cell disease. *Annals of Pharmacotherapy*, 2000. 34(9): p. 1070-4.
[92] Dezube, B.J., Pentoxifylline for the treatment of infection with human immunodeficiency virus. Clin Infect Dis, 1994. 18(3): p. 285-7.
[93] Biswas, D.K., et al., Cooperative inhibition of NF-kappa B and Tat-induced superactivation of human immunodeficiency virus type 1 long terminal repeat. *Proc. Natl. Acad. Sci.* U S A, 1993. 90(23): p. 11044-8.
[94] Clerici, M., et al., Pentoxifylline improves cell-mediated immunity and reduces human immunodeficiency virus (HIV) plasma viremia in asymptomatic HIV-seropositive persons. J Infect Dis, 1997. 175(5): p. 1210-5.

[95] Fazely, F., et al., Pentoxifylline (Trental) decreases the replication of the human immunodeficiency virus type 1 in human peripheral blood mononuclear cells and in cultured T cells. *Blood*, 1991. 77(8): p. 1653-6.
[96] Mhashilkar, A.M., et al., Inhibition of human immunodeficiency virus type 1 replication in vitro by a novel combination of anti-Tat single-chain intrabodies and NF-kappa B antagonists. *J. Virol*, 1997. 71(9): p. 6486-94.
[97] Pimentel-Muinos, F.X., M.A. Munoz-Fernandez, and M. Fresno, Control of T lymphocyte activation and IL-2 receptor expression by endogenously secreted lymphokines. *Journal of Immunology*, 1994. 152(12): p. 5714-22.
[98] Munoz-Fernandez, M.A., et al., Replication of human immunodeficiency virus-1 in primary human T cells is dependent on the autocrine secretion of tumor necrosis factor through the control of nuclear factor-kappa B activation. *Journal of Allergy and Clinical Immunology*, 1997. 100(6 Pt 1): p. 838-45.
[99] Duh, E.J., et al., Tumor necrosis factor alpha activates human immunodeficiency virus type 1 through induction of nuclear factor binding to the NF-kappa B sites in the long terminal repeat. *Proceedings of the National Academy of Sciences of the United States of America*, 1989. 86(15): p. 5974-8.
[100] Osborn, L., S. Kunkel, and G.J. Nabel, Tumor necrosis factor alpha and interleukin 1 stimulate the human immunodeficiency virus enhancer by activation of the nuclear factor kappa B. *Proceedings of the National Academy of Sciences of the United States of America*, 1989. 86(7): p. 2336-40.
[101] Brown, F.L., et al., Inducible transcriptional activation of the human immunodeficiency virus long terminal repeat by protein kinase inhibitors. *Mol. Cell Biol.*, 1993. 13(9): p. 5245-54.
[102] Navarro, J., et al., Pentoxifylline inhibits acute HIV-1 replication in human T cells by a mechanism not involving inhibition of tumour necrosis factor synthesis or nuclear factor-kappa B activation. *Aids*, 1996. 10(5): p. 469-75.
[103] Smith, J.A., et al., Pentoxifylline suppresses transduction by HIV-1-based vectors. *Intervirology*, 2007. 50(5): p. 377-86.
[104] He, J., et al., Human immunodeficiency virus type 1 viral protein R (Vpr) arrests cells in the G2 phase of the cell cycle by inhibiting p34cdc2 activity. *Journal of Virology*, 1995. 69(11): p. 6705-11.
[105] Jowett, J.B., et al., The human immunodeficiency virus type 1 vpr gene arrests infected T cells in the G2 + M phase of the cell cycle. *Journal of Virology*, 1995. 69(10): p. 6304-13.
[106] Re, F., et al., Human immunodeficiency virus type 1 Vpr arrests the cell cycle in G2 by inhibiting the activation of p34cdc2-cyclin B. *Journal of Virology*, 1995. 69(11): p. 6859-64.
[107] Rogel, M.E., L.I. Wu, and M. Emerman, The human immunodeficiency virus type 1 vpr gene prevents cell proliferation during chronic infection. *Journal of Virology*, 1995. 69(2): p. 882-8.
[108] Shostak, L.D., et al., Roles of p53 and caspases in the induction of cell cycle arrest and apoptosis by HIV-1 vpr. *Experimental Cell Research*, 1999. 251(1): p. 156-65.

[109] Stewart, S.A., et al., Human immunodeficiency virus type 1 Vpr induces apoptosis following cell cycle arrest. *Journal of Virology*, 1997. 71(7): p. 5579-92.
[110] Huang, M.B., et al., Effects of extracellular human immunodeficiency virus type 1 vpr protein in primary rat cortical cell cultures.[see comment]. *Journal of Neurovirology*, 2000. 6(3): p. 202-20.
[111] Muthumani, K., et al., HIV-1 Vpr induces apoptosis through caspase 9 in T cells and peripheral blood mononuclear cells. *Journal of Biological Chemistry*, 2002. 277(40): p. 37820-31.
[112] Patel, C.A., M. Mukhtar, and R.J. Pomerantz, Human immunodeficiency virus type 1 Vpr induces apoptosis in human neuronal cells. *Journal of Virology*, 2000. 74(20): p. 9717-26.
[113] Somasundaran, M., et al., Evidence for a cytopathogenicity determinant in HIV-1 Vpr. *Proceedings of the National Academy of Sciences of the United States of America*, 2002. 99(14): p. 9503-8.
[114] Stewart, S.A., et al., Human immunodeficiency virus type 1 vpr induces apoptosis through caspase activation. *Journal of Virology*, 2000. 74(7): p. 3105-11.
[115] Yasuda, J., et al., T cell apoptosis causes peripheral T cell depletion in mice transgenic for the HIV-1 vpr gene. *Virology*, 2001. 285(2): p. 181-92.
[116] Poon, B., et al., Human immunodeficiency virus type 1 vpr gene induces phenotypic effects similar to those of the DNA alkylating agent, nitrogen mustard. *Journal of Virology*, 1997. 71(5): p. 3961-71.
[117] Zhu, Y., et al., Comparison of cell cycle arrest, transactivation, and apoptosis induced by the simian immunodeficiency virus SIVagm and human immunodeficiency virus type 1 vpr genes. *Journal of Virology*, 2001. 75(8): p. 3791-801.
[118] Bartz, S.R., M.E. Rogel, and M. Emerman, Human immunodeficiency virus type 1 cell cycle control: Vpr is cytostatic and mediates G2 accumulation by a mechanism which differs from DNA damage checkpoint control. *Journal of Virology*, 1996. 70(4): p. 2324-31.
[119] Roshal, M., et al., Activation of the ATR-mediated DNA damage response by the HIV-1 viral protein R. *Journal of Biological Chemistry*, 2003. 278(28): p. 25879-86.
[120] Zimmerman, E.S., et al., Human immunodeficiency virus type 1 Vpr-mediated G2 arrest requires Rad17 and Hus1 and induces nuclear BRCA1 and gamma-H2AX focus formation. *Molecular and Cellular Biology*, 2004. 24(21): p. 9286-94.
[121] Ward, I.M. and J. Chen, Histone H2AX is phosphorylated in an ATR-dependent manner in response to replicational stress. *Journal of Biological Chemistry*, 2001. 276(51): p. 47759-62.
[122] Ward, I.M., et al., Accumulation of checkpoint protein 53BP1 at DNA breaks involves its binding to phosphorylated histone H2AX. *Journal of Biological Chemistry*, 2003. 278(22): p. 19579-82.
[123] Tachiwana, H., et al., HIV-1 Vpr induces DNA double-strand breaks. *Cancer Research*, 2006. 66(2): p. 627-31.
[124] Daniel, R., et al., Wortmannin potentiates integrase-mediated killing of lymphocytes and reduces the efficiency of stable transduction by retroviruses. *Mol. Cell Biol.*, 2001. 21(4): p. 1164-72.

In: Caffeine and Health Research
Editor: Kenneth P. Chambers
ISBN 978-1-60456-437-2

Chapter V

Unspecific Effects of Caffeine Consumption: When Does the Mind Overrule the Body?

Rainer Schneider*
University of Osnabrück, Department of Human Sciences,
Differential Psychology and Personality Psychology,
Seminarstr. 20, 49074 Osnabrück, Germany

Abstract

Although much is known about the pharmacokinetics of caffeine (i.e., what the body does to the drug), its pharmacodynamics (i.e., what the drug does to the body) are less well understood. Specifically, the psychological effects associated with caffeine intake may often run counter to what might be expected pharmacologically. Being one of the most consumed stimulants worldwide the instrumental value of caffeine covers a broad range of partially opposing ends. For example, the effect (caffeinated) coffee exerts on human functioning depends to a great deal on the expectation of the consumer. People drink coffee to get started in morning, to enhance performance, or even to unwind after straining experiences. Likewise, the instrumental value of coffee consumption may be bound to psychosocial factors, such as enhancing group coherence. Also, coffee may be consumed for diet-related health issues to prevent diseases like diabetes, cancer, heart diseases, or gastrointestinal problems.

In this chapter, an overview of placebo studies is given to demonstrate the importance of psychological factors. Specifically, results from the so called placebo caffeine paradigm will be discussed to show that the study of the placebo caffeine effect lends itself to a better understanding of the psychological factors involved with caffeine effects. Several ways to methodologically disentangle pharmacologic and psychological effects will be introduced. From this, it will be concluded that the widely employed way

* Tel.: ++49 761 476 67 75, Email: rainer.schneider@kabelbw.de

of testing drug effects (the Randomized Control Trial) is insufficient to fully understand the health effect of caffeine since it is aimed at minimizing psychological factors enhancing the effect (e.g., learning effects, expectation, context). It will be shown that the health effects of caffeine are brought about by synergistically intertwined specific and non-specific factors, which, in real-life situations, always work together and make up the totality of effects. Finally, a functionally oriented psychological theory will be introduced helping to explore the psychological mechanisms associated with unspecific effects.

1. Introduction

Caffeine has a long history of use. Its consumption dates back to early mankind and has taken many forms. In tea, it has been savored in Asia for almost 5,000 years, in coffee humans have consumed it for some 1,000 years. Over the last hundred years, cola drinks, ready-to-drink tea and coffee beverages have steadily gained in popularity. Today, coffee is the second most consumed beverage in the world next to water. The fact that caffeine is the most widely consumed behaviorally active substance in the world has made it subject to vigorous scientific investigation. The biochemical mechanisms underlying the actions of caffeine are well understood. If consumed in doses habitually consumed by humans, caffeine primarily blocks adenosine A_1 and A_{2A} receptors, causing a parallel increase in motor activity and decrease in the expression of genes throughout brain regions like the caudate-putamen and nucleus accumbens (Fredholm, Bättig, Holmén, Nehlig, and Zvartau, 1999; Svenningsson, Nomikos, Ongini, and Fredholm, 1997). Unlike other stimulants (e.g., cocaine), caffeine does not significantly increase the release of dopamine or activate the D_1 neurotransmission in the nucleus accumbens. Rather, it increases transmission through cells equipped with dopamine D_2 receptors in this nucleus and throughout the basal ganglia. Since the effect is inhibitory in nature, the overall activity of this brain region is much less affected by caffeine. Its effects are biphasic with low doses being stimulant and pleasant and high doses being aversive and disturbing. This U-shaped dose-response determines whether caffeine can act as reinforcing agent and thus enhance beneficial effects on subjects.

The behavioral effects of caffeine cover a broad range of phenomena like increased subjective alertness, improved reaction time, and enhanced encoding of novel information. For example, in a series of related studies on central nervous effects (Ruijter, De Ruiter, Snel, and Lorist, 2000; Ruijter, Lorist, and Snel, 1999; Ruijter, Lorist, and Snel, 2000; Ruijter, Lorist, Snel, and Ruiter, 2000) caffeine was found to have increasing properties on arousal sustaining attention and attenuating vigilance decrements. This was evidenced by increased amplitudes of different ERPs (event related potentials) in EEG recordings in fatigued participants, showing for example in the frontal P2 and the parietal P3 component. Caffeine displays its effect in the brain in the working memory and higher level control and co-coordinating functions (prefrontal cortex) as well as heightened information processing (parietal cortex). However, although caffeine is supposed to have a general arousing effect due to the binding of adenosine to its receptor sites resulting in an increase in the levels of other neurotransmitters (e.g., acetylcholine, noradrenaline, dopamine, and serotonin), information processing is more pronouncedly affected under conditions in which availability of energetical resources is insufficient (e.g. tiredness or boredom). Moreover, beneficial effects on tasks involving cognitive performance appear to be mainly expected for tasks of little complexity showing predominantly in the output stage of the information processing (Lorist and Topsa, 2003).

Despite the still growing body of knowledge about the effects of caffeine on, for instance, peripheral physiology (cardiovascular system), sleep, mood, arousal, and pain, the pattern of results is far from being homogeneous. In fact, many findings somewhat contradict the fundamental aspects of psychopharmacology with regard to motor, psychomotor, and cognitive performance. Evidently, there appears to be a dissociation between the pharmacokinetics of caffeine (i.e., what the body does to the drug) and its pharmacodynamics (i.e., what the drug does to the body). This instigated a debate arising in the mid 1990s by James (1994) who contended that studies conducted over several decades contained one fundamental methodological flaw by merely including placebo controls without heeding participants' habitual caffeine intake. According to this line of reasoning, abstinence prior to study participation could result in withdrawal symptoms like headache, sleepiness, or lack of concentration. Hence, the performance and mood effect of caffeine would not reflect a real net gain but rather a restoration of decrements to normal levels of functioning. Therefore, the beneficial effects seen in caffeine would simply be counter-regulating detrimental withdrawal symptoms. In fact, there is empirical evidence for the tenability of this claim (James, 1998; James and Gregg, 2004; James, Gregg, Kane, and Harte, 2005; Phillips-Bute and Lane, 1998; Rogers, Martin, Smith, Heatherley, and Smit, 2003; Yeomans, Ripley, Davies, Rusted, and Rogers, 2002). Interestingly, according to the withdrawal hypothesis, caffeine actually has a detrimental effect on mood quality and cognitive performance.

There are, however, empirical findings which cannot be fully reconciled with the withdrawal effect. For example, Smit and Rogers (2000) demonstrated psychostimulant properties after overnight caffeine abstinence with surprisingly small doses (12.5 mg) for both high and low caffeine consumers. Quite counter-intuitively, the effects found in this study failed to increase as a function of the doses administered, i.e. a dose eight times higher did not show significant increments. In a study including multiple doses of caffeine, regular coffee consumers who were fatigued by carrying out a prolonged testing schedule reported more positive mood and improved performance on a number of different tasks (Smith, Sutherland, and Christopher, 2005). In a series of double-blind, randomized, controlled experiments investigating the role of hidden versus open administration of caffeine in regular coffee consumers involving a caffeine abstinence period of at least 12 hours, very large effects were found for caffeine consumption compared to control groups in primarily cardiovascular measures (Schneider et al., 2006; Schneider and Walach, in preparation). Moreover, in one experiment employing the use of decaffeinated coffee (Experiment 1, Schneider et al., 2006), participants believing to have consumed a strong cup of coffee reported elevated alertness. Post-hoc analyses showed that this effect was not attributable to caffeine cravings or differences in withdrawal symptoms associated with fasting and caffeine abstinence.

Obviously, the impact caffeine has on human health and performance is multifaceted. It is clear from the heterogeneity of the findings that the effects may dissociate significantly depending on the method used. Besides specific effects like drug dose, sample compositions, or drinking habits, so called unspecific effects have thus far been widely neglected.

Unspecific effects refer to the fact that their underlying mechanisms are as yet unknown (Schneider, 2007). Unlike other beverages predominantly serving a more fundamental satisfaction of basic biological needs (e.g., water), consumption of caffeine for instance in the form of coffee, serves many different purposes. These are psychological and psychosocial in nature and thus bound to cognitions (e.g., expectations) and learning experience. For example, an athlete ingesting caffeine prior to working out will ascribe a totally different instrumental value to a cup of coffee than a business manager who socializes with a partner during a meeting. Since large epidemiological studies support the notion that caffeine may have beneficial effects on health, for example as a protective agent in high-risk individuals with liver diseases (American Gastroenterological Association, 2005), caffeine may be assumed to be increasingly consumed for dietary and health care reasons.

In the following, I will outline a fundamental fallacy associated with the thinking that drug effects can unambiguously be reduced to specific effects to understand their modes of action. It will be shown that this mindset is deeply rooted in the belief that placebo administration in experiments is an exclusive way to control for unwanted effects (artifacts) not otherwise regarded meaningful in explaining the drug effect.

2. Placebo Caffeine Effects

The use of placebos in clinical trials dates back to the introduction of the *Randomized Controlled Trial* (RCT) in 1948 (British Medical Journal, 1998). Since then it has become the gold standard and cornerstone of pharmacologic efficacy testing (Biller-Andorno, 2004). The logic behind using placebos is that a pharmacological agent should show its superiority to a "sugar pill" exempt from any specific contents. Administration of placebos grounds on the reasoning that any effects emerging are artificial and therefore neglectable. Such confounds encompass the regression to the mean, the natural course of a disease, or spontaneous fluctuations (Kienle and Kiene, 1997). Clinical testing practice, however, shows that placebo responses may considerably compromise the interpretation of trials. Despite the notorious lack of published negative results (which is referred to as the file drawer problem), reviews of existing data bases, for example from the US pharmacologic industry on depression, show a remarkably high rate of non-superiority of pharmacologic agents over placebo (Kirsch, Scoboria, and Moore, 2002; Thase, 1999). Attempts to minimize placebo effects, for instance by identifying placebo responders in placebo run-in phases of clinical trials, largely fail (Lee, Walker, Jakul, and Sexton, 2004). Because placebo effects are to a great deal difficult to replicate, and hence hard to predict, they are considered unspecific. However, active treatment effects, too, are at times unpredictable and unspecific. For example, surreptitiously administered analgesics sometimes exert smaller or even no specific effects at all (Pollo, Vighetti, Rainero, and Benedetti, 2003). From this it may be concluded that the modern biomedical tradition risks being too overly reductionistic by merely focusing on specific treatment components.

There has been much controversy on the real nature of placebo effects. While there have been overly enthusiastic claims on the powerfulness of placebo effects (Beecher, 1955), in part justified methodological critique has at times been too undifferentiated regarding the conditions which are placebo-responsive and those which are not (Hróbjartsson and Gøtzsche, 2004). There is a growing body of evidence substantiating the therapeutic relevance of placebo effects across a wide range of phenomena (Sauro and Greenberg, 2005; Stolk, ten Berg, Hemels, and Einarson, 2003; ter Riet, de Craen, de Boer, and Kessels, 1998; Turner, Deyo, Loeser, von Korff, and Fordyce, 1994; Vase, Riley, and Price, 2002; Vase, Robinson, Verne, and Price, 2003; Vase, Robinson, and Price, 2005).

Nonetheless, there also has been much confusion. One central misunderstanding regarding placebo effects revolves around definitional clarity. For example, obviously factually wrong definitions attribute to placebos a causative mechanism (cf. Moerman and Jonas, 2002). Fortunately, recent definitions have proven more fruitful. One proposition suggests to regard placebo effects as psychosocial context effects arising from treatment or therapy (Benedetti, 2006). Another related definition points to the meaning of an intervention to which an individual responds (Moerman and Jonas, 2002). These definitions have the advantage to be positive, semiotic, and theory-independent. However, as will be shown later, they do not spell out the psychological mechanisms necessary for placebo effects to show. I will therefore suggest a new definition heeding functional properties.

Much from what has been learned about placebo effects stems from *experimental* placebo research. In a nutshell, experimental placebo designs vary conditions such that the probability of the occurrence of the effect is maximized. Unlike in RCTs where subjective probability for placebo administration is set at .5, participants in experimental placebo research are made to believe to receive an active agent when actually given a placebo. From the many models available, the placebo caffeine paradigm particularly lends itself to study placebo effects mainly due to two reasons. First, the effects can be studied in healthy individuals, and second, people share a common cultural stereotype about how coffee operates and what effects are to be expected. There are a number of findings supporting the usefulness of the placebo caffeine paradigm. For example, Kirsch and Weixel (1988) showed that a deceptive administration of placebo caffeine (i.e. decaffeinated coffee) produced an increase on pulse rate, systolic blood pressure, and subjective mood. The magnitude of this effect was paralleled by participants' confidence that they had in fact consumed caffeine. On the other hand, double-blind administration of decaffeinated coffee produced placebo responses which were approximate mirror images of those found for deceptive placebo administration. Studies varying the expectation about caffeine effects found that positive (enhancing) expectations predicted the placebo effect even when no active agent was administered. Participants who were not instructed, and thus did not have any particular belief about the beverage, did not display any change in psychomotor performance (Fillmore and Vogel-Sprott, 1992; Fillmore, Mulvihill, and Vogel-Sprott, 1994). In a study disentangling expectancy and pharmacologic effects by providing different types of information on the content of the beverages (caffeinated and decaffeinated coffee), different responses were found for different measures. Whilst pharmacologic factors primarily influenced participants' physiology (blood pressure), expectancy about the drug primarily affected self-reported mood and assessment of performance (Fillmore and Blumenthal, 1992). The modulating effects of expectancy were also demonstrated in a study by Fillmore, Roach, and Rice (2002). Alcohol drinkers who expected an antagonist effect of caffeine showed greater impairment in a pursuit rotor task from alcohol than those expecting no such effect.

More importantly, expectancy effects were independent of whether caffeine of placebo caffeine was administered. This finding is interesting inasmuch as little or no actual antagonist effect of caffeine can be expected on alcohol-induced impairment. In a recent study by Anderson & Horne (in press), sleepy participants were given a cup of decaffeinated coffee and verbally primed to suggest caffeinated coffee. Results showed significantly fewer lapses and shorter reaction times compared to a control group. These results are interesting inasmuch as they relativize the withdrawal effect of caffeine mentioned earlier. Specifically, the alleged restoration of decrements to normal levels of functioning is not dependend on caffeine, but can be elicited by means of suggestion.

It should be noted, however, that placebo effects show in different measures to varying degrees and establishing the most sensitive indicators is challenging. For example, two studies failed to demonstrate placebo caffeine effects (Walach, Schmidt, Bihr, and Wiesch, 2001; Walach, Schmidt, Dirhold, and Nosch, 2002). While the reproduction of placebo effects is dependent on many as yet not fully understood boundary conditions (Schneider, 2007), the Walach et al. studies most probably failed due to an insufficient induction of a strong expectation and/or the use of rather insensitive measurements. For example, a series of studies investigating caffeine-associated stimuli and information, administering caffeine or placebo in either orange juice or coffee, caffeine-associated stimuli (taste, smell) increased physiological arousal (Flaten and Blumenthal, 1999; Mikalsen, Bertelsen, and Flaten, 2001). Information about the content of the beverage also modulated arousal in the direction indicated by the information. In two recent experiments disentangling pharmacologic from psychological effects by investigating social stereotypes of decaffeinated coffee (smell and taste), no modulating effect on pharmacologic effects could be found (Schneider et al., 2006a). Rather, stimuli-associated stimuli showed to be an important prerequisite for the placebo effect to show (i.e., decaffeinated coffee produced a placebo effect). This pattern of result was paralleled by two subsequently conducted experiments only administering orange juice which was either caffeinated or not (Schneider et al., in preparation). Yet, despite large pharmacologic effects, misinformed information about the alleged content of the beverage did not suffice to produce placebo effects.

3. Mechanisms of the Placebo Caffeine Effect

Traditionally, two approaches have been put forward to explain placebo effects. According to the mentalistic theory, individuals' cognitions like expectations, meaning, needs, or wishes determine the effect (Kirsch, 1999). According to the conditioning theory, placebo effects are the result of learning processes, i.e. the pairing of unconditioned and conditioned stimuli (Ader, 1993; Wickrameskera, 1980). Figure 1 displays the learning model for placebo caffeine affects. They can be regarded the consequence of the pairing of the unconditioned stimulus [UCS] caffeine with the conditioned stimuli [CS] taste and smell. Hence, the unconditioned reaction [UCR] arousal is elicited by the CS making arousal a conditioned reaction [CR].

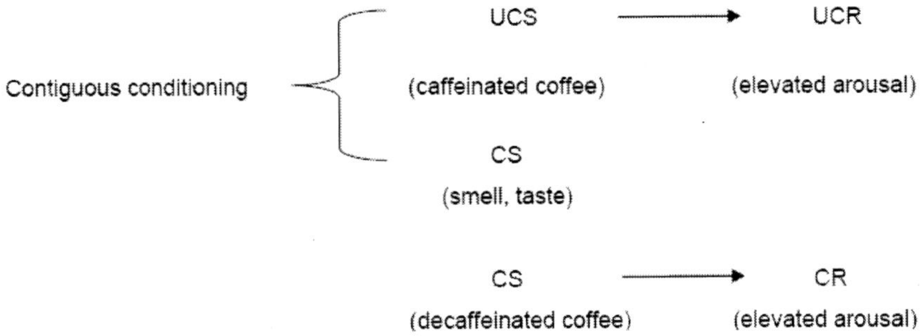

Figure 1. The caffeine placebo effect as a result of conditioned learning.

It should be noted that both approaches are not necessarily mutually exclusive. In fact, they are often synergistic. Unfortunately, unlike other placebo effect phenomena, the neurobiological mechanisms of the caffeine placebo effect have not yet been subjected to investigation. Placebo analgesia, for example, has been found to be maximal when expectation and conditioning are combined (Amanzio and Benedetti, 1999; Colloca and Benedetti, 2006). Yet, expectancy effects have shown to be associated with a different neurological pathway than conditioning effects: Placebo analgesic effects bearing on expectation can be blocked with the opioid antagonist naloxone. Placebo effects brought about by a conditioned treatment (i.e. the injection) with a non-steroid anti-inflammatory drug (ketorolac), have a different pathway because they can't be inhibited. Furthermore, a number of several studies have demonstrated that placebo effects involve different brain areas than pharmacologic effects. These involve subcortical processes (e.g., in pain sensitive neuroanatomical areas via opioid release) and cortical ones (via cognitive appraisal), with the latter occurring after some latency and mostly affecting pain experience (Wager, et. al, 2004; Wager, 2005). Similar findings on the mediating role of the prefrontal cortex in placebo effects have been reported on a broad range of symptoms like depression, irritable bowl syndrome, or chronic pain (cf. Pacheco-Lopez, Engler, Niemi, and Schedlowski, 2006; Schneider, 2007) Consequently, when expectations are engaged, the prefrontal cortex, which maintains evaluative information for control and self-knowledge (Craik et al., 1999; Fuster, 2000), exerts a top-down control modulating experience and physiological processes. It is important to note that expectations need not necessarily be conscious in order to exert a placebo effect (Turner, Jensen, Warms, and Cardenas, 2002). As shown above, from the many effects observed for caffeine ingestion, it may be assumed that in addition to the specific (pharmacologic) effects of caffeine, unspecific (psychological) mechanisms exert an influential role over and above specific ones. This requires a somewhat different methodological approach to fully understand the impact of caffeine on health.

4. Methodological Approaches

Several suggestions have been proposed to study the placebo effect. Benedetti (2006) suggested to surreptitiously administer the pharmacologic agent in order to exempt the treatment form the unspecific effects elicited by the psychosocial context. In so doing, the proportion of the placebo effect can be determined when open and hidden administrations are compared. Although this is a straightforward methodology, it may be questioned whether its ecological validity is sound. For example, to determine bio-availability, absorption rate and pharmacodynamics of caffeine, hidden administration of the agent is likely to have different effects than oral ingestion. Therefore, to study the effects of caffeine under real life conditions this experimental paradigm is not viable.

Another way of studying pharmacologic and psychological factors of caffeine consumption is suggested by the so called balanced placebo design (Marlatt and Rohsenow, 1980). It combines the usual placebo design with an "antiplacebo" design resulting in a 2(drug, placebo) x 2(expectation, no expectation) arrangement. By administering placebo and drug under conditions in which the participants expect to receive an inert substance, independent effects of psychological and pharmacologic effects can be parceled out. As can be seen in Figure 2 (dotted line), a "true" pharmacologic effect would be obtained in an experimental condition were participants are given caffeine but are told to have received placebo.

		Information		
		Caffeine	*Placebo*	*None*
Substance	*Caffeine*	Pharmacological effect + Placebo response	Pharmacological effect	
	Placebo	Placebo response	Confounds	
	None	--	--	Control

Figure 2. The extended balanced placebo design; Placebo effect: Placebo response minus control.

Likewise, when placebo is given but participants are told they ingested caffeine, placebo responses are discernable. It is, however, important to note that the balanced placebo design is only able to unravel placebo *responses* but not placebo *effects*. This is because placebo responses comprise both placebo effects and confounds like artifacts, spontaneous remission, regression effects and the like (Ernst and Resch, 2003; Kirsch and Sapirstein, 1999). Hence, to determine placebo effects the balanced placebo design must be "extended" by including a zero control group with which placebo responses are compared (solid line).

The balanced placebo design has been primarily used in alcohol research with expectancy effects comparable to drug effects (for an overview see Marlatt and Rohsenow, 1980). Since then, it has only seldom been fully employed and somewhat fell into oblivion (for a few exceptions, cf. Juliano and Brandon, 2002; Perkins et al., 2004; Perkins et al., 2008). In placebo caffeine research, this is partly due to the fact that placebo response effects showed as main effects having subsequent researchers focus on comparisons of placebo and control group.

Research on the effects of caffeine on health would benefit greatly from employing the extended balanced placebo design to study the relationship between specific and unspecific effects. However, to understand unspecific effects from a psychological point of view, it may not suffice to primarily focus on conscious thought contents in determining expectations or meaning. This is because people only have limited access to mental processes and cannot fully or adequately explicate (verbalize) them. This is suggested by neurobiological findings showing implicit and parallel-holistic processes of the brain (Beeman, Friedman, Perez, Diamond, and Lindsay, 1994; Beeman and Bowden, 2000; Bowden and Beeman, 1998; Bowers, Regehr, Balthazard, and Parker, 1990; Rumelhart and McClelland, 1986) and that these processes also comprise functional properties like self-regulation, motivation, or affect (Craik et al., 1999; Keenan, Nelson, O'Connor, and Pascual-Leone, 2001; Nadel and Moscovitch, 1997; Quirin, Kazén, Rohrmann, and Kuhl, in press; Quirin, Koole, Baumann, Kazén, and Kuhl, 2007; Rotenberg and Weinberg, 1999; Wheeler, Stuss, and Tulving, 1997). Thus, in placebo research, simply asking people about their cognitions may not suffice when meaning and expectations are assessed. Yet, functional approaches, uncovering subsystems describable in terms of classes of functions, have not been employed in placebo research. In the following, a functionally oriented theory is introduced according to which psychologically important subsystems can be evaluated for their significance of placebo effects.

5. Dynamics of Psychological Functions: Personality-Systems-Interaction Theory

Within the framework of Personality-Systems-Interaction (PSI) Theory a comprehensive functional approach has been developed which lends itself to studying placebo effects (Kuhl, 2000; Kuhl, 2001). The theory comprises two high-level and two low-level systems. These systems may be regarded as complex personality aggregates characterized by distinct functional properties. The two experiential systems generating expectations, and therefore associated with the placebo effect, are extension memory and object recognition. The two behavioral systems are not directly implicated in placebo effects. They are called intention memory and intuitive behavior control with the first being high-inferential and the latter being elementary (see Figure 3). For the sake of simplicity, they will not be further discussed here.

Extension memory is high inferential (complex) and object recognition is low inferential (elementary). Their activational characteristics are antagonistic, that is, activation of extension memory decreases the activation of object recognition and vice versa. This is depicted by the change of colors in the arrows connecting the antagonist systems. Extension memory derives its denomination from the neuronal fabric of the right prefrontal cortex which consists of extended associative networks (Scheibel et al., 1985; Bowden and Beeman, 1998). These allow for a simultaneous, sub-symbolic computation of a vast number of constraints and multiple inputs from both cognitive and affective subsystems through parallel-processing. Extension memory is a central executive system which simultaneously integrates almost unlimited amounts of information. Extension memory also forms the basis for implicit self-representations (so called autonoetic knowledge), that is, integrated representations of internal states, needs, emotions, somatic feelings, or autobiographical experiences (Keenan et al., 2001; McClelland, Koestner, and Weinberger, 1989; Nyberg,

Cabeza, and Tulving, 1996; Wheeler et al., 1997). Moreover, functions of extension memory also encompass attention processes (vigilance) and enhance those perceptual contents which match actual relevant and implicit networks of needs, expectations, and other self-structures. Due to this characteristic, processes of extension memory are not fully conscious. One of the typical functions of extension memory is down-regulation of negative affect elicited by aversive, threatening or unpredictable experiences because extension memory is tightly linked with vegetative and somatosensory processes (Borod and Madigan, 2000; Garavan, Ross, and Stein, 1999; Kapur et al., 1995; Rotenberg, 2004). This is shown as self-relaxation in Figure 3.

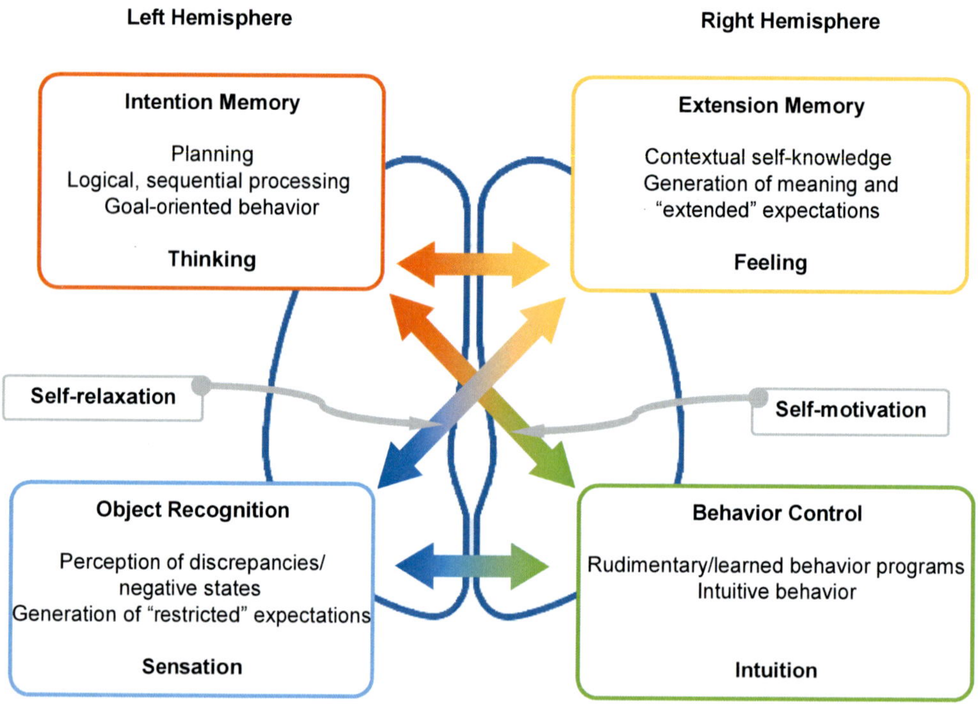

Figure 3. Personality-System-Interaction Theory (PSI).

In contrast, object recognition serves to recognize percepts which can be abstracted (discerned) from their background by specific discrepancy mediating features, for example, concrete things, singular aspects, feelings, sensations etc. Specifically, the system enhances those objects deviating from expectations and self-aspects activated in extension memory. Object recognition is closely linked with one of the cornerstones of cortical pathways (the so-called vision-for-perception stream) where information generated in the primary visual cortex projects into the inferior temporal cortex and further in the prefrontal cortex (Ungerleider and Mishkin, 1982). However, the functional characteristics of object recognition are not limited to these neurological pathways but encompass a number of additional features. As a primarily perceptual system, object recognition focuses on explicit identification and recognition of elementary sensations (e.g., a visual object, an emotion, or semantic category). Characteristic for object recognition (especially in connection with negative affect) is a focus on discrepancies and on sensations that diverge from previously held expectations, wishes and the like. Contrary to the functional properties of extension memory, object recognition allows for an explicit, conscious registration of sensory impressions, which encompasses a relatively rigid analytical categorization (i.e., black/white).

6. The Placebo Effect Revisited: Expectation, Meaning, and Their Functional Significance

According to personality systems interaction (PSI) theory, functional properties determine the powerfulness of placebo-associated expectations and meaning. In other words, different responses follow depending on whether the expectation is generated in extension memory or in the object recognition system. As noted above, strong placebo effects have been found when the meaning of the placebo (treatment) was personally relevant to the participants. This is especially the case for highly aversive states like pain (Zubieta, Yau, Scott, and Stohler, 2006), but basically also holds for placebo caffeine effects (or similar drug effects for that matter). Put differently, only those context factors elicit a placebo effect that are generated and represented in a semantic network of remote associations and coherent complexes of symbolic meaning (extension memory). Furthermore, only expectations generated in extension memory should be accompanied by a placebo effect because extension memory is closely linked with self-regulatory mechanisms affecting a variety of cognitive and somatosensory processes. In contrast, expectations generated in the object recognition system would not suffice to produce significant placebo effects because they lack the connectedness to relevant (meaningful) self-aspects and the network of remote associations requiring (implicit) attention processes (i.e., rare or unexpected effects). Remote associations indeed may be an important prerequisite to elicit placebo effects. For example, Dinnerstein and Halm (1970) and Lyerly, Krugman, and Clyde (1964) found expectancy effects only for experimental conditions where drug effects were introduced as a continuum of possible reactions. Furthermore, as noted above, a number of studies support the notion that placebo effects incorporate self-regulatory mechanisms of the prefrontal cortex which cannot be found for drug effects. This would indicate that active treatment impairs self-regulation whilst placebo treatment fosters it. This implication is supported by leading neuroscientists who recently called for a systematic investigation of self-regulatory factors to psychologically better understand placebo effects (Benedetti, Mayberg, Wager, Stohler, and Zubieta, 2006). Given that placebo caffeine research also found bodily and mental changes when no caffeine was administered, the effects found for caffeinated substances at least in part may bear on such underlying mechanisms. This would explain the somewhat opposing effects found for caffeine: whether a strong cup of coffee exerts an effect on, for instance, cognitive performance, would be mediated by the psychosocial context in which it is consumed and the expectation and meaning which are associated with it. Clearly, the relationship between caffeine and placebo caffeine effects may assume different forms. For example, the psychological mechanisms may supersede or counter-regulate the pharmacologic effects (Fillmore and Blachburne, 2002; Schneider et al., 2006), be neglectable when no expectations are associated with the caffeinated beverage (James, 1998) or be additive when specific and unspecific effects are stressed (Flaten and Blumenthal, 1999).

One corollary derived from PSI Theory is that subsymbolic mechanisms are associated with the placebo effect because expectations and cognitions involved are not fully conscious. Bearing on the findings from hemispheric activation stimulation to activate extension memory (Baumann, Kuhl, and Kazén, 2005) contiguously activating the extension memory, for example, by squeezing a soft ball with the counterlateral hand, upon intake of placebo should ensue much stronger placebo effects. Likewise, since extension memory affords complex cognitive processes, for example the detection of semantic coherences (Baumann and Kuhl, 2002; Bolte, Goschke, and Kuhl, 2003), placebo caffeine effects would comprise coherence perception whilst caffeine effects, which primarily affect relatively simple cognitive processes (Lorist and Topsa, 2003; Ruijter et al., 2000), would not. Hence, when studying (placebo) caffeine effects implicit coherence performance would be enhanced in individuals expecting caffeine to improve coherence perception. Furthermore, if the activation of extension memory is constitutive for the placebo effect, there should be correlations with self-regulatory mechanisms (e.g., affect regulation). This, in turn, would make placebo effects predictable by self-regulatory mechanisms, which, according to PSI theory, are exerted effortlessly and implicitly. Such a relationship should not hold for pharmacological effects because they are, to a much lesser degree, mediated by psychological mechanisms (i.e. self-relevant expectations).

Following this line of reasoning, I suggest the following definition for placebo effects including functional psychological boundary conditions.

Placebo effects are unspecific intervention effects depending on the individulal's implicit competency to construe meaning in the psychosocial context, and to respond to this meaning by means of self-regulation.

Conclusion

The effects caffeine exerts on health cannot be reduced to pharmacological pathways but comprise psychological mechanisms also. The findings on placebo caffeine effects suggest that so called unspecific effects substantially contribute to caffeine effects. The mind in fact may overrule the body when specific expectations with a certain meaning are held. Whether psychological factors exert a significant influence over and above pharmacologic effects is determined by the context in which caffeine is ingested. Disentangling the mediating role of self-regulatory factors in caffeine effects may benefit the understanding of when and how health effects may be expected. To do so, traditional ways of testing caffeine (e.g., employing RCTs) should be complemented with those which allow testing of caffeine and placebo under different conditions (extended balanced placebo design). To better understand psychological factors, functional approaches and methods should be employed (e.g., PSI theory and the diagnostic tools derived from it). Although from a pragmatic point of view a separation of specific and unspecific effects is not necessary (in most cases even disadvantageous), understanding the underlying mechanisms and boundary conditions of the context is important in determining health-related caffeine effects.

References

Ader, R. (1993). Conditioned responses in pharmacotherapy research. *Psychological Medicine, 23,* 297-299.

Amanzio, M. and Benedetti, F. (1999). Neuropharmacological dissection of placebo analgesia: Expectation-activated opioid systems versus conditioning-activated specific subsystems. *Journal of Neuroscience, 19,* 484-494.

American Gastroenterological Association (2005). Coffee and tea can reduce the risk of chronic liver disease. http://www.gastro.org/wmspage.cfm?parm1=1833 [Online].

Anderson, C., and Horne, J. A. (in press). Placebo response to caffeine improves reaction time performance in sleepy people. *Human Psychopharmacology: Clinical and Experimental.*

Baumann, N., Kuhl, J., and Kazén, M. (2005). Left-hemispheric activation and self-infiltration: Testing a neuropsychological model of internalization. *Motivation and Emotion, 29,* 135-163.

Baumann, N. and Kuhl, J. (2002). Intuition, affect, and personality: Unconscious coherence judgments and self-regulation of negative affect. *Journal of Personality and Social Psychology, 83,* 1213-1223.

Beecher, H. K. (1955). The powerful placebo. *Journal of the American Medical Association, 159,* 1602-1606.

Beeman, M. J., Friedman, R. B., Perez, E., Diamond, S., and Lindsay, M. B. (1994). Summation priming and coarse coding in the right hemisphere. *Journal of Cognitive Neuroscience, 6,* 26-45.

Beeman, M. J. and Bowden, E. M. (2000). The right hemisphere maintains solution-related activation for yet-to-be solved problems. *Memory and Cognition, 28,* 1231-1241.

Benedetti, F. (2006). Placebo analgesia. *Neurological Sciences, 27,* S100-S102.

Benedetti, F., Mayberg, H. S., Wager, T. D., Stohler, C. S., and Zubieta, J.-K. (2006). Neurobiological mechanisms of the placebo effect. *Journal of Neuroscience, 25,* 10390-10402.

Biller-Andorno, N. (2004). The use of the placebo effect in clinical medicine - ethical blunder or ethical imperative? *Science and Engineering Ethics, 10,* 43-50.

British Medical Journal (1998). The randomised controlled trial at 50. *British Medical Journal, 7167.*

Bolte, A., Goschke, T., and Kuhl, J. (2003). Emotions and intuition: Effects of positive and negative mood on implicit judgments of semantic coherence. *Psychological Science, 14,* 416-421.

Borod, J. C., and Madigan, N. K. (2000). Neuropsychology of emotion and emotional disorder: An overview and research directions. In J. C. Borod (Ed.), The neuropsychology of emotion (pp. 3-28). New York: Oxford University Press.

Bowden, E. M. and Beeman, M. J. (1998). Getting the right idea: Semantic activation in the right hemisphere. *Psychological Science, 9,* 435-440.

Bowers, K. S., Regehr, G., Balthazard, C., and Parker, K. (1990). Intuition in the context of discovery. *Cognitive Psychology, 22,* 72-110.

Colloca, L. and Benedetti, F. (2006). How prior experience shapes placebo analgesia. *Pain, 124,* 126-133.

Craik, F. I. M., Moroz, T. M., Moscovitch, M., Stuss, D. T., Wincour, G., Tulving, E. et al. (1999). In search of the self: A positron emission tomography study. *Psychological Science, 10,* 26-34.

Dinnerstein, A. L. and Halm, J. (1970). Modification of placebo effects by means of drugs: Effects of aspirin and placebos on self-related moods. *Journal of Abnormal Psychology, 75,* 303-314.

Ernst, E. and Resch, K. L. (2003). Concept of true and perceived placebo effects. *British Medical Journal, 311,* 551-553.

Fillmore, M., Mulvihill, L. E., and Vogel-Sprott, M. (1994). The expected drug and its expected effect interact to determine placebo responses to alcohol and caffeine. *Psychopharmacology, 115,* 383-388.

Fillmore, M., Roach, E., and Rice, J. (2002). Does caffeine counteract alcohol-induced impairment? The ironic effects of expectancy. *Journal of Studies on Alcohol, 63,* 745-754.

Fillmore, M. and Vogel-Sprott, M. (1992). Expected effect of caffeine on motor performance predicts the type of response to placebo. *Psychopharmacology, 106,* 209-214.

Flaten, M. A. and Blumenthal, T. D. (1999). Caffeine-associated stimuli elicit conditioned responses: An experimental model of the placebo effect. *Psychopharmacology, 145,* 105-112.

Fredholm, B. B., Bättig, K., Holmén, J., Nehlig, A., and Zvartau, E. E. (1999). Actions of caffeine in the brain with special reference to factors that contribute to its widespread use. *Pharmacological Reviews, 51,* 83-133.

Fuster, J. M. (2000). Executive frontal functions. *Experimental Brain Research, 133,* 66-70.

Garavan, H., Ross, T. J., and Stein, E. A. (1999). Right hemispheric dominance of inhibitory control: An event-related functional FMRI study. *Proceedings of the National Academy of Sciences USA, 96,* 8301-8306.

Hróbjartsson, A. and Gøtzsche, P. C. (2004). Is the placebo powerless? Update of a systematic review with 52 new randomized trials comparing placebo with no treatment. *Journal of Internal Medicine, 256,* 91-100.

James, J. E. (1994). Does caffeine enhance or merely restore degraded psychomotor performance? *Neuropsychobiology, 30,* 124-125.

James, J. E. (1998). Acute and chronic effects of caffeine on performance, mood, headache, and sleep. *Neuropsychobiology, 38,* 32-41.

James, J. E. and Gregg, M. E. (2004). Effects of dietary caffeine on mood when rested and sleep restricted. *Human Psychopharmacology: Clinical and Experimental, 19,* 333-341.

James, J. E., Gregg, M. E., Kane, M., and Harte, F. (2005). Dietary caffeine, performance and mood: Enhancing and restorative effects after controlling for withdrawal reversal. *Neuropsychology, 52,* 1-10.

Juliano, L. M., and Brandon, T. H. (2002). Effects of nicotine dose, instructional set, and outcome expectancies on the subjective effects of smoking in the presence of a stressor. *Journal of Abnormal Psychology*,111, 88-97.

Kapur, S., Craik, F. I. M., Jones, C., Brown, G. M., Houle, S., and Tulving, E. (1995). Functional role of the prefrontal cortex in retrieval of memories: A PET study. *NeuroReport, 6,* 1880-1884.

Keenan, J. P., Nelson, A., O'Connor, M., and Pascual-Leone, A. (2001). Self-recognition and the right hemisphere. *Nature, 409,* 305.

Kienle, G. S. and Kiene, H. (1997). The powerful placebo effect: Fact or fiction? *Journal of Clinical Epidemiology, 50,* 1311-1318.

Kirsch, I. (1999). *How expectancies shape experience.* Washington, DC: American Psychological Association.

Kirsch, I., Scoboria, A., and Moore, T. J. (2002). Antidepressants and placebos: secrets, revelations, and unanswered questions. Prevention and Treatment [Online]. Available: http://www.journals.apa.org/prevention/volume5/pre0050033r.html.

Kirsch, I., and Sapirstein, G. (1999). Listening to Prozac but hearing placebo: A meta-analysis of antidepressant medications. In: I. Kirsch (Ed.). *How expectancies shape experience* (pp. 303-320), Washington, DC: American Psychological Association.

Kirsch, I. and Weixel, L. J. (1988). Double-blind versus deceptive administration of a placebo. *Behavioral Neuroscience, 102,* 319-323.

Koch, C. and Laurent, G. (1999). Complexity and the nervous system. *Science, 284,* 96-98.

Kuhl, J. (2000). A functional-design approach to motivation and self-regulation: The dynamics of personality systems interaction. In M. Boekaerts, P. R. Pintrich, and M. Zeidner (Eds.), *Handbook of self-regulation* (pp. 111-169). New York: Academic Press.

Kuhl, J. (2001). *Motivation und Persönlichkeit. Interaktionen psychischer Systeme.* Göttingen: Hogrefe.

Kuhl, J. and Kazén, M. (1994). Self-discrimination and memory: State orientation and false self-ascription of assigned activities. *Journal of Personality and Social Psychology, 66,* 1103-1115.

Lee, S., Walker, J. R., Jakul, L., and Sexton, K. (2004). Does elimination of placebo responders in a placebo run-in increase the treatment effect in randomized clinical trials? A meta-analytical evaluation. *Depression and Anxiety, 19,* 10-19.

Lorist, M. M. and Topsa, M. (2003). Caffeine, fatigue, and cognition. *Brain and Cognition, 53,* 82-94.

Lyerly, S. B., Krugman, A. D., and Clyde, D. J. (1964). Drugs and placebos: The effects of instructions upon performance and mood under amphetamine sulphate and chloral hydrate. *Journal of Abnormal and Social Psychology, 68,* 321-327.

Marlatt, G. A. and Rohsenow, D. J. (1980). Cognitive processes in alcohol use: Expectancy and the balanced placebo design. In N. Mello (Ed.), *Advances in Substance Abuse* (pp. 159-199). Greenwich: JAI Press.

McClelland, D. C., Koestner, R., and Weinberger, J. (1989). How do self-attributed and implicit motives differ? *Psychological Review, 96,* 690-702.

Mikalsen, A., Bertelsen, B., and Flaten, M. A. (2001). Effects of caffeine, caffeine-associated stimuli, and caffeine-related information on physiological and psychological arousal. *Psychopharmacology, 157,* 373-380.

Moerman, D. E. and Jonas, W. B. (2002). Deconstructing the placebo effect and finding the meaning response. *Annals of Internal Medicine, 136,* 471-476.

Nadel, L. and Moscovitch, M. (1997). Memory consolidation, retrograde amnesia and the hippocampal complex. *Current Opinion in Neurobiology, 7,* 217-227.

Nyberg, L., Cabeza, R., and Tulving, E. (1996). PET studies of encoding and retrieval: The HERA model. *Psychonomic Bulletin and Review, 3,* 135-148.

Perkins, K. A., Jacobs, L., Ciccocioppo, M., Conklin, C. A., Sayette, M., and Caggiula, A. (2004). The influence of instructions and nicotine dose on the subjective and reinforcing effects of smoking. *Experimental and Clinical Psychopharmacology, 12,* 91-101.

Perkins, K. A., Ciccocioppo, M., Conklin, C. A., Milanak, M. E., Grottenthaler, A., and Sayette, M. (2008). Mood influences on acute smoking responses are independent of nicotine intake and dose expectancy. *Journal of Abnormal Psychology, 117,* 79-93.

Pacheco-Lopez ,G., Engler, H., Niemi, M.-B., and Schedlowski, M. (2006). Expectations and associations that heal: Immunomodulatory placebo effects and its neurobiology. *Brain, Behavior, and Immunity,* 20, 430-446.

Phillips-Bute, B. G. and Lane, J. D. (1998). Caffeine withdrawal symptoms following brief caffeine deprivation. *Physiology and Behavior, 63,* 35-39.

Pollo, A., Vighetti, S., Rainero, I., and Benedetti, F. (2003). Placebo analgesia and the heart. *Pain, 102,* 125-133.

Quirin, M., Kazén, M., Rohrmann, S., and Kuhl, J. (in press). Implicit affectivity predicts reactive and circadian cortisol secretion. *Journal of Personality.*

Quirin, M., Koole, S. L., Baumann, N., Kazén, M., and Kuhl, J. (2007). You can't always remember what you want: The role of cortisol in self-ascription of assigned goals. *Submitted manuscript.*

Rogers, P. J., Martin, J., Smith, C., Heatherley, S. V., and Smit, H. J. (2003). Absence of reinforcing, mood and psychomotor performance effects of caffeine in habitual non-consumers of caffeine. *Psychopharmacology, 167,* 54-62.

Rotenberg, V. S. (2004). The peculiarity of the right-hemisphere function in depression: Solving the paradoxes. *Progress in Neuro-Psychopharmacology and Biological Psychiatry, 28,* 1-13.

Rotenberg, V. S. and Weinberg, I. (1999). Human memory, cerebral hemispheres, and the limbic system: A new approach. *Genetic, Social, and General Psychology Monographs, 125,* 526-532.

Ruijter, J., De Ruiter, M., Snel, J., and Lorist, M. M. (2000). The influence of caffeine on spatial-selective attention: an event-related potential study. *Clinical Neurophysiology, 111,* 2223-2233.

Ruijter, J., Lorist, M. M., and Snel, J. (1999). The influence of different doses of caffeine on visual task performance. *Journal of Psychophysiology, 13,* 37-48.

Ruijter, J., Lorist, M. M., and Snel, J. (2000). The effects of caffeine on visual selective attention to color: An ERP study. *Psychophysiology, 37,* 427-439.

Ruijter, J., Lorist, M. M., Snel, J., and Ruiter, M. B. (2000). The influence of caffeine on sustained attention: An ERP study. *Pharmacology, Biochemistry and Behaviour, 6,* 29-37.

Rumelhart, D. E. and McClelland, J. L. (1986). *Parallel distributed processing: Explorations in the microstructure of cognition.* Cambridge, MA: MIT Press.

Sauro, M. D. and Greenberg, R. P. (2005). Endogenous opiates and the placebo effect. A meta-analytic review. *Journal of Psychosomatic Research, 58,* 115-120.

Scheibel, A. B., Freid, I., Paul, L., Forsythe, A., Tomiyasu, U., Wechsler, A. et al. (1985). Differentiating characteristics of the human speech cortex: A quantitative Golgi study. In D. F. Benson and E. Zaidel (Eds.), *The dual brain.* New York: Guilford Press.

Schneider, R. (2007). The psychology of the placebo effect: Exploring meaning from a functional account. *Journal of Mind and Behavior, 18,* 1-17.

Schneider, R. and Walach, H. (in preparation). Classical and non-classical placebo effect: Testing an experimental model.

Schneider, R., Grüner, M., Heiland, A., Keller, M., Kujanová, Z., Peper, M. et al. (2006). Effects of expectation and caffeine on arousal, well-being, and reaction time. *International Journal of Behavioral Medicine, 13,* 330-339.

Smit, H. J. and Rogers, P. J. (2000). Effects of low doses of caffeine on cognitive performance, mood and thirst in low and higher caffeine consumers. *Psychopharmacology, 152,* 167-173.

Smith, A., Sutherland, D., and Christopher, G. (2005). Effects of repeated doses of caffeine on mood and performance of alert and fatigued volunteers. *Journal of Pharmacology, 19,* 620-626.

Stolk, P., ten Berg, M. J., Hemels, M. E. H., and Einarson, T. R. (2003). Meta-analysis of placebo rates in major depressive disorder trials. *The Annals of Psychotherapy, 37,* 1891-1899.

Svenningsson, P., Nomikos, G. G., Ongini, E., and Fredholm, B. B. (1997). Antagonism of adenosine A2A receptors underlies the behavioural activating effect of caffeine and is associated with reduced expression of messenger RNA for NGFI-A and NGFI-B in caudate-putamen and nucleus accumbens. *Neuroscience, 79,* 753-764.

ter Riet, G., de Craen, A. J. M., de Boer, A., and Kessels, A. G. H. (1998). Is placebo analgesia mediated by endogenous opioids? A systematic review. *Pain, 76,* 273-275.

Thase, M. E. (1999). Randomized clinical trials of treatments for depression? *Journal of Clinical Psychiatry, 60,* 23-31.

Turner, J. A., Deyo, R. A., Loeser, J. D., von Korff, M., and Fordyce, W. E. (1994). The importance of placebo effects in pain treatment and research. *Journal of the American Medical Association, 271,* 1609-1614.

Turner, J. A., Jensen, M. P., Warms, C. A., and Cardenas, D. D. (2002). Blinding effectiveness and association of pretreatment expectations with pain improvement in a double-blind randomized controlled trial. *Pain, 99,* 91-99.

Ungerleider, L. G. and Mishkin, M. (1982). Two visual systems. In D. J .Ingle, M. A. Goodale, and R. J. W. Mansfield (Eds.), *Analysis of visual behavior* (pp. 549-586). Cambridge, MA: MIT Press.

Vase, L., Riley, J. L., and Price, D. D. (2002). A comparison of placebo effects in clinical analgesic trials versus studies of placebo analgesia. *Pain, 99,* 443-452.

Vase, L., Robinson, M. E., and Price, D. D. (2005). Increased placebo analgesia over time in irritable bowel syndrome (IBS) patients is associated with desire and expectation but endogenous opioid mechanisms. *Pain, 115,* 338-347.

Vase, L., Robinson, M. E., Verne, G. N., and Price, D. D. (2003). The contributions of suggestion, desire, and expectation to placebo effects in irritable bowel syndrome patients. An empirical investigation. *Pain, 105,* 17-25.

Wager, T. D., Rilling, J.K., Smith, E.E., Sokolik, A., Casey, K. L., et al. (2004). Placebo-induced changes in fMRI in the anticipation and experience of pain. *Science,* 303, 1162-1167.

Wager, T. D. (2005). The neural bases of placebo effects in anticipation and pain. *Seminars in Pain Medicine, 3,* 22-30.

Walach, H., Schmidt, S., Bihr, Y.-M., and Wiesch, S. (2001). The effects of a caffeine placebo and experimenter expectation on blood pressure, heart rate, well-being, and cognitive performance. *European Psychologist, 6,* 15-25.

Walach, H., Schmidt, S., Dirhold, T., and Nosch, S. (2002). The effects of a caffeine placebo and suggestion on blood pressure, heart rate, well-being and cognitive performance. *International Journal of Psychophysiology, 43,* 247-260.

Wheeler, M. A., Stuss, D. T., and Tulving, E. (1997). Toward a theory of episodic memory: The frontal lobes and autonoetic consciousness. *Psychological Bulletin, 121,* 331-354.

Wickrameskera, I. (1980). A conditioned response model of the placebo effect: Predictions from the model. *Biofeedback and Self Regulation, 5,* 5-18.

Yeomans, M. R., Ripley, T., Davies, L. H., Rusted, J. M., and Rogers, P. J. (2002). Effects of caffeine on performance and mood depend on the level of caffeine abstinence. *Psychopharmacology, 164,* 241-249.

Zubieta, J.-K., Yau, W. Y., Scott, D. J., and Stohler, C. S. (2006). Belief or need? Accounting for individual varitions in the neurochemistry of the placebo effect. *Brain, Behavior, and Immunity, 20,* 15-26.

In: Caffeine and Health Research
Editor: Kenneth P. Chambers

ISBN 978-1-60456-437-2

Chapter VI

Absorption, Distribution, Metabolism and Excretion of Caffeine

***Jhy-Wen Wu*[1,2] *and Tung-Hu Tsai* *[*1,3]**
[1]Institute of Traditional Medicine, School of Medicine,
National Yang-Ming University, Taipei 112, Taiwan
[2]Centers for Disease Control, Department of Health, Taipei, Taiwan
[3]Department of Education and Research, Taipei City Hospital,
Renai Branch, Taipei, Taiwan

Abstract

Pharmacokinetics has had a considerable effect in enhancing our understanding of what happens to drug within the body, and has opened a way to safer and more effective drug administration to the body. Caffeine produces central stimulation because of its effect on the central nervous system. Caffeine is also used for therapeutic purposes, and is included in a wide variety of fixed combination prescription drugs and over-the-counter medications. In the present review we discuss the pharmacokinetics of caffeine. Caffeine is rapidly and completely absorbed from the gastrointestinal tract; peak plasma caffeine concentration reaches in about 15 to 120 min after oral ingestion in humans without any significant first-pass effect. Caffeine is rapidly distributed, which poorly binds to plasma albumin and there is no specific binding to tissue. Caffeine is distributed into all body tissues, rapidly crosses the blood-brain barrier and the placenta, and is also found in breast milk. The human cytochrome p450 monoxygenase metabolizes caffeine yielding trimethyl uric acid, paraxanthine and theobromine. Caffeine is efficiently eliminated through liver biotransformation to several metabolites; only a small percentage of ingested doses in humans are excreted unchanged in urine. People with some liver disorders have a significant prolongation of the half-life and a reduction in plasma clearance. In a healthy subject, the mean elimination half-life of caffeine is

* Fax: (886-2) 2822-5044, Telephone: (886-2) 2826-7115, E-mail: thtsai@ym.edu.tw

around 5 hr. Physiological and environmental factors that alter caffeine metabolism included age, sex, pregnancy, smoking and ingestion of drug.

1. Introduction

Coffee and tea have been the most popular beverages in Western society for several hundred years. Caffeine (1,3,7-trimethylxanthine), which occurs naturally in more than 60 plant species throughout the world is the major pharmacologically active purine present in coffee. Coffee undoubtedly serves as the primary source of caffeine in the adult, but caffeine is also contained in tea and cocoa, and many soft drinks and several drug preparations including over-the-counter stimulants and headache mixture (Newton et al., 1981). Caffeine is probably the most widely ingested natural alkaloid (Newton et al., 1981). Quantitatively, the most important dietary source of caffeine in the United States, accounting for 60% of caffeine consumption; tea is the major dietary source of caffeine in the United Kingdom and in Asia (Berger, 1988).

Caffeine also has been used as a drug to increase wakefulness and as a dietary aid, and it is probably the most widely ingested natural alkaloid (Newton et al., 1981). In Europe and America, caffeine is the most widely consumed drug, and the consequences of caffeine ingestion are potentially profound (Curatolo and Robertson, 1983).

Caffeine also has been used as a dietary aid, it is present in a variety of beverage. In Australia, the mean caffeine content is 80.1 mg/cup, 60.4 mg/cup, and 26.8 mg/cup for brewed coffee, instant coffee, and tea, respectively (Lelo et al., 1986a). The caffeine concentration of the caffeinated energy drinks ranged from 0 to 141.1 mg/12-oz. The caffeine content of the carbonated sodas ranged from none detected to 48.2 mg/12-oz, and the content of the other beverages ranged from 2.7 to 105.7 mg/12-oz. The Food and Drug Administration has included caffeine in the list of substance that are generally recognized as safe and has set the maximum concentration of caffeine in cola beverages at 32.4 mg/6-oz or 65 mg/12-oz (McCusker et al., 2006).

Worldwide consumption of roasted coffee was estimated to be 4.3 million tonnes per year in 1983-87. The average world consumption of caffeine is 70 mg/day for each inhabitant (WHO, 1997). In Australia, the mean daily caffeine consumption was 462.9 mg or 6.8 mg/kg/day (Lelo et al., 1986a), in the United States it was 211 mg/day/person, and in the United Kingdom it was 444 mg/day/person, which is the highest in the world (Donovan and DeVane, 2001). The mean caffeine intake for adults in the total United States population is 3 mg/kg/day and about 7 mg/kg/day (Lelo et al., 1986a) for the heaviest consumer.

Caffeine is a central nervous system stimulant that has been suggested to be effective in the treatment of apnea of premature infants (Aranda et al., 1977). It can significantly increase the risks for spontaneous abortion and the birth of low weight babies if a pregnant women consumes >150 mg/day caffeine (Fernandes et al., 1998). It has been suggested that caffeine might be an ideal teat substance for assessing hepatic function, as it is rapidly and completely absorbed after oral ingestion and is metabolized primarily by P450 (Scott et al., 1989).

2. Absorption of Caffeine

Caffeine absorption from the gastrointestinal tract is rapid and complete in human beings (Newton et al., 1981; Bonati et al., 1982; Axelrod and Reichenthal, 1953; Blanchard and Sawers, 1983a). The pharmacokinetic characteristics revealed no statistical between oral and i.v. routes after 4.9 mg/kg administration (Blanchard and Sawers, 1983a).The rate of absorption more than 99% of the administration dose in about 45 min after 1, 5, or 10 mg/kg of caffeine in water (Bonati et al., 1982). After caffeine 5 mg/kg oral administration, T_{max} was 47.5 min and C_{max} was 8.3 μg/ml (Bonati et al., 1982). After oral administration of 6-9 mg/kg caffeine, the T_{max} of caffeine became 30 min (Santambrogio et al., 1964). After drinking coffee, the mean T_{max} was found to be 50 minutes (Smits et al., 1985). The rate constant of absorption was lower in old than in young rats (Latini et al., 1980).The pharmacokinetics of caffeine administered by inhalation are to a large extent similar to the pharmacokinetics of intravenously administered caffeine. The bioavailability of inhaled caffeine is approximately 60% (Zandvliet et al., 2005). No significant first-pass effect occur following human oral administration of caffeine at a dose of 5 mg/kg (Blanchard and Sawers, 1983a).

The significant prolongation of the time to peak of the plasma caffeine in Type II diabetes may have been due to delayed gastric emptying caused by gastroparesis (Zysset and Wietholtz, 1991). A single oral dose of pure menthol delays caffeine absorption, increase of caffeine T_{max} values from 43.6 min to 76.4 min and a slight decrease of caffeine C_{max}.. Menthol acts by reducing the availability of calcium in gastrointestinal smooth muscle. The relaxant effect of menthol on the gastrointestinal tract could influence the rate of drug absorption by decreasing gastric emptying (Gelal et al., 2003).

3. Distribution of Caffeine

Caffeine is distributed in various tissues in approximate proportion to their water content. The drug passes rapidly into the central nervous system (Axelrod and Reichenthal, 1953; Tsai et al., 2005). It enters the brain rapidly and seems to reach equilibrium within 5 min. The average brain/plasma ratio was 0.64 for old and 0.95 for young rats (Latini et al., 1980). Caffeine enters the brain by a combination of transport mechanism—simple diffusion and carrier-mediated transport (McCall et al., 1982).

After an i.v. dose of 4 mg/kg caffeine in rabbit, the tissue/blood ratio of caffeine in liver and bile were 1.5 and 2.7, respectively. All other tissue except fat and adrenal glands exhibited a tissue/blood ratio approximately 1.0 (Beach et al., 1985). Close correlation between caffeine concentrations has been found in the plasma and saliva of normal subjects after single oral dose of caffeine. Mean saliva/total plasma concentration ratio was 0.79 (Zylber-Katz et al., 1984).

Passive diffusion appears to govern the transfer of caffeine and three of its demethylated metabolites into rabbit milk. The milk-to-serum drug concentration ratio of caffeine was 0.875 (McNamara et al., 1992). Caffeine also can readily cross the placenta and can affect fetal heart rate and breathing (Kaiser and Allen, 2002).

Caffeine binds to albumin to the extent of 37.81%, and in the present case, the binding is essentially constant over the concentration range of 1-20 μg/ml, indicating that only a small fraction of the available binding sites is occupied at these concentrations (Blanchard, 1982). Caffeine was found to bind only about 30% to plasma protein in a health male subject; however, it binds even less (25%) in patients with cirrhosis (Desmond et al., 1980).

4. Metabolism of Caffeine

Caffeine is biotransformed to dimethylxanthines, theobromine, paraxanthine, theophylline, and other metabolites through several enzymatic pathways. Paraxanthine is quantitatively the main demethylation product, followed by theobromine and theophylline respectively (Zandvliet et al., 2005).

However, the P-450 cytochrome oxygenase plays a major role in the primary metabolism of caffeine.

The first biotransformation step in the metabolism of caffeine yields three dimethylxanthines, with paraxanthine representing the main metabolite, followed by theobromine and theophylline. The second biotransformation step in the metabolism of caffeine involves further metabolism of each dimethylxanthine to the corresponding monomethylxanthines, dimethylurates and uracil derivatives. The third biotransformation involves the metabolism of formed monomethylxanthines to the corresponding monomethylurates (Rodopoulos and Norman, 1996).

At physiological concentration of caffeine that 87% of the elimination is due to CYP1A2 (Buters et al., 1996). In human liver microsome, the metabolic profile of caffeine biotransformation by CYP1A2 averaged 81.5% for paraxanthine, 10.8% for theobromine and 5.4% for theophylline formation (Gu et al., 1992).In the clinical study, the mean fractional conversion of caffeine to paraxanthin, theobromine and theophylline was 79.6%, 10.8 % and 3.7 %, respectively (Lelo et al., 1986b). Only caffeine, paraxanthine, theobromine and theophylline were found in plasma during the 24h after ingestion of caffeine, indicating that the metabolites derived from the metabolism of dimethylxanthines are rapidly excreted in urine (Rodopoulos and Norman, 1996). The predominant metabolic pathway of caffeine in man was through paraxanthine (Bonati et al., 1982). The metabolism of caffeine is complex and at least 25 metabolites have been identified in human beings (Rodopoulos et al., 1995). The enzymes involved in these reactions are mainly CYP1A2, CYP2E1, xanthine oxidase, and N-acetyltransferase (Kalow and Tang, 1993). Caffeine also can induce the P-450 system and thus increase its own metabolism (Mitoma et al., 1969).

Regular consumption of caffeine per day may produce pharmacodynamic effects not completely compensated for by the development of tolerance. Mechanisms of tolerance may be overwhelmed by the nonlinear accumulation of caffeine and other methylxanthines in the body when caffeine metabolism becomes saturable (Denaro et al., 1991).

The elimination of caffeine from the body occurs mostly by metabolism. Caffeine is eliminated mainly by metabolism to demethylated and oxidized derivatives (Burg, 1975). The major identifiable urinary metabolites were 1-methyluric acid (46%), 7-methylxanthine

(14%), 3-methylxanthine (12%), 1-methylxanthine (7.5%), 1,7-dimethylxanthine and 1,3-dimethyluric acid (Burg and Stein, 1972; Ullrich et al., 1992).

After 5.5 mg/kg caffeine ingestion, the elimination half-life for the healthy subject was 5.7 hr (Statland and Demas, 1980). It exhibits dose-independent kinetics at a dose of up to 10 mg/kg (Bonati et al., 1982). Caffeine exhibited dose-dependent pharmacokinetics, particularly in subjects with caffeine clearance greater than 1 ml/min/kg after a low dose of caffeine (70 mg). There was a significant decrease in caffeine clearance with increasing dose from 70 mg to 300 mg, indicating saturable caffeine metabolism in the dose from 70 mg to 300 mg (Cheng et al., 1990).

In pregnant women, hormonal influences on the hepatic caffeine metabolizing enzymes might be implicated. During pregnancy, further metabolism of 1,7-dimethylxanthine may be impaired (Scott et al., 1986). Caffeine clearance is impaired in patients with chronic liver disease because of a reduction in hepatic caffeine uptake, and it would be reasonable to advise these patients to moderate their intake of caffeine-containing beverages and medication (Desmond et al., 1980; Scott et al., 1988).

Alcohol is a strong inhibitor of caffeine metabolism. Alcohol intake of 50 g/day significantly prolonged caffeine half-life by 72% and decreased the clearance by 36%. It may be related to alterations in membrane function, NADOH level or inhibition of caffeine binding to cytochromes (George et al., 1986). The caffeine level can be significantly decreased by the pretreatment of rutaecarpine, an extract of *Evodia rutaecarpa* and herbal preparation Wu-Chu-Yu-Tang (a traditional Chinese preparation). Rutaecarpine act as inducers of the CYP1A enzymes (Tsai et al., 2005). Caffeine elimination is stimulated by cigarette smoking. The total body clearance of caffeine was about 55% or 60% greater in smokers than in a nonsmoker. Smokers clear caffeine more rapidly than nonsmokers because of induction of hepatic aryl hydrocarbon hydroxylase activity (Parsons and Neims, 1978; May et al., 1982). Cessation of smoking produced a prolongation of caffeine half-life (29%) and decreased 36% of caffeine clearance, presumably due to the induction of hepatic drug metabolizing enzymes (Murphy et al., 1988). Caffeine elimination is inhibited by cimetidine. Cimetidine in the usual clinical dosage for 3 days induced a 30% to 40% reduction in caffeine total body clearance (May et al., 1982).

Ketoconazole caused prolongation of caffeine elimination, its half-life was prolonged by 16%, and the corresponding clearance was decreased by 9%. Terbinafine influence on the metabolism of caffeine of which was decreased by about 21%, as its elimination half-life was prolonged by about 31% (Wahllander and Paumgartner, 1989).

Concomitant administration of propafenone and caffeine leads to an average 35% increase in the plasma level of caffeine most likely due to a proportional decrease in its metabolic clearance mediated by CYP1A2 (Michaud et al., 2006). Co-administration of ciprofloxacin with caffeine results in a significant increase in plasma caffeine concentration, decrease in the clearance of caffeine by approximately 50%, and a 2.4-fold increase in AUC. This interaction has been attributed to an alteration in the metabolism of caffeine which is due to competitive inhibition of the CYP450 (Mahr et al., 1992; Nicolau et al., 1995). Oral contraceptive steroid markedly altered the pharmacokinetics of caffeine, the half-life was almost twice as long (94% longer), the mean residence time was increased (191%), and the total plasma clearance was 40% less (Patwardhan et al., 1980; Rietveld et al., 1984).

Grapefruit juice contains many flavonoids that are known to inhibit and stimulate hepatic metabolism, but grapefruit juice had no effect on caffeine pharmacokinetics (Maish et al., 1996).

Acute *Plasmodium falciparum* malaria produced significant changes in the disposition of caffeine metabolites. The C_{max} of paraxanthine was significantly lower (about 64%) in malaria than in healthy controls, and the paraxanthine : caffeine area under the plasma concentration time curve ratio, an index of CYP1A2 activity was significantly lower in malaria patients (0.5) than in healthy controls (0.3), the CYP1A2 activity was lower (Akinyinka et al., 2000).

5. Excretion of Caffeine

Caffeine is eliminated in man primarily by metabolic transformation to several methylated xanthine and uric acid metabolites (Tang-Liu et al., 1983). Urinary elimination of caffeine was low and only about 1~1.83 % of the total dose was excreted in the urine (Axelrod and Reichenthal, 1953; Newton et al., 1981). After 5 or 25 mg/kg [^{3}H,^{14}C] caffeine oral administration in male CD-1 mice, 64-90 % total radioactivity was recovered in the urine (Burg and Stein, 1972).

Urinary excretion of caffeine is not affected by urinary PH or plasma concentration (Bonati et al., 1982), whereas it is linearly related to the urine flow rate (Blanchard and Sawers, 1983b). The renal clearance of caffeine, theophylline, paraxanthine and theobromine were all smaller than the glomercular filtration rate and they exhibited urine flow dependence. The clearance of methyluric acid is greater than the glomercular filtration rate and renal secretory mechanisms are likely to be involved in their elimination (Tang-Liu et al., 1983).

Caffeine and its primary demethylation products are excreted into human bile after the oral administration (Holstege et al., 1993). In animal study, the excretion ratio of caffeine from bile-to-blood was 1.24, suggesting that the level of caffeine is higher than those in blood, which indicates that caffeine undergo active hepatobiliary elimination (Tsai et al., 2005).

Conclusion

Although caffeine is not frequently prescribed, caffeine is relatively non-toxic and commonly consumed. Its pharmacokinetics has been well characterized. After oral administration, caffeine is rapidly and completely absorbed.

Caffeine is eliminated primarily by metabolic transformation to several methylated xanthine and uric acid metabolites.

The effect of alcohol or other medicine on caffeine pharmacokinetics has important clinical implications. In patients with cirrhosis, the metabolism of caffeine is significant. Subjects with cirrhosis have impaired elimination of caffeine and it would be reasonable to advise these patients to moderate their intake of caffeine-containing beverages and medication. Inhibition of caffeine metabolism may lead to elevated serum concentrations and subsequently affects the central nervous system.

References

Abernethy DR, Todd EL and Schwartz JB (1985) Caffeine disposition in obesity. *Br. J. Clin. Pharmacol.* 20:61-66.

Akinyinka OO, Sowunmi A, Honeywell R and Renwick AG (2000) The effects of acute falciparum malaria on the disposition of caffeine and the comparison of saliva and plasma-derived pharmacokinetic parameters in adult Nigerians. *Eur. J. Clin. Pharmacol.* 56:159-165.

Aranda JV, Gorman W, Bergsteinsson H and Gunn T (1977) Efficacy of caffeine in treatment of apnea in the low-birth-weight infant. *J. Pediatr.* 90:467-472.

Axelrod J and Reichenthal J (1953) The fate of caffeine in man and a method for its estimation in biological material. *J. Pharmacol. Exp. Ther.* 107:519-523.

Beach CA, Mays DC, Sterman BM and Gerber N (1985) Metabolism, distribution, seminal excretion and pharmacokinetics of caffeine in the rabbit. *J. Pharmacol. Exp. Ther.* 233:18-23.

Berger A (1988) Effects of caffeine consumption on pregnancy outcome. A review. *J. Reprod. Med.* 33:945-956.

Blanchard J (1982) Protein binding of caffeine in young and elderly males. *J. Pharm. Sci.* 71:1415-1418.

Blanchard J and Sawers SJ (1983a) The absolute bioavailability of caffeine in man. *Eur. J. Clin. Pharmacol.* 24:93-98.

Blanchard J and Sawers SJ (1983b) Relationship between urine flow rate and renal clearance of caffeine in man. *J. Clin. Pharmacol.* 23:134-138.

Bonati M, Latini R, Galletti F, Young JF, Tognoni G and Garattini S (1982) Caffeine disposition after oral doses. *Clin. Pharmacol. Ther.* 32:98-106.

Bortolotti A, Jiritano L and Bonati M (1985) Pharmacokinetics of paraxanthine, one of the primary metabolites of caffeine, in the rat. *Drug Metab. Dispos.* 13:227-231.

Burg AW (1975) Physiological disposition of caffeine. *Drug Metab. Rev.* 4:199-228.

Burg AW and Stein ME (1972) Urinary excretion of caffeine and its metabolites in the mouse. *Biochem. Pharmacol.* 21:909-922.

Buters JT, Tang BK, Pineau T, Gelboin HV, Kimura S and Gonzalez FJ (1996) Role of CYP1A2 in caffeine pharmacokinetics and metabolism: studies using mice deficient in CYP1A2. *Pharmacogenetics* 6:291-296.

Cheng WS, Murphy TL, Smith MT, Cooksley WG, Halliday JW and Powell LW (1990) Dose-dependent pharmacokinetics of caffeine in humans: relevance as a test of quantitative liver function. *Clin. Pharmacol. Ther.* 47:516-524.

Curatolo PW and Robertson D (1983) The health consequences of caffeine. *Ann. Intern. Med.* 98:641-653.

Denaro CP, Brown CR, Jacob P, 3rd and Benowitz NL (1991) Effects of caffeine with repeated dosing. *Eur. J. Clin. Pharmacol.* 40:273-278.

Desmond PV, Patwardhan RV, Johnson RF and Schenker S (1980) Impaired elimination of caffeine in cirrhosis. *Dig Dis Sci* 25:193-197.

Donovan JL and DeVane CL (2001) A primer on caffeine pharmacology and its drug interactions in clinical psychopharmacology. *Psychopharmacol Bull* 35:30-48.

Fernandes O, Sabharwal M, Smiley T, Pastuszak A, Koren G and Einarson T (1998) Moderate to heavy caffeine consumption during pregnancy and relationship to spontaneous abortion and abnormal fetal growth: a meta-analysis. *Reprod. Toxicol.* 12:435-444.

Gelal A, Guven H, Balkan D, Artok L and Benowitz NL (2003) Influence of menthol on caffeine disposition and pharmacodynamics in healthy female volunteers. *Eur. J. Clin. Pharmacol* 59:417-422.

George J, Murphy T, Roberts R, Cooksley WG, Halliday JW and Powell LW (1986) Influence of alcohol and caffeine consumption on caffeine elimination. *Clin. Exp. Pharmacol. Physiol.* 13:731-736.

Gu L, Gonzalez FJ, Kalow W and Tang BK (1992) Biotransformation of caffeine, paraxanthine, theobromine and theophylline by cDNA-expressed human CYP1A2 and CYP2E1. *Pharmacogenetics* 2:73-77.

Holstege A, Kurz M, Weinbeck M and Gerok W (1993) Excretion of caffeine and its primary degradation products into bile. *J. Hepatol.* 17:67-73.

Kaiser LL and Allen L (2002) Position of the American Dietetic Association: nutrition and lifestyle for a healthy pregnancy outcome. *J. Am. Diet. Assoc.* 102:1479-1490.

Latini R, Bonati M, Marzi E, Tacconi MT, Sadurska B and Bizzi A (1980) Caffeine disposition and effects in young and one-year old rats. *J. Pharm. Pharmacol.* 32:596-599.

Lelo A, Miners JO, Robson R and Birkett DJ (1986a) Assessment of caffeine exposure: caffeine content of beverages, caffeine intake, and plasma concentrations of methylxanthines. *Clin. Pharmacol. Ther.* 39:54-59.

Lelo A, Miners JO, Robson RA and Birkett DJ (1986b) Quantitative assessment of caffeine partial clearances in man. *Br. J. Clin. Pharmacol.* 22:183-186.

Mahr G, Sorgel F, Granneman GR, Kinzig M, Muth P, Patterson K, Fuhr U, Nickel P and Stephan U (1992) Effects of temafloxacin and ciprofloxacin on the pharmacokinetics of caffeine. *Clin. Pharmacokinet.* 22 Suppl 1:90-97.

Maish WA, Hampton EM, Whitsett TL, Shepard JD and Lovallo WR (1996) Influence of grapefruit juice on caffeine pharmacokinetics and pharmacodynamics. *Pharmacotherapy* 16:1046-1052.

May DC, Jarboe CH, VanBakel AB and Williams WM (1982) Effects of cimetidine on caffeine disposition in smokers and nonsmokers. *Clin. Pharmacol. Ther.* 31:656-661.

McCall AL, Millington WR and Wurtman RJ (1982) Blood-brain barrier transport of caffeine: dose-related restriction of adenine transport. *Life Sci.* 31:2709-2715.

McCusker RR, Goldberger BA and Cone EJ (2006) Caffeine content of energy drinks, carbonated sodas, and other beverages. *J. Anal. Toxicol.* 30:112-114.

McNamara PJ, Burgio D and Yoo SD (1992) Pharmacokinetics of caffeine and its demethylated metabolites in lactating adult rabbits and neonatal offspring. Predictions of breast milk to serum concentration ratios. *Drug Metab. Dispos.* 20:302-308.

Michaud V, Mouksassi MS, Labbe L, Belanger PM, Ferron LA, Gilbert M, Grech-Belanger O and Turgeon J (2006) Inhibitory effects of propafenone on the pharmacokinetics of caffeine in humans. *Ther. Drug Monit.* 28:779-783.

Mitoma C, Lombrozo L, LeValley SE and Dehn F (1969) Nature of the effect of caffeine on the drug-metabolizing enzymes. *Arch. Biochem. Biophys.* 134:434-441.

Murphy TL, McIvor C, Yap A, Cooksley WG, Halliday JW and Powell LW (1988) The effect of smoking on caffeine elimination: implications for its use as a semiquantitative test of liver function. *Clin. Exp. Pharmacol. Physiol.* 15:9-13.

Newton R, Broughton LJ, Lind MJ, Morrison PJ, Rogers HJ and Bradbrook ID (1981) Plasma and salivary pharmacokinetics of caffeine in man. *Eur. J. Clin. Pharmacol.* 21:45-52.

Nicolau DP, Nightingale CH, Tessier PR, Fu Q, Xuan DW, Esguerra EM and Quintiliani R (1995) The effect of fleroxacin and ciprofloxacin on the pharmacokinetics of multiple dose caffeine. *Drugs* 49 Suppl 2:357-359.

Parsons WD and Neims AH (1978) Effect of smoking on caffeine clearance. *Clin. Pharmacol. Ther.* 24:40-45.

Patwardhan RV, Desmond PV, Johnson RF and Schenker S (1980) Impaired elimination of caffeine by oral contraceptive steroids. *J. Lab. Clin. Med.* 95:603-608.

Rietveld EC, Broekman MM, Houben JJ, Eskes TK and van Rossum JM (1984) Rapid onset of an increase in caffeine residence time in young women due to oral contraceptive steroids. *Eur. J. Clin. Pharmacol.* 26:371-373.

Rodopoulos N and Norman A (1996) Assessment of dimethylxanthine formation from caffeine in healthy adults: comparison between plasma and saliva concentrations and urinary excretion of metabolites. *Scand. J. Clin. Lab. Invest.* 56:259-268.

Santambrogio G, Mognoni P and Ventrella L (1964) Plasma Levels of Caffeine after Oral, Intramuscular and Intravenous Administration. *Arch. Int. Pharmacodyn. Ther.* 150:259-263.

Scott NR, Chakraborty J and Marks V (1986) Urinary metabolites of caffeine in pregnant women. *Br. J. Clin. Pharmacol.* 22:475-478.

Scott NR, Stambuk D, Chakraborty J, Marks V and Morgan MY (1988) Caffeine clearance and biotransformation in patients with chronic liver disease. *Clin. Sci. (Lond)* 74:377-384.

Scott NR, Stambuk D, Chakraborty J, Marks V and Morgan MY (1989) The pharmacokinetics of caffeine and its dimethylxanthine metabolites in patients with chronic liver disease. *Br. J. Clin. Pharmacol.* 27:205-213.

Smits P, Thien T and van't Laar A (1985) Circulatory effects of coffee in relation to the pharmacokinetics of caffeine. *Am. J. Cardiol.* 56:958-963.

Statland BE and Demas TJ (1980) Serum caffeine half-lives. Healthy subjects vs. patients having alcoholic hepatic disease. *Am. J. Clin. Pathol.* 73:390-393.

Tang-Liu DD, Williams RL and Riegelman S (1983) Disposition of caffeine and its metabolites in man. *J. Pharmacol. Exp. Ther.* 224:180-185.

Tsai TH, Chang CH and Lin LC (2005) Effects of Evodia rutaecarpa and rutaecarpine on the pharmacokinetics of caffeine in rats. *Planta Med.* 71:640-645.

Ullrich D, Compagnone D, Munch B, Brandes A, Hille H and Bircher J (1992) Urinary caffeine metabolites in man. Age-dependent changes and pattern in various clinical situations. *Eur. J. Clin. Pharmacol.* 43:167-172.

Wahllander A and Paumgartner G (1989) Effect of ketoconazole and terbinafine on the pharmacokinetics of caffeine in healthy volunteers. *Eur J Clin Pharmacol* 37:279-283.

WHO (1997) Coffee, tea, mate, methylxanthines and methylglyoxal. IARC Working Group on the Evaluation of Carcinogenic Risks to Humans. Lyon, 27 February to 6 March 1990, in: *IARC Monographs on the Evaluation of Carcinogenic Risks to Humans*.

Zandvliet AS, Huitema AD, de Jonge ME, den Hoed R, Sparidans RW, Hendriks VM, van den Brink W, van Ree JM and Beijnen JH (2005) Population pharmacokinetics of caffeine and its metabolites theobromine, paraxanthine and theophylline after inhalation in combination with diacetylmorphine. *Basic Clin. Pharmacol. Toxicol.* 96:71-79.

Zylber-Katz E, Granit L and Levy M (1984) Relationship between caffeine concentrations in plasma and saliva. *Clin. Pharmacol. Ther.* 36:133-137.

Zysset T and Wietholtz H (1991) Pharmacokinetics of caffeine in patients with decompensated type I and type II diabetes mellitus. *Eur. J. Clin. Pharmacol.* 41:449-452.

In: Caffeine and Health Research
Editor: Kenneth P. Chambers
ISBN 978-1-60456-437-2

Chapter VII

Topographic Brain Mapping of Caffeine Use and Caffeine Withdrawal

***Roy R. Reeves*[1] *and Frederick A. Struve*[2]**
[1]Department of Mental Health at the G.V. (Sonny) Montgomery VA Medical Center at the University of Mississippi School of Medicine
[2] Department of Psychiatry at Yale University School of Medicine and the New Haven VA Connecticut Healthcare System.

Abstract

Caffeine is a widely used psychoactive substance consumed daily by the majority of Americans. Saletu showed that 250 mg of caffeine can produce a transient reduction of EEG total absolute power in normal persons. Additional studies have confirmed this phenomenon. Overall, however, studies of EEG changes following caffeine exposure have reported variable results. Studies have been done in individuals who are not caffeine naïve and the effect of previous caffeine usage (often for years) on EEG is unknown. It is postulated that this confound may contribute to the variations in results between studies of caffeine exposure.

Several studies have shown that persons consuming even low or moderate amounts of caffeine (in some cases, as low as 100 mg per day) may develop a withdrawal syndrome with caffeine cessation with symptoms such as headaches, lethargy, muscle pain, impaired concentration, and physiological complaints such as nausea or yawning. Preliminary studies of individuals abstaining from caffeine have demonstrated significant changes relative to when they were consuming the drug in a number of EEG variables, including: 1.) increases in theta absolute power over all cortical areas, 2.) increases in delta absolute power over the frontal cortex, 3.) decreases in the mean frequency of both the alpha and beta rhythm, 4.) increase in theta relative power and decrease in beta relative power, and 5.) significant changes in interhemispheric coherence. Additionally, caffeine cessation appears to increase firing rates of diffuse paroxysmal dysrhythmias in some individuals. Preliminary data also suggests that caffeine withdrawal has some effect on cognitive P300 auditory and visual evoked potentials.

Introduction

Caffeine, a naturally occurring member of the methylxanthine family with a chemical structure similar to theophylline, is generally believed to be the most widely consumed psychoactive agent in the world. It is ingested daily by millions of people in a variety of forms, and often in large quantities [1]. The amount consumed annually in the world probably exceeds several billion kilograms. Yet for most of the last century, caffeine seemed to interest neither clinicians nor investigators and was considered a relatively innocuous agent. Although history indicates that it has been consumed for a thousand years or more, it was not until the 1970s that attention began to be called to caffeine's pharmacological consequences.

Caffeine is easily available to most individuals, including children, and may be ingested in a variety of forms, including brewed coffee (100 mg per 6 oz); instant coffee (65 mg per 6 oz); tea (40 mg per 6 oz); carbonated soft drinks (50 mg per 6 oz); over the counter stimulants, analgesics, antihistamines, and weight loss aids (50 to 200 mg per tablet); and prescription analgesics and migraine medications (30 to 100 mg per tablet). Individuals taking over the counter medications are often unaware of their caffeine content. In North America 80 to 90% of adults use caffeine regularly, with almost half of them ingesting caffeine from multiple sources [2]. Average daily intake of caffeine consumers in the United States is approximately 280 mg per day with higher intakes estimated in some European countries [3]. Occasionally, however, patients are encountered who report intake as high as 2,000 to 5,000 mg per day [4]. After oral ingestion caffeine is rapidly and completely absorbed, with peak blood levels generally reached in 30 to 45 minutes [5] and is rapidly eliminated with a half life of 4 to 6 hours [6]. Once absorbed, caffeine is poorly bound (10 to 30%) to plasma albumin, promptly crosses the blood-brain barrier, and enters into relative equilibrium between the plasma and brain [7].

The primary mechanism of action of caffeine is antagonism of adenosine receptors. Adenosine receptors activate an inhibitory G protein, inhibiting the formation of the second messenger cyclic adenosine monophosphate (cAMP). Caffeine intake therefore results in an increase in intraneuronal cAMP concentrations in neurons that have adenosine receptors [8]. Caffeine, especially at high doses, may enhance dopamine activity and affect noradrenergic neurons [9]. It has been shown to elevate brain lactate among caffeine intolerant subjects [10]. Many studies [11-15] have found that caffeine causes global vasoconstriction, although this may not occur in the elderly. Tolerance does not develop to the vasoconstrictive effects, and cerebral blood flow shows a rebound effect after withdrawal from caffeine. In a placebo double blind study [16] in which subjects abstaining from caffeine were given either caffeine or placebo capsules, subjects receiving placebo had significantly increased mean velocity, systolic velocity, and diastolic velocity in all four cerebral arteries.

Caffeine produces a variety of physiological effects, including effects on the cerebral vascular system, blood pressure, respiratory functioning, gastric and colonic activity, urine volume, and exercise performance. Low to moderate doses of caffeine (20 to 200 mg) produce reports of increased well being, happiness, energy, alertness, and sociability, whereas higher doses are more likely to produce reports of anxiety, jitteriness, and upset stomach [17]. Physical dependence on caffeine has been documented in both pre-clinical and clinical research, and the physiological basis has been postulated to be increased functional sensitivity to endogenous adenosine [18]. Persons using caffeine regularly may develop a withdrawal syndrome 12-24 hours after abrupt caffeine cessation; this has been demonstrated using placebo double blind methods in which regular caffeine consumers were given either caffeine or placebo and monitored for signs and symptoms of withdrawal [19]. "Withdrawal" refers to time-limited effects due to cessation of a drug. Symptoms of caffeine withdrawal have been described in the literature for more than 170 years. A variety of symptoms occurring with caffeine withdrawal have been cited, including headache, tiredness/fatigue, decreased energy/activeness, decreased alertness, drowsiness/sleepiness, decreased contentedness/well being, decreased desire to socialize, flu-like symptoms, depressed mood, difficulty concentrating, irritability, lack of motivation for work, foggy/not clearheaded feelings, yawning, decreased self confidence, confusion/bewilderment, nausea/vomiting, muscle pain/stiffness, anxiety/nervousness, heavy feelings in arms and legs, increased night time sleep duration, need for analgesic use, craving for caffeine, blurred vision, lightheadedness/dizziness, anger/hostility, hot and cold spells, rhinorrhea, diaphoresis, and limb tremor [20]. Symptoms have occurred in some persons after cessation of doses as low as 100 mg of caffeine per day [21]. So significant has been the literature on the occurrence of withdrawal symptoms that it has been proposed that caffeine withdrawal be included in the Diagnostic and Statistical Manual of Mental Disorders (DSM) and the International Classification of Diseases (ICD) [22] (currently the DSM lists specific criteria for a diagnosis of caffeine intoxication). A recent excellent comprehensive review [20] identifies and summarizes a total of 57 experimental and 9 survey studies of caffeine withdrawal.

It is evident from the volume of both basic science and clinical research and literature that has accumlated that caffeine is likely to have a significant affect on neurophysiological functioning. This chapter will review electrophysiological studies of exposure to caffeine and of caffeine withdrawal.

The EEG during Caffeine Exposure

EEG variables are sensitive to the CNS effects of numerous pharmacological compounds, and interest in the effects of caffeine on the EEG began in the 1960s. In 1963, Goldstein and associates [23] showed that caffeine ingestion may decrease EEG voltage. Saletu [24] later demonstrated that a 250 mg caffeine dose can produce a transient reduction of EEG total power (in frequencies from 1.3 to 35 Hz) in normal healthy volunteers and Bruce et al [25] reported similar findings with 250 mg and 500 mg doses of caffeine. Kaplan et al [26] found that 250 mg of caffeine (a dose producing favorable subjective effects such as elation, peacefulness, and pleasantness) and 500 mg (a dose producing unpleasant effects such as tension, nervousness, anxiety, excitement, irritability, nausea, palpitations, and restlessness) both reduced electroencephalographic amplitude over the 4 Hz to 30 Hz spectrum, as well as in the alpha (8 to 11 Hz) and beta (12 to 30 Hz) ranges. However, these effects were not dose dependent. Seipman and Kirch [27] described total EEG power reduction over both hemispheres by 200 mg of caffeine with the effect more pronounced when the subjects had their eyes open than when they had their eyes closed. Gilbert et al [28] found that caffeine decreased EEG power across all conditions they studied and produced a wider range of EEG power decrease than did nicotine.

Patat et al [29] found that a 600 mg slow release caffeine formulation produced a significant decrease in delta and theta relative power and a significant increase in alpha and beta (12-40 Hz) relative power. Lundolt et al [30] found that administration of 200 mg of caffeine in the morning reduced sleep time and efficiency and EEG power the subsequent night. In another study conducted by Newman and associates [31], caffeine was associated with a significant increase in peak occipital alpha frequency and significant decreases in occipital alpha amplitude, central beta amplitude, and central theta amplitude both in subjects with panic disorder (who have been demonstrated to be more sensitive than normal individuals to the anxiogenic effects of caffeine) and in normal control subjects. Studies published in languages other than English by Krapivin and Veronina (drop in the absolute power of all frequency ranges) [32] and Kunkel (highly significant reduction of theta amplitude, decreased theta frequency, decreased alpha amplititude, and increased alpha frequency) [33, 34] also reported EEG power reduction secondary to caffeine exposure.

However, several other studies of EEG changes secondary to caffeine exposure have not yielded the same results. Pritchard and colleagues [35] using a dose of less than 200 mg found little in the way of caffeine effects on EEG. In an investigation of the physiological effects of smoking and caffeine, Hasenfratz and Battig [36] reported that caffeine increased blood pressure, finger vasoconstriction, motor activity, frontal EMG, and EEG theta power and decreased heart rate and EEG beta power. Dimfel [37] et al presented data that suggested that caffeine dependent decreases in theta power and delta power occurred under relaxation conditions after exposure to 400 mg of caffeine, but that these same EEG changes did not occur if subjects were engaged in the performance of tasks requiring mental concentration. Other studies of EEG change following caffeine exposure by Sule et al [38], Clubley et al [39], and Pollock et al [40] reported minimal or inconsistent effects.

Why should some studies of caffeine exposure show changes in EEG power while others did not? The reason is uncertain but a reasonable explanation might be related to the fact that the subjects exposed to caffeine were not caffeine naïve. In general, studies used subjects who had previously consumed caffeine and then underwent a period of abstinence during which they were exposed to caffeine for the EEG studies. The effect of previous caffeine usage (often in variable amounts and often for years) on EEG is unknown. It is postulated that this confound may contribute to the variations in results between studies of the effects of caffeine exposure on EEG. The ideal situation to assess the effects of caffeine exposure on EEG would be to find individuals who did not consume caffeine and study them during exposure to the drug. However, finding adults who have had no or minimal use of caffeine to consent to such studies is difficult (and possibly unethical according to some scientists and clinicians who believe caffeine to possess addictive potential).

The Quantitative EEG during Caffeine Withdrawal

An approach which avoid the confounds of previous caffeine use is to study subjects who regularly consume caffeine during abstinence or withdrawal from the drug. Two studies involving EEG have utilized this approach. Both studies have limitations and in a sense could be considered preliminary investigations, but both reveal pertinent neurophysiological findings. Jones and associates [16] investigated cerebral blood flow and quantitative EEG in caffeine withdrawal in a double blind study, but EEG applications were relatively limited. Reeves and colleagues [41, 42] performed a comprehensive analysis of EEG variables, but used an open (versus double blind) investigation.

Jones and associates [16] examined the effect of caffeine withdrawal on cerebral blood flow and quantitative EEG. Ten volunteers reporting moderate caffeine intake (mean 333 mg per day) participated in this double blind study. Subjects were studied while maintaining their normal diet (baseline period) and during two 1-day periods during which they consumed caffeine free diets and received capsules containing placebo (placebo test session) or caffeine (caffeine test session) in amounts equal to their baseline daily caffeine consumption. Blood flow velocity was determined for right and left middle cerebral arteries and right and left anterior cerebral arteries using pulsed transcranial Doppler sonography. Placebo (i.e., the caffeine withdrawal state) significantly increased the mean velocity, systolic velocity, and diastolic velocity in all four cerebral arteries.

Three minutes of EEG were recorded from eight electrode sites and assessment of theta power differences between the placebo condition and the caffeine condition were performed. A significant limitation of the EEG methodology used would be the relatively short recording time and the use of eight versus a larger number of electrodes. However, even in these short recordings the placebo condition (caffeine withdrawal) demonstrated significantly increased EEG theta power.

Reeves and colleagues [41, 42] investigated caffeine withdrawal focusing primarily on comprehensive assessment of EEG variables using an open study. EEGs utilized recording from 21 electrode sites for 30-45 minutes. Thirteen subjects who consumed 300 mg or more of caffeine daily underwent quantitative EEG studies during their usual caffeine consumption (baseline). They then underwent a 4-day period of abstinence from caffeine and were studied on days 1, 2, and 4 of abstinence. The severity of withdrawal was rated at each visit on a scale of 1+ to 4+. Serum caffeine levels were performed on the day of each study to verify abstinence. The project was conducted as an open study and was not a double blind protocol, although the individual who performed analyses of the EEGs was not aware of whether the EEGs were obtained from subjects consuming caffeine or at some point in the period of abstinence. Each subject served as his or her own control with EEG data obtained on caffeine abstinence days compared to the pre-withdrawal baseline measures. In addition to the EEGs obtained at baseline and on days 1, 2, and 4 of abstinence, 10 of the subjects underwent a second EEG on day 4 after being given caffeine. To accomplish this, the final EEG of the abstinence period was obtained, and with the EEG electrodes still in place, the subject was given 2 cups of brewed coffee (200 mg of caffeine) over 15 minutes. Afterward EEG was recorded for an additional 30 minutes.

For each EEG, 25 artifact free 2.5 second epochs were selected for analysis. An analog to digital conversion digitized each epoch into 512 individual points and multiple epochs were averaged together. Spectra subdivision into four basic EEG bandwidths was accomplished with a Fast Fourier Transform. A comprehensive analysis of multiple quantitative variables, including estimates of absolute power, relative power, and mean frequency for the four major

EEG frequency bands (alpha: 7.5 to 12.5 Hz; beta: greater than 12.5 Hz; theta: 3.5 to 7.5 Hz; and delta: less than 3.5 Hz) was performed for each EEG study during the abstinence period and compared to the variables obtained at baseline for each subject. Interhemispheric coherence and power asymmetry were also obtained for the four standard EEG frequency bands using homologous central, posterior, temporal, parietal, and occipital electrode pairs, and the baseline and withdrawal conditions compared.

Even before quantitative analysis was performed, changes in the analog (visual) could be seen, demonstrating an effect from caffeine abstinence and resumption. Generalized increase of alpha and theta voltage, particularly over the frontal cortex was observable during withdrawal from caffeine. Figure 1 demonstrates samples of raw analog EEG tracings from a subject showing representative voltage increases from baseline to a point during caffeine withdrawal, and then again approximately 30 minutes after resumption of caffeine consumption. As seen here, in most cases it was possible to visually recognize voltage increases during caffeine withdrawal and a return of voltage to previous levels with caffeine resumption.

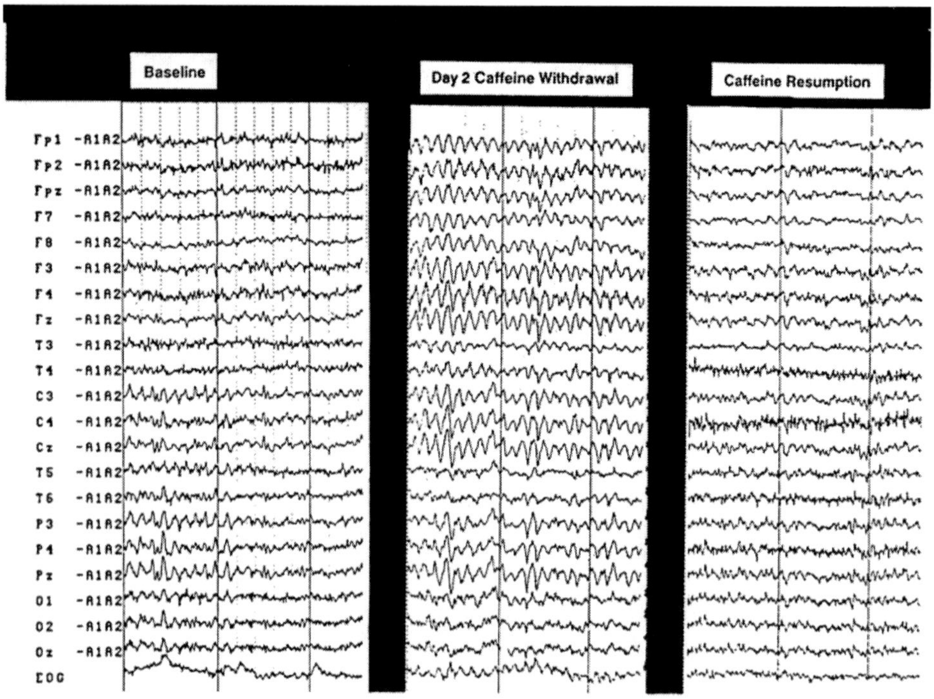

Figure 1. Analog EEG samples during baseline, caffeine withdrawal, and caffeine resumption.

For the results of the quantitative EEG comparisons, the most striking changes occurred with the absolute power of theta. 38.5% of subjects showed statistically significant increases of theta power on withdrawal day 1 and this nearly doubled to 76.9% on withdrawal day 2. Fully 92.3% of subjects showed statistically significant increases of theta absolute power over the frontal cortex at some point during caffeine withdrawal. Significant voltage increase of theta activity following caffeine withdrawal appears to be a highly robust effect. This finding was confirmed by the study by Jones et al [16] mentioned above showing increased theta power during 1-day periods of caffeine abstinence. Caffeine's effect is dramatically illustrated by topographic maps of change in theta absolute power (in Standard Deviation units) on days 1, 2, and 4 relative to baseline conditions (Figure 2). Caffeine abstinence-induced increase in theta voltage is particularly noticeable over the frontal cortex and is most marked on day 2. Topographic maps of EEGs recorded within only 30 minutes of caffeine reintroduction demonstrate return to near baseline conditions in almost all instances.

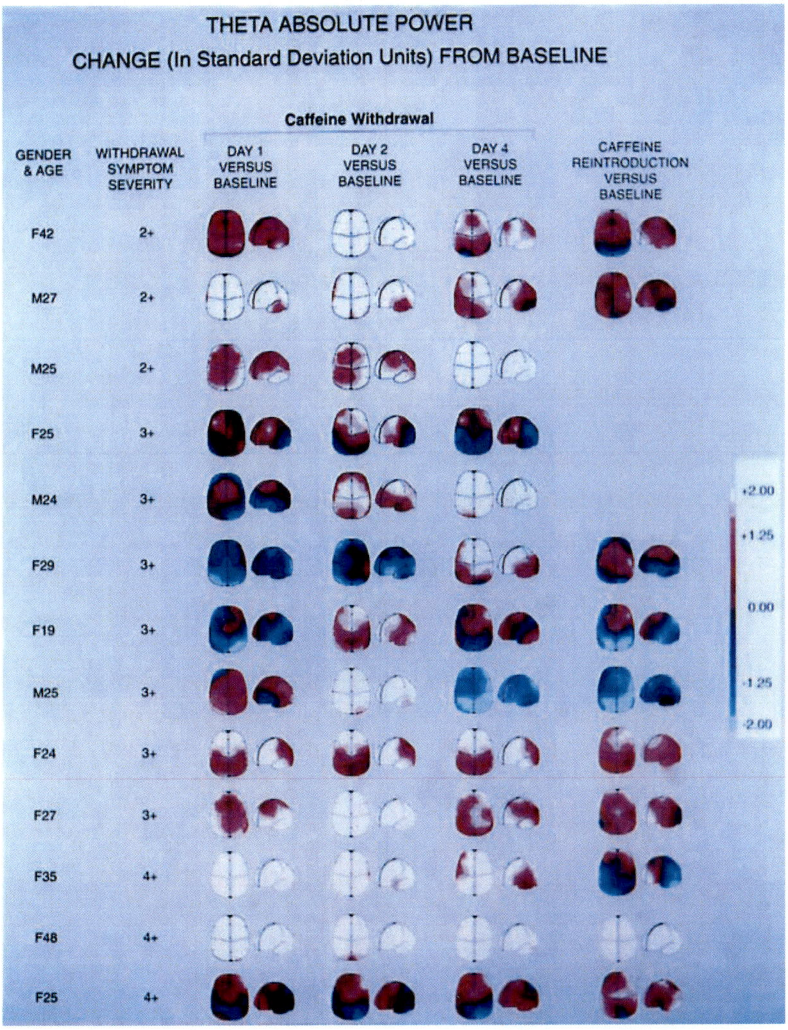

Figure 2. Changes in theta absolute power (in Standard Deviation Units) relative to baseline during caffeine withdrawal and with caffeine reintroduction.

For absolute power of delta, significant changes were confined primarily to increases at the bilateral frontal electrodes, with a single additional electrode, the left posterior temporal, also showing a significant decrease in delta voltage over time. Group statistical analyses from baseline across the withdrawal period indicated no significant changes in alpha absolute power or beta absolute power as a function of caffeine withdrawal. For alpha absolute power considerable intersubject variation occurred, with some subjects showing a marked EEG change while others showed little or no change. Because the intersubject variability in alpha power attenuated the EEG effect for collapsed group data, mean changes in alpha absolute power during caffeine withdrawal were not significant for the group as a whole.

Neither alpha relative power nor delta relative power showed significant change during the period of caffeine withdrawal when compared with pre-abstinent baseline measures. There was a substantial increase of theta relative power for the subjects as a whole. Beta relative power tended to substantially decrease during caffeine withdrawal days as opposed to baseline values.

Withdrawal from caffeine appears to be associated with significant reductions in the frequency of the alpha rhythm (alpha slowing). At all 21 electrode sites the mean alpha frequency decreased throughout the caffeine withdrawal days as contrasted with baseline measures. As with theta absolute power, for most subjects who underwent QEEG after the reinstitution of caffeine on day 4, the mean frequency of the alpha returned to baseline values within 30 minutes. With the exception of only a few electrode sites (FP_1, F_8, and O_2), there was a small but significant decrease in mean beta frequency as a function of caffeine withdrawal. There were no significant changes in mean frequency across caffeine withdrawal days for either theta frequency bands or delta frequency bands.

Interhemispheric coherence measures, expressed as Z-score departures from normative database means were obtained across baseline and caffeine withdrawal periods. Eight (25%) of the 32 coherence measures showed significant change with caffeine withdrawal. Of interest is the observation that coherence values increased during caffeine withdrawal over the frontal cortex but decreased over the posterior cortex. Both alpha coherence and theta coherence increased sharply over the frontal cortex (FP_1/FP_2 and F_3/F_4) throughout the first two days of caffeine abstinence and moved back toward baseline levels by day 4 of caffeine withdrawal. When coherence data following caffeine reinstitution was compared with baseline values, no significant differences were obtained. This suggests that coherence values that did undergo significant change had returned to baseline levels. Both theta coherence (T_5/T_6, P_3/P_4), and delta coherence (C_3/C_4 and O_1/O_2) decreased significantly over posterior cortex during the caffeine withdrawal period. As before, when caffeine was reintroduced following the withdrawal period, coherence measures were no longer significantly different from baseline values.

Interhemispheric asymmetry as a function of caffeine withdrawal was examined for the four traditional EEG frequency bands at all 21 electrode sites. These analyses did not reveal any significant differences between baseline and withdrawal or reinstitution parameters. This suggests that caffeine withdrawal does not produce significant changes in interhemispheric symmetry for any of the frequency bands at any of the cortical regions.

Other EEG Occurrences during Caffeine Withdrawal

In addition to the findings described above, it was observed that patients who have diffuse paroxysmal slowing (DPS) on EEG may have increased bursts of DPS during caffeine withdrawal [43]. DPS is a minor EEG dysrhythmia that is sometimes seen in normal individuals and may be more common in persons with migraine. In six individuals with DPS at baseline (normal consumption), bursts of slowing increased by 88.3% on day 1 of caffeine abstinence, and peaked on day 2 at a 106.4% increase. After the subjects were given caffeine on day 4, the DPS firing rate for all subjects returned to, or below baseline levels.

Cognitive Evoked Potential and Caffeine Withdrawal

The only study currently in the literature on the effects of caffeine withdrawal on cognitive evoked potentials is an extention of the 4 day EEG study of caffeine withdrawal described above. On the same days these subjects underwent quantitative EEG studies, cognitive auditory and visual P300 evoked potentials were also performed. Results [44] indicated that there were no significant differences in auditory P300 latencies from baseline through caffeine withdrawal days 1, 2, and 4. However, there were significant decreases in auditory P300 amplitudes across the caffeine withdrawal days. In contrast to the results from the auditory P300 measures, caffeine withdrawal produced a different effect on visual P300 measurements. Findings indicated a statistically significant decrease in the visual P300 latency and no differences in P300 amplitude as a function of caffeine withdrawal. Why there would be differences in the types of responses of auditory and visual evoked potentials to the caffeine withdrawal state remains to be explained.

Significance of Electrophysiological Effects of Caffeine Exposure and Withdrawal

A number (but not all) of EEG studies of caffeine exposure demonstrate decreased power (voltage). The lack of this finding by some studies is postulated to be related to the confound of the effect of previous usage of caffeine among subjects. In spite of these inconsistencies, there appear to be adequate studies [23-34] supporting decreased EEG power with caffeine exposure to conclude that this is a valid phenomenon. Supporting this finding are a number of SPECT and PET studies [11-15] demonstrating cerebral blood flow decreases following caffeine exposure. It is easily plausible that decreased EEG voltage could occur as a result of decreased cerebral blood flow caused by vasoconstriction induced by caffeine exposure.

Quantitative EEG parameters that show significant changes as a result of caffeine withdrawal can be summarized as follows: 1.) increases in theta absolute power over all cortical areas; 2.) increases in delta absolute power over the frontal cortex; 3.) decreases in the mean frequency of both the alpha and beta rhythm; 4.) increase in theta relative power and decrease in beta relative power; and 5.) significant changes in interhemispheric coherence. Since caffeine exposure can result in alpha frequency increase [30], decreases in mean alpha frequency during withdrawal would not be unexpected. Increased EEG voltage during caffeine withdrawal is consistent with the postulate that caffeine exposure causes cerebral vasoconstriction followed by rebound cerebral vasodilitation during caffeine withdrawal. In fact, decreased cerebral blood flow during caffeine withdrawal has been shown to be reversed within 2 hours after caffeine intake [16]. These findings would be consistent with the report of occurrence of headache in 77% of studies of caffeine withdrawal [20]. It would appear that, at least in some cases, these headaches may be vascular in nature. The increase in DPS dysththymia [43] in some individuals may then be related to vascular headache as DPS occurs more often in migraine sufferers than in the general population.

Caffeine withdrawal related vasodilitation would appear, at least for some individuals, to be reversed with caffeine consumption. In addition to the cerebral blood low study mentioned above, Reeves et al [42] showed that, in most cases theta absolute power quickly returns to essentially baseline conditions within 30 minutes of caffeine resumption (see Figure 2). However, this vascular phenomenon may be limited to younger persons as it did not occur in the single patient in their study who was over 30 years old (age 48).

EEG changes including relative power as well as mean frequency measures are less clearly understood in terms of a vasodilitation hypothesis. The implications of caffeine withdrawal induced changes in interhemispheric coherence, particularly the directional differentiation of change between the anterior and posterior cortex remain obscure. Similarly, the findings of decreases in auditory P300 evoked potentials amplitudes and no significant differences in auditory latencies, but decreases in visual P300 latencies and no significant differences in visual amplitudes during caffeine withdrawal are difficult to explain. The anatomic and/or neurophysiological substrate involved in the regulation of coherence during caffeine withdrawal are not well understood.

The fact that in nearly every case reinstitution of caffeine following withdrawal tended to return altered QEEG values to baseline levels supports the contention that caffeine withdrawal was truly the operative variable in the EEG changes seen in the studies of caffeine withdrawal discussed here. It is interesting that despite the fact that post-caffeine reintroduction QEEGs were completed before peak levels of caffeine were likely to have been obtained (i.e., 30 to 45 minutes post ingestion), the majority of EEG variables did return to baseline following caffeine reintroduction [42]. More importantly, for most subjects, at all electrode sites the caffeine withdrawal changes in alpha rhythm returned completely to baseline levels within 30 minutes following caffeine reintroduction. This was also true for all electrodes for which beta mean frequency was altered by caffeine withdrawal. Thus it appears that caffeine withdrawal is a detectable and to some degree measureable phenomenon which can be reversed at some levels by reinstitution of caffeine. However, in spite of EEG or cerebral blood flow normalization with caffeine reinstitution, many of the clinical symptoms of caffeine withdrawal may not immediately resolve.

Conclusions

There would seem to be little question that caffeine exposure and caffeine withdrawal have neurophysiological effects which are detectable and quantifiable by EEG methods. A number of physiological responses to caffeine exposure and caffeine withdrawal may be theoretically explained by the phenomenon of cerebral vasoconstriction during caffeine exposure and rebound cerebral vasodilitation with abrupt cessation of caffeine. However, some of the effects of caffeine and its withdrawal are poorly understood, and for some effects (e.g., differences in directional changes in interhemispheric coherence in different areas of the brain and differences in effects on amplitudes and latencies of auditory and visual cognitive evoked potentials during caffeine withdrawal), no explanation is available as to why they occur.

Although there is a signicant collection of research on the electrophysiological effects of caffeine exposure, studies of caffeine withdrawal done to date could at best be described as preliminary. These studies present fascinating data but are limited in design and numbers of subjects. A number of needs and possibilities for further research are readily obvious. Particularly important would be placebo double blind studies to confirm data from previous open studies. Future work should attempt to extend the caffeine abstinence over additional days as this would permit assessment of the duration of neurophysiological caffeine withdrawal effects over longer periods of time. In addition, assessment of caffeine reinstitution should be done in a double blind paradigm with placebo or measurable doses of caffeine given in tablet form, and the time period of response should be carefully recorded and be sufficiently long (i.e., over 30 to 45 minutes) to allow peak caffeine blood levels to be obtained. It might be particularly interesting in view of previous findings to combine a cerebral blood flow study with a comprehensive quantitative EEG and evoked potentials study using a double blind placebo protocol for caffeine withdrawal and reinstitution. Assessing EEG parameters in combination with other research tool such as magnetic resonance spectroscopy could also be of value. For example, a proton spectroscopic study [10] has demonstrated globally and regionally specific brain lactate increases in caffeine intolerant subjects when they were exposed to caffeine; quantitative EEG changes in combination with spectroscopic data in such individuals could provide further insight into caffeine's effects. Finally, the relevance of the EEG findings to date, if confirmed, might largely depend on whether or not subjective symptoms of caffeine withdrawal can be shown to significantly co-vary over time with alterations of electrophysiological measures.

References

[1] Gilbert RM. Caffeine consumption. In: Spiller GA, editor. The Methylxanthine Beverages and Foods: Chemistry, Consumption, and Health Effects. New York: Alan R. Liss; 1984, pp 185-213.

[2] Hughes JR, Oliveto AH. A systematic survey of caffeine intake in Vermont. Exp Clin Psychopharmacol 1997; 5:393-398.
[3] Barone JJ, Roberts HR. Caffeine consumption. Food Chem Toxicol 1996; 34:119-129.
[4] Molde DA. Diagnosing caffeineism. Am J Psychiatry 1975; 132:202-205.
[5] Mumford GK, Benowita NL, Evans SM. Kaminski BJ, Preston KL, Sannerud CA, Silverman K, Griffiths RR. Absorption rates of methylxanthines following capsules, cola, and chocolate. Euro J Clin Pharmacol 1996 ; 51 :319-325.
[6] Liguori A, Hughes JR, Grass JA. Absorption and subjective effects of caffeine from coffee, cola, and capsules. Pharmacol Biochem Behav 1997; 58:721-726.
[7] Kaplan GB, Greenblatt DJ, LeDuc BW, Thompson ML, Shader RI. Relationships of plasma and brain concentrations of caffeine and metabolites to benzodiazepine receptor binding and locomotor activity. J Pharmacol Exp Ther 1989; 248:1078-1083.
[8] Snyder SS, Katims JJ, Annau Z. Adenosine receptors and behavioral actions of methylxanthines. Proc Natl Acad Sci USA 1981; 78:3260-3264.
[9] Goldstein A, Kaiser S, Whitby O. Psychotropic effects of caffeine in man. IV. Quantitative and qualitative differences associated with habituation to caffeine. Clin Pharmacol Ther 1969; 10:489.
[10] Dager SR, Layton ME, Strauss W, Richards TL, Heide A, Friedman SD, Artru AA, Hayes CE, Posse S. Human brain metabolic response to caffeine and the effects of tolerance. Am J Psychiatry 1999; 156:229-237.
[11] Cameron OG, Model JG, Hariharan M. Caffeine and human cerebral blood flow: A positron emission topographic study. Life Sci 1990; 47:1141-1146.
[12] Mathew RJ, Wilson WH. Caffeine-induced changes in cerebral circulation. Stroke 1985; 16:814-817.
[13] Mathew RJ, Wilson WH. Caffeine consumption, withdrawal and cerebral blood flow. Headache 1985; 25:305-309.
[14] Mathew RJ, Barr DL, Weinman ML. Caffeine and cerebral blood flow. Brit J Psychiatry 1983; 143:604-608.
[15] Couterier ECM, Laman DM, van Dujin MAJ, van Dujin H. Influence of caffeine and caffeine withdrawal on headache and cerebral flow velocities. Cephalgia 1997; 17:188-190.
[16] Jones HE, Herning RI, Cadet JL, Griffiths RR. Caffeine withdrawal increases cerebral blood flow and alters quantitative electroencephalography (EEG) activity. Psychopharmacol 2000; 147:371-377.
[17] Griffiths RR, Juliano LM, Chausmer AL. Caffeine pharmacology and clinical effects. In: Graham AW, Schultz TK, Mayo-Smith M, Ries K, Wilford BB, editors. Principles of Addiction Medicine, 3rd edition. Chevy Chase: American Society of Addiction Medicine; pp 193-224.
[18] Griffiths RR, Mumford GK. Caffeine reinforcement, discrimination, tolerance, and physical dependence in laboratory animals and humans. In: Schuster CR, Kuhar MJ, editors. Pharmacological Aspects of Drug Dependence: Toward an Integrated Neurobehavioral Approach (Handbook of Experimental Pharmacology). Berlin Heidelberg New York: Springer; pp 315-341.

[19] Silverman K, Evans SM, Strain EC, Griffiths RR. Withdrawal syndrome after the double-blind cessation of caffeine consumption. New Eng J Med 1992; 327:1109-1114.

[20] Juliano LM, Griffiths RR. A critical review of caffeine withdrawal: empirical validation of symptoms and signs, incidence, severity, and associated features. Psychopharmacology (Berl) 2004; 76:1-29.

[21] Griffiths RR, Evans SM, Heightman SJ. Low-dose caffeine dependence in humans. J Pharmacol Exp 1990; 225:1123-1132.

[22] Hughes JR, Oliveto AH, Helzer JE, Higgins ST, Bickel WK. Should caffeine abuse, dependence, or withdrawal be added to DSM-IV and ICD-10? Am J Psychiatry 1992; 149:33-40.

[23] Goldstein L, Murphree HB, Pfeiffer CC. Quantitative electroencephalography in man as a measure of CNS stimulation. Ann NY Acad Sci 1963; 107:1045-1056.

[24] Saletu B. EEG imaging of brain activity in clinical psychopharmacology. In: Mauer K, editor. Topographic Brain Mapping of EEG and Evoked Potentials. New York: Springer Verlag; 1989, pp 482-506.

[25] BruceM, Scott N, Ladner M, Marks V. The psychopharmacological and electrophysiological effects of single doses of caffeine in human subjects. Br J Pharmacol 1986; 22:81-87.

[26] Kaplan GB, Greenblatt DJ, Ehrenberg BL, Goddard JE, Cotreau MM, Harmatz JS, Shader RI. Dose-dependent pharmacokinetics and psychomotor effects of caffeine in humans. J Clin Pharmacol 1997; 37:693-703.

[27] Seipman M, Kirch W. Effects of caffeine on topographic quantitative EEG. Neuropsychobiology 2002; 45:161-166.

[28] Gilbert DG, Dibb WD, Plath LC, Hiyane SG. Effects of nicotine and caffeine, separately and in combination, on EEG topography, mood, heart rate, cortisol, and vigilance. Psychophysiology 2000; 37:583-595.

[29] Patat A, Rosenzweig P, Enslen M, Trocherie S, Miget N, Bozon MC, Allain H, Gandon JM. Effects of a new slow release formulation of caffeine on EEG, psychomotor and cognitive functions in sleep-deprived subjects. Hum Psychopharmacol 2000; 15:153-170.

[30] Landolt HP, Werth E, Borbely AA, Dijik DJ. Caffeine intake (200 mg) in the morning affects human sleep and EEG power spectra at night. Brain Res 1995; 675:67-74.

[31] Newman F, Stein MB, Trettau JR, Coppola R, Uhde TW. Quantitative electroencephalographic effects of caffeine in panic disorder. Psychiatric Res 1992; 45:105-113.

[32] Krapivin SV, Voronina TA. Comparative quantitative pharmacological-EEG anakysis of the effects of psychostimulants [article in Russian]. Vestn Ross Akad Med Nauk 1995; 6:7-16.

[33] Kunkel H. EEG spectral analysis of caffeine effects [article in German]. Arzneimittelforschung 1976; 26:462-465.

[34] Kunkel H. Multichannel EEG spectral analysis of the caffeine effect [article in German]. Z Ernahrungswiss 1976; 15:71-79.

[35] Pritchard WS, Robinson JH, DeBethizy JD, Davis RA, Stiles MF. Caffeine and smoking: subjective performance and psychophysiological effects. Psychophysiology 1995; 32:19-27.

[36] Hasenfratz M, Battig K. Action profiles of smoking and caffeine: Stroop effect, EEG, and peripheral physiology. Pharmacol Biochem Behavior 1992; 42:155-161.

[37] Dimfel W, Schober F, Spuler M. The influence of caffeine on human EEG under resting conditions and during mental loads. Clin Investig 1993; 71:197-207.

[38] Sule J, Brozek G, Cmiral J. Neurophysiological effects of small doses of caffeine in man. Activitas Nervosa Superior (Praha) 1974; 16:217-218.

[39] Clubley M, Bye CE, Henson TA, Peck AW, Riddington CJ. Effects of caffeine and cyclizine alone and in combination on human performance, subjective effects, and EEG activity. Brit J Pharmacol 1979; 7:157-163.

[40] Pollock VE, Teasdale T, Stern J. Effects of caffeine on resting EEG and response to sine wave modulated light. Electroencephalogr Clin Neurophysiol 1981; 51:470-476.

[41] Reeves RR, Stuve FA, Patrick G, Bullen JA. Topographic quantitative EEG measures of alpha and theta power changes during caffeine withdrawal: Preliminary findings from normal subjects. Clin Electroencephalogr 1995; 26:154-162.

[42] Reeves RR, Struve FA, Patrick G. Topographic quantitative EEG response to acute caffeine withdrawal: A comprehensive analysis of multiple quantitative variables. Clin Electroencephalogr 2002; 178-188.

[43] Patrick G, Reeves RR, Struve FA. Does caffeine cessation increase firing rates of diffuse of diffuse paroxysmal slowing dysrhythmia? A serendipitous observation. Clin Electroencephalogr 1996; 27:78-83.

[44] Reeves RR, Struve FA, Patrick G. The effects of caffeine withdrawal on cognitive P300 auditory and visual evoked potentials. Clin Electroencephalogr 1999; 30:24-27.

In: Caffeine and Health Research
Editor: Kenneth P. Chambers
ISBN 978-1-60456-437-2

Chapter VIII

"Coffee or Tea? From the Historically Alleged Curative Properties of Common Beverages to Their Current Evidence-Based Benefits on Human Health"

Andrea A. Conti[*]
Dipartimento di Area Critica Medico Chirurgica,
Università degli Studi di Firenze.
Fondazione Don Carlo Gnocchi, IRCCS Firenze
Centro Italiano per la Medicina Basata sulle Prove,
Firenze, Italy

Abstract

Various positive effects on the human body have been attributed through time to diverse beverages commonly consumed in the Western world. The purpose of this paper is to examine the extent to which popular beliefs regarding certain drinks have a scientific basis. A historical description of the putative therapeutic and/or preventive characteristics of four widely consumed beverages will be presented, followed by a discussion of the state-of-the-art biomedical knowledge regarding them. The importance of wine on human health has been affirmed from time immemorial, and today, in an evidence-based nutritional perspective, the beneficial properties on the vascular system of red wine consumed in moderate quantities have been confirmed both on pathophysiological and clinical grounds. The relevance of voices of the past claiming the favourable effects of coffee, tea and chocolate on human health is also examined. Current evidence documents the beneficial effects, not only on the cardiocirculatory system, but

[*] Author for correspondence: Andrea Alberto Conti, MD, MPH, PhD. Dipartimento di Area Critica Medico Chirurgica, Università degli Studi di Firenze. Viale Morgagni 85, I-50134, Firenze, Italy. Tel.: +39-055-7949357; Fax: +39-055-7947608; E-mail: aa.conti@dac.unifi.it

also on other human apparati, including the respiratory and the gastrointestinal ones, of the methylxanthines, polyphenols and flavonoids contained in coffee, green tea and chocolate when assumed by healthy subjects in appropriate dosages.

This historical perspective evidences the continuing pertinence of past traditions regarding major beverages, even when compared with up-dated scientific information. The adage that one never learns enough from the past therefore holds true, though the learning may be as easy as drinking a glass of wine, sipping a cup of tea or enjoying a cup of coffee or chocolate.

Key words: Adults; cardiovascular system; chocolate; coffee; elderly; evidence based medicine; history of medicine; nutrition; tea; wine

Introduction

Various positive effects on the human body have been attributed through time to diverse beverages commonly consumed in the Western world. The purpose of this paper is to examine the extent to which popular beliefs regarding certain drinks have a scientific basis, and to give a balanced view of the favourable properties of wine, coffee, tea and chocolate. Given that many aliments, if assumed in an excessive way, may be harmful for humans, in this article the positive effects on adult and also elderly healthy subjects of four drinks consumed in moderate quantities will be described. In many cases, these evidence-based beneficial effects interestingly confirm the historically alleged curative properties of the four beverages considered, and, therefore, for each of them, a historical description of the putative therapeutic and/or preventive characteristics is presented, followed by a discussion of the pertinent state-of-the-art biomedical knowledge.

Wine

Wine is an alcoholic beverage derived from the fermentation of the juice of grapes. The importance of wine on human health has been affirmed from time immemorial. The Old Testament documents Noah's knowledge of the fermentation of grapes, while the first miracle of Jesus described in the New Testament is the turning of water into wine. With regard to the Western world, the medical properties of wine were already documented in the Greek epic poems, the *Iliad* and the *Odyssey*. In ancient Egypt, as in many other cultures, the role of wine was central in rites and in religious ceremonies. In the Roman empire wine constituted a fundamental part of the diet, and, given the extent of this empire, the drinking of wine also had enormous impact on the development of viticulture and oenology in Roman-held territories. Furthermore, wine tended to be considered the preferable liquid medium for containing curative substances and, consequently, medicinal wines, meaning wines with different principles added in order to treat different disorders, were already largely in use in Roman times. It may be noted that even today popular medicine continues to make provision for the addition of specific substances to wine for curative purposes (sage for toothache, iron filings for anaemia).

Through time, however, it was essentially the intrinsic positive effects on human health of wine alone that were evidenced. This is confirmed by proverbs, that represent so-called popular wisdom: in Italy, for example, wine is commonly said "to make good blood". In fact, probably because of its appearance as a red fluid, wine was associated to blood in various ways: the common denominator of popular wisdom was that wine assumption, particularly if moderate and during meals, favourably influenced blood composition and circulation [1,2]. It is also important to remember that in Italy as well as in other Mediterranean countries wine has always been considered essential in pharmacopoeia, having been adopted for a wide array of needs, ranging from the cleaning and disinfection of wounds to the procuring of rudimental anaesthesia.

At the present time and in an evidence-based nutritional perspective, granted that an excessive use of wine is dangerous for human health, and that, exactly as for many other substances, wine may become toxic according to its dosage, consistent epidemiological evidence, confirming popular tradition, indicates that regular and moderate red wine intake reduces cardiovascular risk and total mortality in adult and elderly healthy subjects [3,4]. The recommendation of moderation has a clear scientific rationale, since an excess of a level of consumption that has been quantified in one-two glasses of red wine a day for men and one glass of red wine a day for women, has harmful effects on multiple human organs and systems, including the cardiovascular one. Popular recommendations are also correct with regard to the modality of assumption of wine; thus, its parcelled intake with meals has been shown to exert more favourable effects than its autonomous assumption far from meals, and this on account of the tempering effect of food on the rate of its metabolism [5]. With respect to non-drinkers of wine, moderate healthy drinkers usually have higher levels of HDL cholesterol (the so-called "good cholesterol"), lower fibrinogen values and lower PAI-1 (plasminogen activator inhibitor 1) levels [6]. In fact, the pattern of protection of wine on the cardiovascular system is J-shaped, implicating that no and high consumption are less favourable for human health than a moderate intake. The daily regular consumption of 150 ml of wine had been shown to reduce cardiovascular diseases by around 32% [7]. Moreover, today red wine is considered more protective than white wine, as different studies indicate that the positive effects of wine are largely determined by polyphenols, and in particular resveratrol, of which red wine is rich [8]. The neuroprotective, anti-viral and anti-proliferative properties of trans-resveratrol have also been shown [9]. Among other described beneficial effects of resveratrol, mechanisms leading to an increase in nitric oxide, a decrease in the activity of angiotensin II and a decrease in platelet aggregation [6,8] appear interesting. Furthermore, anti-ischemic effects, including the decrease in LDL-oxidation and the enhancement of pro-survival paths, have been documented [10]. Therefore, on evidence-based grounds, it can effectively be said that, for its favourable effects on the cardiovascular and on the coagulation systems, "a little wine makes good blood".

Coffee

Coffee and tea provide further good examples of the relevance of the voices of the past claiming the favourable effects of these beverages on human health. Current evidence well documents the beneficial activity, not only on the cardiocirculatory system but also on other human apparati, including the respiratory and the gastrointestinal ones, of the methylxanthines, polyphenols and flavonoids contained in coffee and green tea assumed by adult and elderly healthy subjects in moderate dosages [11,12].

Coffee originated from Africa, and precisely from Abyssinia, where it was already cultivated in the VII century. By the XI century coffee was widely recognized as a stimulating beverage, sharing with wine the attributed characteristic of producing euphoria. However, since the consumption of wine was forbidden in the Islamic world, coffee there became its substitute and underwent a rapid diffusion. In the XI century the great Persian physician Avicenna described the different positive effects of coffee on the human neurological and cardiovascular systems, and, convinced of its therapeutic value, he prescribed it as a drug. In the XVI century the first coffee shops were opened in Constantinople, from where it was imported to Italy by Venetian merchants. In the first half of the XVII century the first coffee shop was opened in Italy, and, in the course of less than 150 years, more than 200 coffee shops appeared in Venice. At the beginning of the XVIII century the Dutch took coffee to Brazil, and soon after South America became the world's leading area for coffee production.

Although the pharmacological properties of coffee were first described in Europe by the voyager Prospero Alpino at the end of the XVI century (*De plantis Aegypti*, Venice 1592), it was only in the XIX century that the stimulating character of coffee, related to caffeine, was quantitatively defined in Western world. At that time coffee was used both in medical settings and in empirical contexts as an activator drink for the central nervous system, a remedy for headache and a diuretic beverage [2, 13].

Coffee contains caffeine, a methylxanthine, similar to the theofilline characteristic of tea and the theobromine of chocolate. Methylxanthines have various biological effects on different systems and organs, including a positive inotropic and chronotropic influence on the heart. In the cardiovascular system they cause dilation in the coronary, peripheral and renal vessels, and vasoconstriction of the cerebral circulation, a mechanism that partly explains the effective favourable role of caffeine on headaches [11, 12]. Methylxanthines inhibit platelet aggregation, cause bronchodilation, provoke the stimulation of renin release and bring about a general diuretic effect [12]. Coffee therefore not only has activating and stimulating effects on the nervous system, in accordance with popular ideas, but also exerts many other relevant biological actions [14]. It should be stressed that coffee not only contains caffeine, which in effect accounts for merely 2-3% of the total biological activity of this beverage, but also hundreds of different substances with definite effects, including diterpens (fats), magnesium and fenolic acids [11]. Diterpens increase cholesterol, while magnesium increases the sensitivity of human peripheral tissues to insulin. Fenolic acids increase homocysteine, decrease LDL oxidation, platelet aggregation and glucose absorption. The overall importance of coffee in human nutrition is confirmed by the fact that, in many and different populations

(Germany, Norway, Spain), coffee is, on a theoretical basis, the single most important dietetic source of precious antioxidants [11, 15].

In synthesis, coffee is a complex aliment, that might be defined as a "variety of beverages", containing numerous and diverse active substances. Their overall action depends on their reciprocal quantitative and qualitative balance, on the method of preparation, on the rhythm and entity of consumption and on the dietetic habits and lifestyle patterns in which the consumption itself is embedded [16]. In past decades coffee has sometimes been accused of being potentially dangerous for the cardiovascular system, and in particular for the heart. A recent comprehensive meta-analysis by our group has on the contrary shown that a moderate daily consumption (1-3 espresso cups a day) in adult and elderly healthy subjects, if included in a correct and balanced diet and within an appropriate lifestyle scheme, does not increase the risk of coronary heart disease [17].

Tea

Camellia sinensis, the technical definition of tea, derives from the Eastern world, as indicated by the adjective "sinensis" (Chinese). Already in the VI century tea was cultivated in China, where it was a very popular beverage, well reputed for its healing and therapeutic qualities. About the middle of the XVI century Giovanbattista Ramusio, the famous Italian humanist, wrote that tea could make fever, headache, stomach ache and joint pain disappear, provided it was assumed as hot as possible. A century later tea was imported into Europe by the Portuguese and Dutch. In Great Britain the consumption of this beverage grew and spread rapidly. Though at first confined to the higher classes, it subsequently gained popularity in every rank of society, becoming the national English drink (as coffee is for Italy). Indeed, it may be said that in England drinking tea became, and still is, almost a ritual. The medical properties of tea had already been observed in the fifteen hundreds, when it was considered a remedy for a wide range of health problems, given that it was retained to accelerate metabolism, to depurate the body, to calm inflammation, to render blood circulation more fluent, and to reduce the sensation of fatigue. In the XIX century its pharmacological effects began to be defined in a precise way, this being particularly true for the diuretic and vasodilatative effects of theophilline, an alkaloid of which tea is rich. If coffee has always been considered a drink useful in activating the human mind, tea has been considered a beverage effective in relaxing the human body. In reality, the alkaloids contained in tea are stimulating substances, and tea contains caffeine as well. It is true, however, as believed in the past, that tea has antioxidant, vasodilatative and diuretic properties, which will now be briefly illustrated [18, 19].

In recent times many biological characteristics of tea, and in particular of green tea, have been documented and their effects with regard to the human organism and human health have been evidenced [20]. The overall positive effects of green tea probably derive from the interaction of polyphenols, and especially of flavonoids and epigallocatechin gallate [21]. Flavonoids have indeed anti-inflammatory, anti-oxidant and anti-thrombogenic properties, which are responsible for their cardioprotective impact [22]. The xanthines and polyphenols contained in tea produce lipolitic and diuretic activity, while catechins have been shown to produce antiatherosclerotic effects. In vitro, in fact, they prevent LDL cholesterol oxidation (the so-called "bad cholesterol") [23].

Evidence is also growing with regard to the fact that tea polyphenols containing a galloyl group may favourably interfere with many different pathways of signal transduction, in particular in cardiovascular system cells. The prompting of pleiotropic effects on the part of green tea may play a key role in the prevention and therapy of cardiovascular diseases, and further extensive research may confirm the impact of tea components on human cells [18]. Green tea catechins also have effects on the molecular mechanisms involved in multi-drug resistance, in the regulation of cellular death and in angiogenesis [24]. Some Japanese researchers have consequently proposed green tea as a preventive beverage for cancer, suggesting the disseminated prophylactic assumption of ten cups per day [25]. However, such a powerful preventive and therapeutic role for tea needs further structured experimentation, as some data need diffuse, in vivo confirmation. Globally, however, up-dated knowledge is extremely promising and confirms many of the alleged properties attributed to tea in the past.

Chocolate

Chocolate is the name given to a drink made by mixing the powder (cocoa) obtained from the crushed seeds of the cacao tree with hot water or milk. It is thought that more than 2,500 years ago Mayans drank chocolate, as suggested by chocolate residues traced in ancient Mayan pots, while the Aztecs linked chocolate with Xochiquetzal, the goddess of fertility. In pre-Columbian America the native populations dried the seeds of the cacao plant, prepared them on the fire, and, after powdering them, mixed this powder with water. They consumed the resulting cocoa as a spicy and bitter drink called xocoatl, seasoned with pepper and vanilla, but not milk. This is interesting, since it has now been established that the maximum positive effects of chocolate on the cardiovascular system are connected to the dark, and not the milk, variety. Spanish conquerors came into contact with the cacao plant in America when the New World was discovered, and the introduction of chocolate into Europe is therefore successive to 1492. In the XVI century in Mexico Fernando Cortez was taken to be the god Quatzcoalt by the natives, and therefore the inhabitants of that region, in his honour, called the cocoa beverage Cacahualt, which later became Chocolatlla, from whence the name.

One of the first documentations in Europe of the use of chocolate as a medical remedy is to be found in the "Ragionamenti del mio viaggio intorno al mondo" ("Reflections on my voyage around the world"), of the Italian voyager Francesco Carletti, who, at the end of the XVI century, wrote that chocolate was then drunk as a real medicine. In a later period, although some exponents of the Catholic Church for some time considered chocolate a voluptuous and transgressive aliment, pope Pius V formally refused to sanction a requested prohibition of chocolate consumption. In effect, it is retained that it was most probably in convents that, at this time, the preparation of chocolate was altered, and its recipe, previously containing hot pepper and spices, was modified in the direction of current taste. Precisely on account of this improvement in flavour, chocolate was also called "theobroma", "the food of the gods". From the word "theobroma" comes the term theobromine, later assigned to the major alkaloid contained in chocolate. The XVII century was the period in which large amounts of chocolate began to be produced in paste form in many European areas, especially in Spain and Flanders, thus testifying to the constantly growing attraction exercised by the substance. In the XIX century, to the generalized recognition of chocolate's pleasing and pleasant qualities, as also of its ability to bring about a good mood and its capacity to cause vasodilation with consequent beneficial effects on the heart and vessels, there was added the scientific confirmation of its diuretic features [2, 26].

As has been said, chocolate derives from the cocoa bean, which is one of the most concentrated sources of flavonoids. The specific antioxidants of chocolate include flavanol molecules, such as catechin and epicatechin, similar to the antioxidants contained in grapes, and consequently in wine, and in tea. Flavonoids reduce platelet activation and aggregation, induce nitric-oxide-dependent vasodilation in healthy humans and prompt the generation of eicosanoids, confirming the historically alleged beneficial effects of chocolate on the vascular apparatus [27]. Flavonoid-rich dark chocolate is a powerful ex vivo and in vivo antioxidant and an anti-atherosclerotic agent in animal models [28]. It may be noted that in the United States chocolate is the third highest individual source of antioxidants, after coffee and tea [29]. Flavonoids also improve the endothelial function by increasing plasma catechins, and decrease vascular cell adhesion molecules in hypercholesterolemic women [30]. These multiple positive effects of chocolate on the cardiovascular system are more specific in dark chocolate and, in general, the darker the chocolate the more likely its favourable effects on the cardiovascular apparatus. In effect, according to the authors of an elegant recent study, the secondary links established between chocolate flavonoids and milk proteins (in milk chocolate) determine a reduced biological availability of flavonoids and an overall reduction of the in vivo antioxidant positive characteristics of chocolate [31]. Recent evidence also indicates that cocoa intake has a favourable effect in reducing arterial pressure [32], thus again confirming popular adages. In elderly individuals with systolic arterial hypertension, 100 mg of dark chocolate a day reduces systolic blood pressure levels by 5.1 mm Hg and diastolic values by 1.8 mm Hg, corresponding to a decrease in cardiovascular events of more than 20% [33]. The mechanisms through which chocolate may decrease blood pressure are likely to be multiple, but, overall, probably linked to its capacity to facilitate the synthesis of nitric oxide. Chocolate has also been proved to lower, at least in animal models, cholesterol and triglycerides. The optimal dosage for the beneficial effects on the cardiovascular system has still to be identified and it currently represents a major area of study for basic and clinical researchers. However, it has already been reported that 50 grams of dark chocolate (1-2 cups a day) may reduce the risk of the insurgence and development of cardiovascular diseases by approximately 10% [34].

Conclusion

This historical perspective evidences the continuing pertinence of past traditions regarding major beverages, even when compared with up-dated scientific information [35]. Although a major challenge for current and future studies consists in identifying the optimal dosage in the assumption of beverages such as tea and chocolate, with regard to wine and coffee dosages, their assumption limits now seem reasonably clear. Best current evidence on wine and coffee indicates that, in adult and elderly healthy people and with specific reference to the cardiovascular system, moderate use is not only better than a higher intake, but also appears more protective than no use at all [36]. The history of medicine thus documents how popular wisdom has proved to be correct and may be summarised by the Latin adage "Est modus in rebus" ("Measure in things") [37].

One therefore never learns enough from the past, though the learning may be as easy as drinking a glass of wine, sipping a cup of tea or enjoying a cup of coffee or chocolate.

Acknowledgements

The Author would like to thank Professor Luisa Camaiora, B.A., M.Phil., for her correction of the English.

References

[1] Foulkes, C. *Larousse Encyclopedia of Wine*. Paris: Larousse; 2001.

[2] Cosmacini, G; Gaudenzi, G; Satolli, R. *Dizionario di storia della salute*. Torino: Einaudi; 1996.

[3] Opie, LH; Lecour, S. The red wine hypothesis: from concepts to protective signalling molecules. *European Heart Journal,* 2007; 28: 1683-93.

[4] Tolstrup, J; Jensen, MK; Tjonneland, A; et al. Prospective study of alcohol drinking patterns and coronary heart disease in women and men. *BMJ,* 2006; 332: 1244-8.

[5] Mukamal, KJ; Jensen, MK; Gronbaek, M; et al. Drinking frequency, mediating biomarkers, and risk of myocardial infarction in women and men. *Circulation*, 2005; 112: 1406-13.

[6] Bradamante, S; Barenghi, L; Piccinini, F; et al. Resveratrol provides late-phase cardioprotection by means of a nitric oxide- and adenosine-mediated mechanism. *Eur. J. Pharmacol.*, 2003; 465: 115-23.

[7] Di Castelnuovo, A; Rotondo, S; Iacoviello, D; Donati, MB; De Gaetano, G. Meta-analysis of wine and beer consumption in relation to vascular risk. *Circulation*, 2002; 105: 2836-44.

[8] Stef, G; Csiszar, A; Lerea, K; et al. Resveratrol inhibits aggregation of platelets from high-risk cardiac patients with aspirin resistance. *J. Cardiovasc. Pharmacol.*, 2006; 48: 1-5.

[9] Palamara, AT; Nencioni, L; Aquilano, K. Inhibition of influenza A virus replication by resveratrol. *J. Infectious. Diseases*, 2005; 191: 1719-29.

[10] Scalbert, A; Manach, C; Morand, C; Remesy, C; Jimenez L. Dietary polyphenols and the prevention of diseases. *Crit. Rev. Food Sci. Nutr.*, 2005; 45: 287-306.

[11] Natella, F; Ghiselli, A; Rossi, L; Sette, S; D'Amicis, A. Caffè e cuore. Roma: INRAN; 2005.

[12] D'Amicis, A; Ghiselli, A; Rossi, L; Sette, S. Caffè e salute. Roma: INRAN; 2005.

[13] Gensini, GF; Conti, AA. Does coffee consumption represent a coronary risk factor? *Recenti Prog. Med.*, 2004; 95: 563-5.
[14] Garattini, S. Caffeine, coffee and health (8th edition). New York: Raven Press; 1993.
[15] Nawrot, P; Jordan, S; Eastwood, J; Rotstein, J; Hugenholtz, A; Feeley, M. Effects of caffeine on human health. *Food Addit. Contam.*, 2003; 20: 1-30.
[16] Tavani, A; Bertuzzi, M; Negri, E; Sorbara, L; La Vecchia, C. Alcohol, smoking, coffee and risk of non-fatal acute myocardial infarction in Italy. *Eur. J. Epidemiol.*, 2001; 17: 1131-7.
[17] Sofi, F; Conti, AA; Gori, AM; Luisi, MLE; Casini, A; Abbate, R; Gensini, GF. Coffee consumption and risk of coronary heart disease: a meta-analysis. *Nutr. Metab. Cardiovasc. Dis.*, 2007; 17: 209-23.
[18] Gensini, GF; Lippi, D; Conti, AA. Past, present and future of green tea: from pleasant beverage to drug in pills? *Recenti Prog. Med.*, 2007; 98: 347-51.
[19] Heiss, ML; Heiss, RJ. *The story of tea: a cultural history and drinking guide*. Ten Speed Press; 2007.
[20] Graham, HN. Green tea composition, consumption, and polyphenol chemistry. *Prev. Med.*, 1992; 21: 334-50.
[21] Cabrera, C; Artacho, R; Gimenez, R. Beneficial effects of green tea. A review. *J. Am. Coll. Nutr.*, 2006; 25: 79-99.
[22] Stangl, V; Dreger, H; Stangl, K; Lorenz, M. Molecular targets of tea polyphenols in the cardiovascular system. *Cardiovasc. Res.*, 2007; 73: 348-58.
[23] Peters, U; Poole, C; Arab, L. Does tea affect cardiovascular disease? A meta-analysis. *Am. J. Epidemiol.*, 2001; 154: 495-503.
[24] Fraser, ML; Mok, GS; Lee, AH. Green tea and stroke prevention: emerging evidence. *Complement. Ther. Med.*, 2007; 15: 46-53.
[25] Fujiki, H; Suganuma, M; Imai, K; Nakachi K. Green tea: cancer preventive beverage and/or drug. *Cancer Letters*, 2002; 188: 9-13.
[26] Coe, SD; Coe, MD. The true history of chocolate. London: Thames and Hudson Ltd.; 1996.
[27] Ding, EL; Hutfless, SM; Ding, X; Girotra S. Chocolate and prevention of cardiovascular disease: a systematic review. *Nutrition and Metabolism*, 2006; 3: 2.
[28] Vinson, JA; Proch, J; Bose, P; et al. Chocolate is a powerful ex vivo and in vivo antioxidant, an anti-atherosclerotic agent in an animal model, and significant contributor to antioxidants in European and American diets. *J. Agric. Food Chem.*, 2006; 54: 8071-6.
[29] Alspach, G. The truth is often bittersweet. Chocolate does a heart good. *Critical Care Nurse*, 2007; 27: 11-5.
[30] Wang-Polagruto, JF; Villablanca, AC; Polagruto, JA; et al. Chronic consumption of flavanol-rich cocoa improves endothelial function and decreases vascular cell adhesion molecules in hypercholesterolemic postmenopausal women. *J. Cardiovasc. Pharmacol.*, 2006; 47 (suppl 2): S177-S186.
[31] Murphy, KJ; Chronopoulos, AK; Singh, I; et al. Dietary flavanols and procyanidin oligomer from cocoa (Theobroma cacao) inhibit platelet function. *Am. J. Clin. Nutr.*, 2003; 77: 1466-73.

[32] Buijsse, B; Feskens, EJM; Kok, FJ; Kromhout D. Cocoa intake, blood pressure and cardiovascular mortality: the Zutphen elderly study. *Arch. Intern. Med.*, 2006; 166: 411-7.

[33] Taubert, D; Berkels, R; Roesen, R; Klaus, W. Chocolate and blood pressure in elderly individuals with isolated systolic hypertension. *JAMA*, 2003; 290: 1029-30.

[34] Franco, OH; Bonneux, L; de Laet, C; Peeters, A; Steyerberg, EW; Mackenbach, JP. The Polymeal: a more natural, safer, and probably tastier (than the Polypill) strategy to reduce cardiovascular disease by more than 75%. *BMJ*, 2004; 329: 1447-50.

[35] Gensini, GF; Conti, AA. From cardiovascular prevention to cardiovascular rehabilitation: statins and Evidence Based Medicine. *Ital. Heart J.*, 2002 Suppl 3: 91-4.

[36] Marcucci, R; Gori, AM; Bertuccioli, M; Gensini, GF; Abbate, R. In vivo effect of Chianti red wine on tissue factor, tissue factor pathway inhibitor and homocysteine levels. *Thromb. Haemost.*, 2005; 94; 689-90.

[37] Conti, AA; Galanti, C; Gensini, GF. Is evidence-based medicine really a craze? Surely it is fashionable to criticize it. A methodologic comment from the Italian Center for Evidence Based Medicine. *Ital. Heart J.*, 2000 Suppl 1(9):1192-5.

Index

E

F

G

H

I

J

K

L

N

O

P

S

T

X

Y

Z